AF840128

VOLUME EIGHTY FIVE

ADVANCES IN PHARMACOLOGY

VOLUME EIGHTY FIVE

ADVANCES IN PHARMACOLOGY

Drug-induced Liver Injury

Edited by

ANUP RAMACHANDRAN

Department of Pharmacology, Toxicology, and Therapeutics, University of Kansas Medical Center, Kansas City, KS, United States

HARTMUT JAESCHKE

Department of Pharmacology, Toxicology, and Therapeutics, University of Kansas Medical Center, Kansas City, KS, United States

Serial Editor

S.J. ENNA

University of Kansas Medical Center, Kansas City, KS, United States

Managing Editor

LYNN LeCOUNT

University of Kansas Medical Center, School of Medicine, Kansas City, KS, United States

ELSEVIER

ACADEMIC PRESS

An imprint of Elsevier

Academic Press is an imprint of Elsevier
50 Hampshire Street, 5th Floor, Cambridge, MA 02139, United States
525 B Street, Suite 1650, San Diego, CA 92101, United States
The Boulevard, Langford Lane, Kidlington, Oxford OX5 1GB, United Kingdom
125 London Wall, London, EC2Y 5AS, United Kingdom

First edition 2019

Copyright © 2019 Elsevier Inc. All rights reserved.

No part of this publication may be reproduced or transmitted in any form or by any means, electronic or mechanical, including photocopying, recording, or any information storage and retrieval system, without permission in writing from the publisher. Details on how to seek permission, further information about the Publisher's permissions policies and our arrangements with organizations such as the Copyright Clearance Center and the Copyright Licensing Agency, can be found at our website: www.elsevier.com/permissions.

This book and the individual contributions contained in it are protected under copyright by the Publisher (other than as may be noted herein).

Notices
Knowledge and best practice in this field are constantly changing. As new research and experience broaden our understanding, changes in research methods, professional practices, or medical treatment may become necessary.

Practitioners and researchers must always rely on their own experience and knowledge in evaluating and using any information, methods, compounds, or experiments described herein. In using such information or methods they should be mindful of their own safety and the safety of others, including parties for whom they have a professional responsibility.

To the fullest extent of the law, neither the Publisher nor the authors, contributors, or editors, assume any liability for any injury and/or damage to persons or property as a matter of products liability, negligence or otherwise, or from any use or operation of any methods, products, instructions, or ideas contained in the material herein.

ISBN: 978-0-12-816759-5
ISSN: 1054-3589

For information on all Academic Press publications
visit our website at https://www.elsevier.com/books-and-journals

Publisher: Zoe Kruze
Acquisition Editor: Zoe Kruze
Editorial Project Manager: Shellie Bryant
Production Project Manager: Vignesh Tamil
Cover Designer: Alan Studholme

Typeset by SPi Global, India

Working together to grow libraries in developing countries

www.elsevier.com • www.bookaid.org

Contents

Contributors

Julien Allard
INSERM, Univ. Rennes, INRA, Institut NUMECAN (Nutrition Metabolisms and Cancer) UMR_A 1341, UMR_S 1241, Rennes, France

Pieter Annaert
Drug Delivery and Disposition, KU Leuven Department of Pharmaceutical and Pharmacological Sciences, Leuven, Belgium

Udayan Apte
Department of Pharmacology, Toxicology, and Therapeutics, University of Kansas Medical Center, Kansas City, KS, United States

Steven Ballet
Research Group of Organic Chemistry, Departments of Chemistry and Bioengineering Sciences, Vrije Universiteit Brussel, Brussels, Belgium

Karima Begriche
INSERM, Univ. Rennes, INRA, Institut NUMECAN (Nutrition Metabolisms and Cancer) UMR_A 1341, UMR_S 1241, Rennes, France

Xiaojuan Chao
Department of Pharmacology, Toxicology and Therapeutics, University of Kansas Medical Center, Kansas City, KS, United States

Melissa M. Clemens
Interdisciplinary Biomedical Sciences Graduate Program, University of Arkansas for Medical Sciences, Little Rock, AR, United States

Bruno Cogliati
Department of Pathology, School of Veterinary Medicine and Animal Science, University of São Paulo, São Paulo, Brazil

Axelle Cooreman
Department of *In Vitro* Toxicology and Dermato-Cosmetology, Vrije Universiteit Brussel, Brussels, Belgium

Steven C. Curry
Department of Medical Toxicology, Banner—University Medical Center Phoenix; Division of Clinical Data Analytics and Decision Support; Division of Medical Toxicology and Precision Medicine, University of Arizona College of Medicine—Phoenix, Phoenix, AZ, United States

Lily Dara
Division of Gastrointestinal and Liver Diseases, Department of Medicine, Keck School of Medicine; Research Center for Liver Disease, Keck School of Medicine, University of Southern California, Los Angeles, CA, United States

Wen-Xing Ding
Department of Pharmacology, Toxicology and Therapeutics, University of Kansas Medical Center, Kansas City, KS, United States

Erik S. Fisher
Department of Medical Toxicology, Banner—University Medical Center Phoenix; Division of Clinical Data Analytics and Decision Support; Division of Medical Toxicology and Precision Medicine, University of Arizona College of Medicine—Phoenix, Phoenix, AZ, United States

Bernard Fromenty
INSERM, Univ. Rennes, INRA, Institut NUMECAN (Nutrition Metabolisms and Cancer) UMR_A 1341, UMR_S 1241, Rennes, France

Eva Gijbels
Department of *In Vitro* Toxicology and Dermato-Cosmetology, Vrije Universiteit Brussel, Brussels, Belgium

Emma Gustafson
Department of *In Vitro* Toxicology and Dermato-Cosmetology, Vrije Universiteit Brussel, Brussels, Belgium

Andrea Iorga
Division of Gastrointestinal and Liver Diseases, Department of Medicine, Keck School of Medicine; Research Center for Liver Disease, Keck School of Medicine, University of Southern California, Los Angeles, CA, United States

Hartmut Jaeschke
Department of Pharmacology, Toxicology, and Therapeutics, University of Kansas Medical Center, Kansas City, KS, United States

Dounia Le Guillou
INSERM, Univ. Rennes, INRA, Institut NUMECAN (Nutrition Metabolisms and Cancer) UMR_A 1341, UMR_S 1241, Rennes, France

Mitchell R. McGill
Department of Environmental and Occupational Health, Fay W. Boozman College of Public Health; Department of Pharmacology and Toxicology, College of Medicine, University of Arkansas for Medical Sciences, Little Rock, AR, United States

Anup Ramachandran
Department of Pharmacology, Toxicology, and Therapeutics, University of Kansas Medical Center, Kansas City, KS, United States

Jack Uetrecht
Faculties of Pharmacy and Medicine, University of Toronto, Toronto, ON, Canada

Raf Van Campenhout
Department of *In Vitro* Toxicology and Dermato-Cosmetology, Vrije Universiteit Brussel, Brussels, Belgium

Vânia Vilas-Boas
Department of *In Vitro* Toxicology and Dermato-Cosmetology, Vrije Universiteit Brussel, Brussels, Belgium

Mathieu Vinken
Department of *In Vitro* Toxicology and Dermato-Cosmetology, Vrije Universiteit Brussel, Brussels, Belgium

Paul B. Watkins
Eshelman School of Pharmacy, Institute for Drug Safety Sciences, University of North Carolina, Chapel Hill, NC, United States

Preface

Drug-induced liver injury (DILI) is an important clinical problem with an estimated annual incidence between 10 and 15 cases per 10,000–100,000 individuals and DILI is the most common cause of acute liver failure in the Western World. In addition, DILI is also a major concern for drug development in the pharmaceutical industry. Fundamentally, two types of DILI can be distinguished. One is dose-dependent and predictable across many different species. Compounds causing this type of DILI are increasingly recognized today during routine preclinical drug safety assessment and their development is prevented. However, some older compounds, such as acetaminophen (APAP), cause dose-dependent DILI, albeit only after an overdose. APAP hepatotoxicity is clinically relevant due to the >60,000 intentional or unintentional overdose cases that are hospitalized every year in the United States alone. APAP emerged also as the most mechanistically studied DILI compound and as such is increasingly used as a model toxin to evaluate potential hepatoprotective drugs especially natural products. The second class of DILI compounds causes idiosyncratic toxicity, which means that these drugs only trigger liver injury in very few individuals, generally less than 1 in 10,000 people who mostly took therapeutic doses. The challenge here is early identification of compounds with idiosyncratic DILI potential during the drug development process and determining causality in patients with adverse drug reactions.

In the current volume of *Advances in Pharmacology*, experts in DILI research discuss the latest basic and clinical findings in this field. The first chapter begins with an examination of various in vitro techniques using cultured primary hepatocytes to evaluate DILI and their relevance to the drug development pipeline. Dr. Mathieu Vinken and colleagues discuss liver architecture and its reproduction in the in vitro milieu as well as mechanisms involved in loss of hepatocyte drug metabolic functions after isolation and methods to minimize these changes. They then summarize these issues by using an example of testing for drug-induced cholestatic liver injury in primary hepatocyte cultures. Next, Drs. Lily Dara and Andrea Iorga delve into mechanisms of cell death caused by various DILI-inducing agents. The main types of cell death relevant to DILI, namely, apoptosis and necrosis, are discussed in the context of idiosyncratic liver injury and APAP hepatotoxicity. Current understanding of cell signaling involved in the pathophysiology is elaborated and their relevance to DILI is analyzed. In addition, the authors also touch upon autophagy as well as other modes of cell death such as pyroptosis and ferroptosis, which could be relevant in DILI. Following up with a clinically important aspect of DILI, Dr. Bernard Fromenty and colleagues discuss DILI on a background of obesity and nonalcoholic fatty liver disease (NAFLD). The authors start with an introduction to the pathophysiology of NAFLD and touch upon the various relevant animal models being used to investigate the condition. They subsequently discuss various DILI-causing agents including APAP, methotrexate, and tamoxifen among others and evaluate the role NAFLD plays in modulating their hepatotoxic properties.

The next chapter by Dr. Wen-Xing Ding and Xiaojuan Chao focuses on alcoholic liver disease (ALD) and the role of autophagy in the pathogenesis. After introducing the disorder and discussing alcohol metabolism, the authors explain molecular mechanisms involved in the process of autophagy within the cell and go on to compare findings from various animal models of ALD including chronic consumption as well as binge drinking models. Finally, therapeutic aspects of targeting autophagy are discussed, with a focus on removal of damaged mitochondria (mitophagy), lipid droplets, and protein aggregates by autophagy.

The next two chapters deal with idiosyncratic DILI with the first by Dr. Jack Uetrecht focusing on the various mechanisms which could play a role in the process and link reactive metabolite formation with induction of the immune response. After an introduction to the clinical characteristics of idiosyncratic DILI, he discusses the involvement of reactive metabolite formation and its modulation of the immune response. Other proposed mechanisms including mitochondrial injury as well as endoplasmic reticulum stress are then evaluated, followed by examination of animal models that are useful in mechanistic studies of idiosyncratic DILI. In closing, he touches upon implications for prevention and treatment of idiosyncratic DILI with a discussion on prediction of patient susceptibility as well as screening for potential idiosyncratic DILI of drug candidates. These basic mechanistic aspects of idiosyncratic DILI are extended to the clinical scenario in the next chapter by Dr. Paul Watkins. He discusses diverse clinical presentations of idiosyncratic DILI, which have been classified into various phenotypes, including acute hepatitis, cholestatic hepatitis, etc. He then focuses on the immune phenotype, which is the most common in idiosyncratic DILI. Further, various clinical outcomes are explored, followed by a discussion of the diagnosis of idiosyncratic DILI and prediction of its course in patients.

The chapter then concludes with a discussion of the relevance of idiosyncratic DILI in drug discovery, with particular focus on FDA approaches to assessing liver safety in clinical trials.

The next series of chapters focus on the most common cause of acute liver failure in the United States, namely, APAP overdose, and begin with our chapter examining molecular mechanisms involved in APAP-induced hepatotoxicity with a focus on the role of the mitochondria. The etiology of hepatocyte injury with the importance of reactive metabolite formation and the role of mitochondrial protein adduct formation and subsequent mitochondrial oxidative and nitrosative stress are discussed. This is followed by a critical evaluation of the impact of MAP kinase activation and amplification of mitochondrial dysfunction in inducing hepatocyte necrosis. The role of mitochondria in adaptation and recovery from APAP-induced liver injury is then examined and the relevance of these mitochondrial changes to the clinical condition is discussed. The next chapter by Drs. McGill and myself examines the progress in biomarker research for DILI diagnosis, prognosis, and prediction. In addition, mechanistic insight in human DILI based on circulating biomarkers is discussed. Despite the significant advance in knowledge in this area, many challenges remain. In the chapter on liver repair and recovery, Dr. Udayan Apte and coworkers compare the signaling mechanisms of liver regeneration after partial hepatectomy and DILI with focus on APAP hepatotoxicity. Commonality and differences between the signaling mechanisms are discussed. In addition, the emerging field of liver regeneration biomarkers is reviewed. The final chapter by Drs. Fisher and Curry reviews clinical aspects of APAP poisoning, beginning with the clinical course of acute acetaminophen ingestion, followed by aspects of diagnosis and determination of risk of toxicity as well as typical treatment modalities. Finally, overdose due to chronic APAP oral ingestion is also touched upon.

Together, the chapters in this volume provide an updated overview of basic mechanisms of DILI and recovery together with its clinical translation.

Anup Ramachandran and Hartmut Jaeschke

CHAPTER ONE

Primary hepatocytes and their cultures for the testing of drug-induced liver injury

Vânia Vilas-Boas*,[2], Axelle Cooreman*,[2], Eva Gijbels*, Raf Van Campenhout*, Emma Gustafson*, Steven Ballet†, Pieter Annaert‡, Bruno Cogliati§, Mathieu Vinken*,[1]

*Department of *In Vitro* Toxicology and Dermato-Cosmetology, Vrije Universiteit Brussel, Brussels, Belgium
†Research Group of Organic Chemistry, Departments of Chemistry and Bioengineering Sciences, Vrije Universiteit Brussel, Brussels, Belgium
‡Drug Delivery and Disposition, KU Leuven Department of Pharmaceutical and Pharmacological Sciences, Leuven, Belgium
§Department of Pathology, School of Veterinary Medicine and Animal Science, University of São Paulo, São Paulo, Brazil
[1]Corresponding author: e-mail address: mvinken@vub.ac.be

Contents

Abstract

Drug-induced liver injury is a major reason for discontinuation of drug development and withdrawal of drugs from the market. Intensive efforts in the last decades have focused on the establishment and finetuning of liver-based *in vitro* models for reliable

[2] Equally contributing first authors.

Advances in Pharmacology, Volume 85
ISSN 1054-3589
https://doi.org/10.1016/bs.apha.2018.08.001
© 2019 Elsevier Inc.
All rights reserved.

prediction of hepatotoxicity triggered by drug candidates. Of those, primary hepatocytes and their cultures still are considered the gold standard, as they provide an acceptable reflection of the hepatic *in vivo* situation. Nevertheless, these *in vitro* systems cope with gradual deterioration of the differentiated morphological and functional phenotype. The present paper gives an overview of traditional and more recently introduced strategies to counteract this dedifferentiation process in an attempt to set up culture models that can be used for long-term testing purposes. The relevance and applicability of such optimized cultures of primary hepatocytes for the testing of drug-induced cholestatic liver injury is demonstrated.

1. Introduction

Drug-induced liver injury is a significant reason for drug failure through all phases of drug development and marketing, accounting for as much as a third of all drug withdrawals (Lee, 2013; Van den Hof et al., 2015). Besides its importance for pharmaceutical industry, drug-induced liver injury is equally of clinical relevance. In this respect, drug-induced liver injury develops in 1 out of 100 patients upon hospitalization, but is regularly misdiagnosed (Meier et al., 2005). In addition, drug-induced liver injury underlies more than half of all clinical cases of acute liver failure (Goldberg et al., 2015). Preclinical animal models only allow to predict up to 60% of human drug-induced liver injuries, which obviously is due to interspecies differences (Laverty et al., 2010; Xu, Diaz, & O'Brien, 2004). A number of state-of-the-art human-based *in vitro* models to study hepatotoxicity induced by chemicals is available today, namely liver-derived *in vitro* models and stem cell-derived *in vitro* models. The latter seem promising for predicting steatotic drug-induced liver injury (Pradip et al., 2016; Rodrigues et al., 2014). However, although some groups showed their relevance (Ghodsizadeh et al., 2010; Imagawa et al., 2017), liver cells obtained from induced pluripotent stem cells are not the most appropriate *in vitro* systems for picking up cholestatic drugs (Bell et al., 2017). Liver-derived *in vitro* models are more suitable tools for drug-induced liver injury screening (Godoy et al., 2013). These liver-derived *in vitro* models range from whole isolated perfused livers over liver slices, primary hepatocytes and liver-derived cell lines all up to subcellular liver fractions. Obviously, all these systems differ in complexity and longevity, and all have their own specific strengths and flaws (Table 1). Among those, isolated primary hepatocytes and their cultures are still considered the gold standard liver-based *in vitro* model, as they provide a good reflection of the hepatic

Table 1 Liver-derived *in vitro* models.

Strengths	**Limitations**
Whole isolated perfused liver	
– Preservation of entire liver structure – Highly *in vivo* representative	– Mainly suitable to small livers – Limited viability
Liver slices	
– Preservation of entire lobular structure – Highly *in vivo* representative	– Requires high technical skills – Limited viability
Adherent cultures of primary hepatocytes	
– May be cryopreserved – Highly *in vivo* representative	– No preservation of liver structure – Cope with progressive dedifferentiation
Liver-derived cell lines	
– Unlimited – Highly reproducible test results	– Originate from one single donor – May be dedifferentiated
Subcellular liver fractions	
– Readily available – Easy to use	– No preservation of liver structure – Poorly *in vivo* representative

Strengths and limitations of each of the models are listed.

in vivo situation. However, they cope with gradual loss of the differentiated phenotype, which limits their use (Godoy et al., 2013). In this paper, focus will be put on primary hepatocyte cultures as prominent tools for drug-induced liver injury testing. In a first part, the complex architecture of the liver will be discussed as being the overall reference for *in vitro* modeling. Thereafter, mechanisms involved in the loss of *in vivo*-like morphology and functionality upon isolation of primary hepatocytes from liver will be presented, followed by an overview of strategies to counteract this process. In a final part, the use of primary hepatocyte cultures for screening drug-induced cholestatic liver injury will be exemplified.

2. Hepatic architecture as the benchmark for liver-based *in vitro* modeling

The liver is the second biggest organ of the human body, constituting 2–3% of total body weight. It is located in the upper right quadrant of the abdominal cavity under the diaphragm and consists of four lobes of different size and shape (Abdel-Misih & Bloomston, 2010; Rutkauskas, Gedrimas, Pundzius, Barauskas, & Basevicius, 2006). The liver receives blood *via* the portal vein and the hepatic artery, while the blood is drained through the hepatic vein. The hepatic artery carries oxygen-rich blood from the aorta, whereas the portal vein conveys blood rich in digested nutrients from the entire gastrointestinal tract as well as from the spleen and pancreas (Bismuth, 1982). These blood vessels subdivide into small capillaries known as liver sinusoids, which lead to a lobule, being the morphological unit of the liver (Fig. 1). Liver lobules have a hexagonal structure and are built up by plates of hepatocytes that are segregated by sinusoids. Liver sinusoids are enlarged capillaries through which blood from the portal vein and hepatic artery enters *via* the portal triads and subsequently drains to the central hepatic vein (Ishibashi, Nakamura, Komori, Migita, & Shimoda, 2009; Malarkey, Johnson, Ryan, Boorman, & Maronpot, 2005). The acinus is the functional unit of the liver. This roughly elliptical region consists of hepatocytes from two neighboring lobules. The acinus represents the population of hepatocytes supplied by one portal triad. It is divided into zones that correspond to the distance from the arterial blood supply, in particular the periportal, the midlobular and the perivenous areas (Jungermann, 1986). The hepatocytes

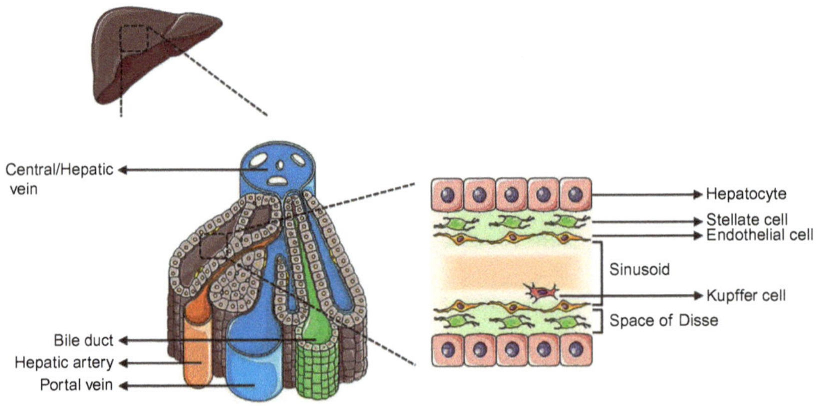

Fig. 1 Hepatic architecture. The liver consists of thousands of liver lobules, in which cells are organized radially around a branch of the central/hepatic vein. The contact area between adjacent lobules is called the portal triad and is composed of branches of the hepatic artery, the portal vein and the bile duct. Different cell types populate the liver, namely parenchymal (*i.e.*, hepatocytes) and non-parenchymal cells. The latter include liver sinusoidal endothelial cells, which create the space of Disse, stellate cells and different immune cell types in the blood circulation (*i.e.*, sinusoids), such as Kupffer cells.

in the periportal zone benefit from the highest oxygen and nutrient supply, because the blood is unidirectionally drained from the portal venules to the central vein. As a consequence, hepatocytes are exposed to a spatial biochemical gradient, which underlies the differential and thus regional expression of biotransformation enzymes and other factors. This phenomenon is also known as functional zonation (Jungermann & Kietzmann, 1996).

The liver performs a number of vital functions, such as carbohydrate metabolism, lipid metabolism, detoxification of endobiotics and xenobiotics, bile acid production, immunological protection and the production of essential proteins, including albumin and blood coagulation factors, of which most are carried out by hepatocytes (Ishibashi et al., 2009). Hepatocytes are large polygonal cells, averaging about 25–30 μm in cross section. They are the most abundant cells in the liver parenchyma, forming 60% of the total amount of cells present in the liver. Hepatocytes are arranged in plates and are large polarized epithelial cells with a complex structural organization of the plasma membrane in three different domains, namely the sinusoidal, the lateral and the canalicular areas. The sinusoidal or basal membrane pole is in contact with liver sinusoidal endothelial cells, while the canalicular or apical membrane area aligns with bile canaliculi. About 15% of the hepatocellular volume is attributed to smooth and rough endoplasmic reticulum, and there are about 30 lysosomes and 500 peroxisomes per hepatocyte. Hepatocytes are endowed with mitochondria and accommodate numerous free ribosomes, Golgi complexes, cytoskeleton elements, such as microfilaments, intermediate filaments and microtubules, and varying levels of cytoplasmic lipid and glycogen (Weibel, Stäubli, Gnägi, & Hess, 1969).

Liver sinusoidal endothelial cells represent up to 20% of all liver cells. They are a unique type of endothelial cells because they possess *fenestrae*, lack a basal lamina and can transfer molecules and particles by endocytosis (Braet & Wisse, 2002). Liver sinusoidal endothelial cells form a continuous line of liver sinusoids. In this way, they act as a barrier and filter between the blood and the space of Disse (De Leeuw, Brouwer, & Knook, 1990). Indeed, high permeability of capillary endothelium to macromolecules, solutes and water is driven by special transporting systems, such as vesicles, channels, diaphragms and *fenestrae*. Endothelial transport is a very complex process, in which substances are transported according to their size, charge and chemical properties (Irie & Tavassoli, 1991).

Hepatic stellate cells, also known as perisinusoidal cells or Ito cells, make up about 5% of the total liver cell number. Hepatic stellate cells normally produce extracellular matrix components, control microvascular tone, and store vitamin A and triglycerides. In normal liver, hepatic stellate cells are in a quiescent state. They may become activated upon liver damage, where they transform into myofibroblast-like cells, in which desmin and smooth muscle actin filaments are typically expressed (Trautwein, Friedman, Schuppan, & Pinzani, 2015). Activated stellate cells are also responsible for secreting collagen. Because of these characteristics, they are key players in the pathogenesis of liver fibrosis and cirrhosis (Friedman, 2015; Lee, Wallace, & Friedman, 2015).

Kupffer cells make up around 2% of the liver volume and 15% of the liver cell number. They are located within the sinusoidal lumen. Kupffer cells present an irregular shape and are held in place by loose arrangements to the sinusoidal endothelium. Kupffer cells possess an important phagocytic function for the clearance of relatively large particles, such as bacteria, damaged hepatocytes and erythrocytes (Smedsrød et al., 1994). Moreover, these cells produce and secrete a number of chemokines and cytokines (Smedsrød, 2004). Together with Kupffer cells, a large number of other immunological cells, including T lymphocytes, natural killer cells and dendritic cells, are found in the liver, located along sinusoids and in portal tracts (Parker & Picut, 2005).

3. Induction of dedifferentiation during primary hepatocyte isolation

The two-step collagenase perfusion technique is the most commonly used procedure to isolate hepatocytes from liver tissue of rodent and human origin (Papeleu et al., 2006; Seglen, 1976). It is based upon the notion that calcium ions are critical for maintaining cellular adhesion. Thus, the freshly removed liver is perfused with a calcium-free medium in a first run in order to disrupt cell–cell junctions. In a second step, the liver is further perfused with a collagenase-containing buffer to eradicate cell–extracellular matrix interactions (Alpini, Phillips, Vroman, & LaRusso, 1994; Berry, Grivell, Grivell, & Phillips, 1997; Papeleu et al., 2006; Seglen, 1976). The abolishment of the entire repertoire of cellular contacts triggers a proliferative response mediated by mitogen-activated protein kinase. The hepatocytes are hereby forced to re-enter the cell cycle from their quiescent G0 status into the G1 phase, a process evidenced by the production of proto-oncogenes, such as *c*-jun and *c*-fos. Simultaneously, an inflammatory reaction is induced, with nuclear factor-kappa beta as master regulator, and is associated with the production of a plethora of cytokines. This is equally promoted by the occurrence of an ischemia/reperfusion event as well as by the presence of impurities in the collagenase, such as lipopolysaccharide, used during the hepatocyte isolation procedure (Elaut et al., 2006; Paine & Andreakos, 2004).

The proliferative and inflammatory processes that are activated during the two-step collagenase perfusion technique negatively affect hepatocyte morphology and functionality, a process designated dedifferentiation. This implies that differentiation-related genes, including those that code for phase I and phase II biotransformation enzymes as well as liver-enriched transcription factors, are strongly and rapidly downregulated (Baker et al., 2001; Beigel, Fella, Kramer, Kroeger, & Hewitt, 2008; Boess et al., 2003; de Longueville et al., 2003). These alterations at the transcriptional level become already detectable a few hours after plating of the cells, yet they are most pronounced between 24 and 48 h of culture (Beigel et al., 2008; Boess et al., 2003; Rodriguez-Antona et al., 2002). The drastic disruption of hepatocellular homeostasis during and following the two-step collagenase perfusion method ultimately burgeons into the occurrence of cell death, mainly apoptosis (Elaut et al., 2006; Paine & Andreakos, 2004; Vinken et al., 2006). An essential determinant of spontaneous cell death progression in primary hepatocyte cultures is cell density (Bresgen et al., 2008; Qiao & Farrell, 1999; Shinzawa, Watanabe, & Akaike, 1995). In this respect, hepatocytes plated at low density (*i.e.*, 0.35×10^5 cells per cm^2) display less apoptotic activity compared with their counterparts seeded at high density (*i.e.*, 1.4×10^5 cells per cm^2), which is about half of the *in vivo* density (*i.e.*, $2–3 \times 10^5$ cells per cm^2) in liver tissue (Qiao & Farrell, 1999). However, unlike cell survival, cell density positively correlates with the functional status of the cultured hepatocytes (Hamilton et al., 2001). Another critical parameter of cell survival in freshly isolated hepatocytes relates to the composition of the cell culture medium. A comparison of a number of commonly used and commercially available hepatocyte culture media revealed that Williams' E medium and *N*-2-hydroxyethylpiperazine-*N*′-2-ethanesulfonic acid buffer offer the lowest background of spontaneous apoptotic and necrotic cell death for freshly isolated rat hepatocytes in suspension culture (Elaut, Vanhaecke, Heyden, & Rogiers, 2005). More specific cell culture media, such as the University of Wisconsin solution, also are efficient in counteracting self-generated cell death in isolated hepatocytes (Fu et al., 2001).

4. Counteracting dedifferentiation during primary hepatocyte cultivation

The dedifferentiation response that is triggered during the two-step collagenase perfusion technique is pursued and amplified upon subsequent seeding and cultivation of the freshly isolated primary hepatocytes. Consequently, conventional cultures of primary hepatocytes have a limited lifespan, typically 2–3 days, and hence can only be used for short-term pharmaco-toxicological purposes, although differences exist between species (Elaut et al., 2006; Paine & Andreakos, 2004; Papeleu et al., 2006; Vinken et al., 2006). However, for studying many types of toxicity, including those related to drug-induced liver injury, longer cultivation regimes are required. For this reason, considerable attention has been paid over the past decades, and is still being paid, to the development and optimization of primary hepatocyte cultures eligible for the toxicity testing during extended periods of time. Today, two strategies are followed in this respect. A first strategy, commonly called the classical anti-dedifferentiation approaches, aims at counteracting the consequences of dedifferentiation by mimicking the natural hepatocyte microenvironment *in vitro*. The second strategy, collectively designated the novel anti-dedifferentiation approaches, includes tackling the actual causes of dedifferentiation at the most upstream regulatory level of this deteriorative process (Fig. 2) (Table 2).

4.1 Classical anti-dedifferentiation approaches

4.1.1 Addition of soluble differentiation-promoting compounds to the cell culture medium

Glucocorticoids. Dexamethasone and hydrocortisone are routinely added to hepatocyte culture media. They boost liver-specific functionality *via* enhancing expression and activity of liver-enriched transcription factors and biotransformation enzymes (Elaut et al., 2006; Matsuno et al., 1996; Vinken et al., 2006). Glucocorticoids act by binding to glucocorticoid nuclear receptors, which then translocate to the nucleus, where they bind to glucocorticoid response elements within the promoter regions of specific genes, including those coding for albumin. Furthermore, glucocorticoids interfere with mitogen-activated protein kinase and nuclear factor-kappa beta signaling, and positively affect the maintenance of the *in vivo*-like polygonal hepatocyte shape and bile canaliculi-like structures (Garside et al., 2004; Sidhu, Liu, & Omiecinski, 2004). Dexamethasone also suppresses spontaneous

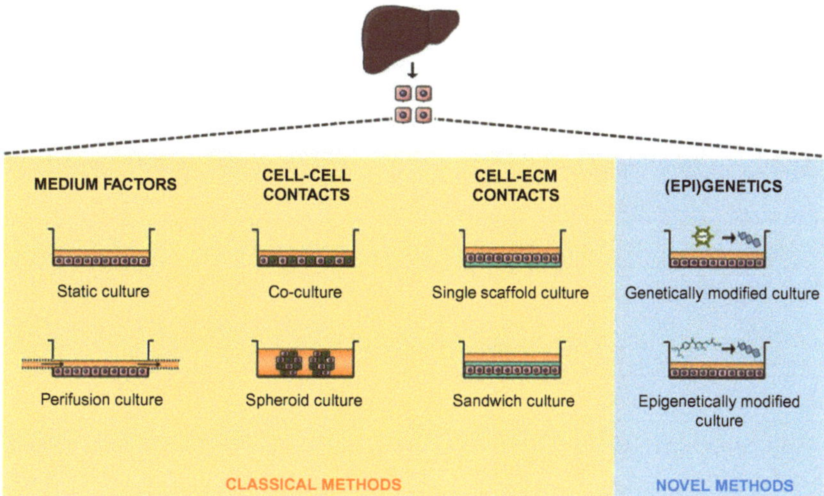

Fig. 2 Primary hepatocyte anti-dedifferentiation strategies. Different strategies can be used to counteract dedifferentiation in cultures of freshly isolated primary hepatocytes. Classical methods typically focus on recreating the *in vivo* hepatocellular micro-environment by (i) adding differentiation-promoting compounds to the cell culture medium either in a static or dynamic way, (ii) co-culturing with another cell type either in a two- or three-dimensional configuration, and (iii) restoring cell–extracellular matrix (ECM) contacts by seeding cells on single layer or between two layers of extracellular matrix components. Novel methods include (i) genetic alteration by transfecting with genes encoding liver-specific proteins, and (ii) epigenetic alteration using chromatin remodeling agents to promote expression of liver-specific proteins.

apoptotic cell death in primary hepatocyte cultures (Bailly-Maitre et al., 2002; Bresgen et al., 2008).

Insulin and glucagon. Insulin and glucagon are added to hepatocyte culture media because of their positive effects on hepatocyte attachment and morphology, activation of liver-specific expression and cell survival (Elaut et al., 2006; Matsuno et al., 1996). The beneficial outcome of insulin on carbohydrate metabolism is mediated by the binding to its receptor. Insulin is also able to bind to insulin-like growth factor receptors (Kim, Park, Kido, & Accili, 2001). Additional effects of insulin include improvement of lipogenesis, amino acid transport and protein synthesis. Insulin is essential for maintaining albumin synthesis in primary hepatocyte cultures (LeCluyse, Bullock, & Parkinson, 1996). Glucagon is included in cell culture media formulations together with glucocorticoids and insulin. Positive effects exerted by glucagon include enhancement of gluconeogenesis and the activity of pyruvate kinase, glucokinase and lactate dehydrogenase

Table 2 Primary hepatocyte anti-dedifferentiation strategies.

Strengths	**Limitations**
Addition of soluble differentiation-promoting compounds to the cell culture medium	
– Easy to apply	– Reduces consequences of dedifferentiation – Does not suffice as a stand-alone method
The restoration of cell–cell contacts	
– Repairs cellular interactions	– Reduces consequences of dedifferentiation – Analysis may be hampered because of the presence of a second cell type
The re-establishment of cell–extracellular matrix contacts	
– Cells adopt three-dimensional configuration	– Reduces consequences of dedifferentiation – Test compounds may absorb to or poorly penetrate through the extracellular matrix
– Novel anti-dedifferentiation approaches	
Interfering with transcriptional regulation	
– Tackles causes of dedifferentiation – Specific boost of gene transcription	– Effects may be transient – Primary hepatocytes are notoriously hard to transfect
Interfering with epigenetic regulation	
– Tackles causes of dedifferentiation – Easy to apply	– Non-specific boost of gene transcription – Epigenetic modifiers may interfere with test compounds

Strengths and limitations of each of the approaches are listed.

(Dich, Vind, & Grunnet, 1988; Guguen-Guillouzo & Guillouzo, 1983). Both insulin and glucagon reduce apoptosis in primary hepatocyte cultures (Bresgen et al., 2008; Fladmark, Gjertsen, Doskeland, & Vintermyr, 1997).

Epidermal growth factor and fetal bovine serum. Epidermal growth factor increases the survival of cultured hepatocytes (Ethier, Raymond, Musallam, Houle, & Bilodeau, 2003; Musallam, Ethier, Haddad, & Bilodeau, 2001). However, because of its mitogenic activity, epidermal growth factor negatively affects the differentiated phenotype, including expression of biotransformation enzymes (Papeleu et al., 2004). Similar observations have been described regarding fetal bovine serum supplementation of hepatocyte culture media. Fetal bovine serum promotes hepatocyte attachment and survival, yet it also destabilizes bile canaliculi-like networks, disrupts hepatocellular polarization and negatively influences biotransformation activity (Tuschl, Hrach, Walter, Hewitt, & Mueller, 2009). Some of these effects are due to the presence of epidermal growth factor and other growth hormones, including hepatocyte growth factor. The latter triggers mitogen-activated protein kinase signaling and counteracts apoptosis (Gomez-Quiroz et al., 2008; Schulze-Bergkamen et al., 2004).

Nicotinamide. Because the intracellular nicotinamide adenosine dinucleotide pool is rapidly depleted in primary hepatocytes, culture media can be supplemented with nicotinamide or its derivatives to compensate for its loss. This was found to enhance albumin secretion and cell survival in primary hepatocytes. Nicotinamide also boosts biotransformation capacity (Inoue, Yamamoto, Nakamura, Ichihara, & Okamoto, 1989). These effects are mediated by favoring gene transcription and by delaying protein catabolism (Edwards, Glistak, Lucas, & Wilson, 1984).

Dimethylsulfoxide. The oxygen radical scavenger dimethylsulfoxide exerts many anti-dedifferentiation effects, including the maintenance of *in vivo*-like hepatocyte morphology, enhanced expression of biotransformation enzymes and liver-enriched transcription factors, and increased secretion of albumin (Su & Waxman, 2004). Some of these effects can result from the ability to inhibit hepatocellular growth by inducing cell cycle arrests (Elaut et al., 2006). Furthermore, dimethylsulfoxide suppresses apoptosis in primary hepatocyte cultures (Banic, Nipic, Suput, & Milisav, 2011; Gilot et al., 2002).

Supplementation of all of the abovementioned soluble factors to hepatocyte culture media can be done either in a static or in a dynamic manner (Fig. 2). Simple two-dimensional static culture systems require daily media changes because of accumulation of potentially toxic metabolites. A precise control of the hepatocyte micro-environment is challenging, since cell culture parameters, such as temperature, pH and oxygen concentration, are not easy to monitor in real-time in conventional culture dishes or multi-well plates. In addition, oxygen is supplied by passive diffusion through the cell culture medium considering the impermeability of plastic cell culture dishes. Consequently, a hypoxic environment is created, forcing the cells to fulfill their energetic needs through anaerobic glycolysis (Goral & Yuen, 2011). Hepatocytes adopt high oxygen uptake rates upon cell attachment. Hence, appropriate availability of oxygen is critical to sustain liver-specific functionality *in vitro* (Goral & Yuen, 2011; Leite et al., 2011). This can be overcome by using perifusion systems that reproduce the dynamic *in vivo* liver blood flow, including continuous supply of nutrients and oxygen, and instant removal of waste. It has been shown on many occasions that cell survival, secretory activity of albumin and the expression and activity of a number of biotransformation enzymes are significantly enhanced in perfused cultures of primary hepatocytes as compared to static counterparts (Goral et al., 2010; Leite et al., 2011; Vinci et al., 2011). In such set-ups, primary hepatocytes are cultured in bioreactors furnished with pumps, which generate culture medium flow, and in-built sensors that enable accurate control of hepatocyte culture conditions. A critical parameter in such experimental systems is shear stress (Goral & Yuen, 2011). High cell culture medium flow rates deteriorate hepatocellular functionality, affect cellular architecture and may induce cell death (Nakatsuka et al., 2006; Tanaka, Sato, Yamato, Okano, & Kitamori, 2006). Miniaturization of perfused hepatocyte culture systems to a chip format has been facilitated by implementing microfluidics, which enables monitoring and handling of small volume of cell culture media (Baudoin, Corlu, Griscom, Legallais, & Leclerc, 2007; Kang, Chung, Langer, & Khademhosseini, 2008). Indeed, cultivation of primary hepatocytes in microcapillaries that are linked to a microfluidic device considerably reduces cell culture media volumes, while increasing throughput. In turn, this allows incorporation into "lab-on-a-chip" and "micro-total-analysis-system" tools (Baudoin et al., 2007; El-Ali, Sorger, & Jensen, 2006; Prot et al., 2011).

4.1.2 The restoration of cell–cell contacts

A second factor that controls hepatocyte functionality is the presence of cell–cell contacts. In this light, a multitude of hepatic and non-hepatic cell types has been tested as co-cultivation partners for primary hepatocytes (Fig. 2) (Guguen-Guillouzo et al., 1983; Khetani & Bhatia, 2008). The beneficial effects of such co-cultivation techniques on hepatocyte functionality are brought about by membrane-associated proteins provided by the cultivation partners as well as secreted soluble factors, such as cytokines (Leite et al., 2011; Vinken et al., 2006). Cell–cell contacts underlie restoration of hepatocyte polarity and *in vivo*-like morphology, and improve biotransformation functionality and secretion of albumin (Caperna, Blomberg, Garrett, & Talbot, 2011; Evenou, Hamon, Fujii, Takeuchi, & Sakai, 2011). Furthermore, co-cultured hepatocytes display an extended life span (Auth et al., 2005; Mesnil, Fraslin, Piccoli, Yamasaki, & Guguen-Guillouzo, 1987). Importantly, the presence of non-parenchymal liver cells, such as Kupffer cells, in hepatocyte cultures may assist in triggering more *in vivo*-like mechanisms of drug-induced liver injury. Among the hepatic co-cultivation partners for hepatocytes that have been tested are stellate cells, Kupffer cells, liver sinusoidal endothelial cells and rat liver epithelial cells of biliary origin (Kasuya, Sudo, Mitaka, Ikeda, & Tanishita, 2011; Kim & Rajagopalan, 2010). Liver sinusoidal endothelial cells perform a number of metabolic activities and, like hepatocytes, are prone to toxic insults (McCuskey, 2008). Several groups reported strategies to recreate the space of Disse in liver sinusoidal endothelial cell-hepatocyte co-cultures, thereby delaying hepatocyte dedifferentiation (Kim & Rajagopalan, 2010; Rajagopalan et al., 2006). Rat liver epithelial cells of biliary origin produce several liver extracellular matrix components. These cells equally express liver-regulating protein, which is believed to drive signal transduction cascades that control transcription of liver-specific genes in hepatocytes (Corlu et al., 1997; Corlu et al., 1998). A number of non-hepatic partners have been used to establish hepatocyte co-cultures, including fibroblastic cell lines (Evenou et al., 2011; Leite et al., 2011). These cells abundantly produce growth factors and extracellular matrix components, and are essential for the processes of tissue repair and remodeling (Hiramatsu et al., 2005). Hepatocytes alone or together with co-cultivation partners can be cultured in a three-dimensional configuration, such as in so-called spheroids (Fig. 2), which maximize interaction between adjacent cells. Spheroids can be generated by impeding cell attachment to cell culture plates by use of cell-repelling surfaces as well as by continuous rotation. Such advanced three-dimensional cultures maintain hepatocellular functionality to a higher extent compared to two-dimensional set-ups (Bell et al., 2016; Bell et al., 2017; Bell et al., 2018; Hendriks, Fredriksson Puigvert, Messner, Mortiz, & Ingelman-Sundberg, 2016; Vorrink et al., 2017; Vorrink, Zhou, Ingelman-Sundberg, & Lauschke, 2018).

4.1.3 The re-establishment of cell–extracellular matrix contacts

The re-establishment of cell–extracellular matrix interactions *in vitro* is indispensable to restore structural and functional polarization in hepatocytes. *In vivo*, hepatocytes face the space of Disse at the sinusoidal membrane pole, where they also interact with the extracellular matrix. The latter is composed of collagens type I to IV and glycoproteins, such as laminin and fibronectin, and proteoglycans, mainly heparan sulfate (LeCluyse et al., 1996). As such, the extracellular matrix provides anchorage and support for the liver cells. The interaction of surface receptors with extracellular matrix components controls hepatocellular functionality through integrin-based signaling.

Extracellular matrix binding prevents apoptosis and cell cycling of hepatocytes (Elaut et al., 2006). Several scaffolds, both of natural and synthetic origin, have been used to restore cell–extracellular matrix contacts *in vitro*. Collagen is the most frequently applied natural physiological scaffold for primary hepatocytes. Coating cell culture dishes with collagen I favors hepatocyte survival and attachment, and enhances the maintenance of the differentiated phenotype (Skett, 1994; Skett & Bayliss, 1996). In recent years, the entire physiological liver-derived extracellular matrix, obtained by decellularization of whole liver, has been explored as a cultivation setting (De Kock et al., 2011; Lang et al., 2011). Decellularized liver matrices keep critical extracellular matrix components, including collagen I and IV, laminin and fibronectin, as well as extracellular matrix-bound growth factors, such as vascular endothelial growth factor. Moreover, microvasculature of the decellularized liver matrix remains intact and is capable of withstanding fluid flows in the three hepatic circular systems (De Kock et al., 2011). A popular non-physiological scaffold for hepatocytes is Matrigel®, a mouse sarcoma-derived extracellular matrix containing mainly collagen IV, laminin and entactin (Hughes, Postovit, & Lajoie, 2010). Hepatocytes cultured on a Matrigel® layer adopt an *in vivo*-like polarity and morphology. Concomitantly, Matrigel® promotes cellular differentiation by positively affecting liver-enriched transcription factors (Elaut et al., 2006). Furthermore, a plethora of biomaterials, including polymers and peptides as hydrogels or nanofibers, has been introduced as synthetic support matrices for primary hepatocytes (Lu, Wang, & Young, 2011; Schutte et al., 2011; Williams et al., 2011). These synthetic materials were found to enhance albumin secretion as well as expression of liver-enriched transcription factors and biotransformation enzymes (Bhadriraju & Hansen, 2000; Genove et al., 2009). In addition to acting as a simple cultivation scaffold, natural or synthetic matrices can be used as an overlay (*i.e.*, the sandwich method) or as part of a cell encapsulation approach (*i.e.*, the immobilization method) (Dunn, Tompkins, & Yarmush, 1991) (Fig. 2). The three-dimensional aspect introduced by these techniques foresees ample anchorage sites for primary hepatocytes and therefore greatly promotes cell polarity and differentiation (Tuschl et al., 2009; Tuschl & Mueller, 2006). This becomes especially manifested after several days in culture, when hepatocytes cultured in a monolayer configuration present a morphology reminiscent of fibroblasts, while hepatocytes seeded between two layers of collagen show a cuboidal shape with bile canaliculi-like structures (Tuschl & Mueller, 2006).

Furthermore, hepatocytes cultured in a collagen sandwich system have a higher viability and albumin secretion, improved expression of biotransformation enzymes as well as enhanced production of the respective transcriptional regulators (Dunn et al., 1991; Farkas, Bhat, Mandapati, Wishnok, & Tannenbaum, 2005; Farkas & Tannenbaum, 2005; Tuschl & Mueller, 2006).

4.2 Novel anti-dedifferentiation approaches

4.2.1 Interfering with transcriptional regulation

Liver-enriched transcription factors are a family of transcription factors that are particularly abundant in liver. Among the liver-enriched transcription factors characterized thus far are those coding for hepatocyte nuclear factors, including hepatocyte nuclear factor 1, 2, 3, 4 and 6 (Hwang-Verslues & Sladek, 2010; Kaestner, 2010). Liver-enriched transcription factors underlie the commitment of the hepatic phenotype during embryogenesis and are goalkeepers of the maintenance of the differentiated status during the postnatal stage. Liver-enriched transcription factors play an indispensable role by controlling the expression of a diverse spectrum of genes, including those encoding for mediators of urea cycling and intermediary metabolism, biotransformation enzymes, plasma proteins and blood coagulation factors (Cereghini, 1996; Gonzalez, 2008). Hence, it is not surprising that the loss of hepatocyte-specific functions during primary hepatocyte cultivation is paralleled by simultaneous deterioration of liver-enriched transcription factor production (Mizuguchi, Mitaka, Hirata, Oda, & Mochizuki, 1998; Rodriguez-Antona et al., 2002). Accordingly, restoration of liver-enriched transcription factor expression seems an interesting strategy to counteract dedifferentiation in primary hepatocyte cultures (Fig. 2). In this respect, transduction of primary rat hepatocytes with an adenoviral vector carrying the FOXA3 gene, being a prominent liver-enriched transcription factor, led to improved hepatocyte morphology and albumin secretion (Nakamura et al., 1998). Overexpression of hepatocyte nuclear factor 4 alpha in primary hepatocyte cultures does not induce re-expression of biotransformation enzymes, but promotes mitochondrial function and urea removal, and enhances cell viability (Naiki, Nagaki, Asano, Kimata, & Moriwaki, 2005).

4.2.2 Interfering with epigenetic regulation

Like in other organs, critical aspects of liver homeostasis are associated with alterations in chromatin structure and consequently in epigenetic regulation of gene expression patterns. Major determinants of the epigenome are reversible histone modifications, DNA methylation and microRNA-related control. Regarding the former, histone acetylation is typically associated with active gene expression, while the inverse holds true for histone deacetylation (Vinken, 2016). Histone deacetylase inhibitors, with trichostatin A as a prototype, reduce spontaneous apoptosis in primary hepatocyte cultures, as evidenced by decreased caspase 3 activity and lowered Bid steady-state protein levels (Vanhaecke, Henkens, Kass, & Rogiers, 2004). At the same time, trichostatin A effectively stabilizes liver-specific functionality (Henkens et al., 2007). The trichostatin A structural analogue 5-(4-dimethylaminobenzoyl)aminovaleric acid hydroxamide also delays the onset of spontaneous apoptosis in primary hepatocyte cultures (Papeleu et al., 2007). The DNA methylation inhibitor decitabine, whether or not in combination with histone deacetylase inhibitors, improves hepatic functionality, namely secretion of albumin and expression of biotransformation enzymes, in primary hepatocyte cultures (Fraczek, Vinken, Tourwé, Vanhaecke, & Rogiers, 2011) (Fig. 2). MicroRNA expression in cultured hepatocytes undergoes drastic changes following seeding. Trichostatin A was found to have positive effects on miR-122, a liver-specific microRNA species, in primary hepatocyte cultures. Furthermore, trichostatin A affects a number of other microRNA members, including miR-143 and miR-379, which have been associated with inhibition of the proliferative response (Bolleyn et al., 2011).

5. Testing of drug-induced cholestatic liver injury in primary hepatocyte cultures

5.1 Mechanisms and relevance of drug-induced cholestatic liver injury

Cholestasis originates from the Greek words *chole* indicating bile and *stasis* meaning halting (Noor, 2015), and refers to any situation of reduced bile secretion with concurrent accumulation of bile acids in the liver and/or in the blood. Cholestasis may be caused by a wide diversity of factors, including metabolic pathologies, infectious diseases, genetic disorders, immunogenic stimuli and drugs (Gossard & Talwalkar, 2014; Nguyen, Sundaram, & Ayoub, 2014). Drugs can induce either acute or chronic cholestasis. In acute drug-induced cholestasis, symptoms disappear upon drug withdrawal, while they persevere for periods over 6 months despite drug retraction in case of chronic drug-induced cholestasis. Acute drug-induced cholestasis is observed most frequently and presents either with or without hepatocellular and inflammatory injury, and is accompanied by indistinct symptoms, such as fatigue, malaise, nausea, and anorexia. Chronic drug-induced cholestasis takes place following injury to bile ductules or ducts with clinical hallmarks, such as pruritus, jaundice, xanthoma and melanoderma formation (Bhamidimarri & Schiff, 2013; Gossard & Talwalkar, 2014).

Drug-induced cholestasis defines a subclass of drug-induced liver injury. As such, 12–20% and 20–40% of drug-induced liver injury patients show mixed hepatocellular/cholestatic injury and pure cholestatic pattern, respectively (Bhamidimarri & Schiff, 2013). Men over 60 years old seem particularly prone to cholestatic drug-induced liver injury (Meier et al., 2005). In general, the drug-induced liver injury mortality rate associated with cholestasis is 2.5–7.8% (Bhamidimarri & Schiff, 2013; Björnsson & Olsson, 2005; Noor, 2015). Despite the fact that more than one drug can be involved in drug-induced liver injury, single prescription medication is responsible for 73% of all drug-induced cholestasis cases. As much as 1000 drugs have been linked to cholestatic liver injury, including anti-inflammatory drugs, antidiabetics, anti-infectious drugs, cardiovascular drugs, psychotropic drugs and steroids (Bhamidimarri & Schiff, 2013; Parmentier et al., 2017).

Mechanistically, cholestatic drug-induced liver injury can be induced through three types of triggers. (i) Reduced functionality, expression and/or aberrant subcellular localization of transporters responsible for conveying bile acids and/or drugs, such as the bile salt export pump, multidrug resistance-associated protein 2/3/4 and multidrug resistance protein 3. (ii) Various hepatocellular changes, including compromised cytoskeletal architecture, disruption of tight junctions and decreased membrane fluidity. (iii) Altered bile canaliculi dynamics. These three types of cholestatic stimuli induce two cellular responses, each typified by a number of key events. (i) An adverse response triggered by bile acid accumulation and characterized by the occurrence of mitochondrial impairment, endoplasmic reticulum stress with unfolded protein responses, oxidative stress, inflammation and different cell death modes, including necrosis, apoptosis, necroptosis and autophagy. (ii) An adaptive response aimed at decreasing the uptake and increasing the export of bile acids into and from hepatocytes, respectively, which relies on the activation of nuclear receptors, including the farnesoid X receptor, the pregnane X receptor and the constitutive androstane receptor (Vinken, 2018; Vinken et al., 2013) (Fig. 3).

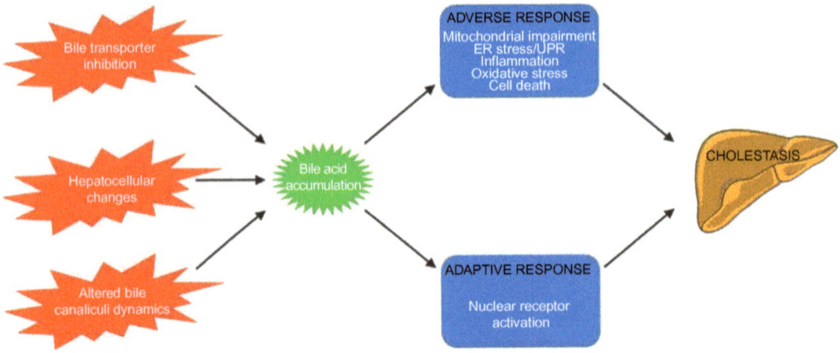

Fig. 3 Mechanisms of drug-induced cholestatic liver injury. Drug-induced cholestatic liver injury can be induced through three types of triggers, namely (i) reduced functionality, expression and/or aberrant subcellular localization of bile transporters, (ii) various hepatocellular changes, including compromised cytoskeletal architecture, disruption of tight junctions and decreased membrane fluidity, and (iii) altered bile canaliculi dynamics. These three types of cholestatic stimuli induce two cellular responses, being (i) an adverse response characterized by the occurrence of mitochondrial impairment, endoplasmic reticulum (ER) stress with unfolded protein responses (UPR), oxidative stress, inflammation and different cell death modes, and (ii) an adaptive response relying on the activation of nuclear receptors.

5.2 Sandwich and spheroid cultures of primary hepatocytes as tools to test drug-induced cholestatic liver injury

Because of their longevity, the presence of an *in vivo*-like three-dimensional cellular configuration and cellular interactions as well as of bile ductules, sandwich and spheroid cultures of primary hepatocytes are currently considered as the best performing *in vitro* systems to detect cholestatic compounds (Vinken, 2018). A typical protocol used to sensitize hepatocytes in both culture systems to cholestatic insults includes co-incubation with a cholestatic drug and bile acids. Serum bile acid pool concentrations typically increase by 50-fold during human cholestasis compared to healthy conditions (Humbert et al., 2012; Tagliacozzi et al., 2003). Therefore, a 30–50 times concentrated mixture of the five most abundant bile acids present in serum is typically added to cell culture media of primary hepatocytes in sandwich (Oorts, Richert, & Annaert, 2015) and spheroid cultures (Hendriks et al., 2016). When exposing human and rat hepatocytes in sandwich cultures to hepatotoxic drugs in the presence of such concentrated bile acid mixture for 24–48 h, a distinction can be made between those that act in a cholestatic or in a non-cholestatic way. This relies on the so-called drug-induced cholestasis index, defined as hepatocyte viability, based on measurement of urea formation after exposure of primary hepatocytes in sandwich culture to a combination of the drug and the concentrated bile acid mixture over hepatocyte functionality after exposure of primary hepatocytes in sandwich culture to the drug alone. Unlike non-cholestatic hepatotoxic drugs, cholestatic counterparts, such as nefazodone and troglitazone, are characterized by drug-induced cholestasis indices below 0.8. For those drugs, a safety margin can be further calculated as the ratio of the lowest *in vitro* concentration resulting in drug-induced cholestasis index values below 0.8 over the total maximum plasma concentration, and do not exceed 30. In fact, the safety margin values in sandwich cultures of human hepatocytes correlate well with the incidence of clinical drug-induced cholestasis (Chatterjee, Richert, Augustijns, & Annaert, 2014; Oorts et al., 2016). Microarray analysis of primary human hepatocytes in sandwich culture following exposure to cholestatic drugs in therapeutic concentrations yielded a transcriptomic signature of cholestatic liver injury. Interestingly, the degree of transcriptomic changes induced by drugs, such as cyclosporine A, after short (*i.e.*, 1–3 days) and long-term (*i.e.*, 14 days) treatment can be directly related to the expression of nuclear receptors, drug and bile acid transporters as well as metabolizing enzymes (Parmentier et al., 2017). This reflects the occurrence of the typical adaptive response to cholestatic insult, which is rather difficult to pick up with other liver-based *in vitro* models. At the phenotypic level, bile canaliculi kinetics and dynamics seem reliable and fast parameters to predict the cholestatic potential of drugs in sandwich cultures of primary hepatocytes. In this context, inhibition of bile canaliculi network formation, such as by benzbromarone, in this *in vitro* setting was found to correlate with clinical cholestatic liability (Takemura, Izaki, Sekine, & Ito, 2016). This equally holds true when using hepatic uptake, biliary excretion and biliary clearance as read-outs (Ansede, Smith, Perry, St Claire, & Brouwer, 2010). Such experimental approaches can be fully automated and quantified, rendering them promising screening tools for pharmaceutical industry (Reif et al., 2015).

A recent interlaboratory study showed that spheroid cultures of primary hepatocytes are more sensitive to hepatotoxic compounds, including cholestatic drugs, like bosentan, compared to sandwich cultures of primary hepatocytes, in particular upon long-term (*i.e.*, 14 days) exposures (Bell et al., 2018). Spheroid cultures of primary hepatocytes remain phenotypically stable and retain morphology, viability as well as hepatocyte-specific functions for culture periods of at least 5 weeks (Bell et al., 2016; Vorrink et al., 2017). In fact, by repeatedly co-exposing spheroid cultures of primary hepatocytes to drugs with different mechanisms of hepatotoxicity and a concentrated bile acid mixture for 8 days, a selective synergistic toxicity of drugs known to cause cholestatic or mixed cholestatic/hepatocellular toxicity and the bile acid mixture compared to exposure to the drugs alone is observed. This phenomenon becomes even more pronounced after extending the exposure time to 14 days and can be expressed in the cholestatic index, a parameter similar to the drug-induced cholestasis index in sandwich cultures of primary hepatocytes, albeit using adenosine triphosphate content and not urea formation as a read-out (Bell et al., 2016). As a matter of fact, exposure of spheroid cultures of primary human hepatocytes for 14 days to more than 100 drugs showed that adenosine triphosphate content can be used as a single endpoint to distinguish hepatotoxic from non-hepatotoxic compounds with 100% specificity (Vorrink et al., 2018).

6. Conclusion

Because of its unique function and localization in the body, the liver is a primary target of toxicity induced by xenobiotics, *in casu* drugs. Drug-induced liver injury can be manifested in a number of ways, such as cholestasis, steatosis and fibrosis, and is a major reason for discontinuation of drug development and withdrawal of drugs from the market. Nevertheless, it still remains challenging to detect drug-induced liver injury. Indeed, standard animal studies conducted during routine drug development usually pick up merely 50–60% of all human hepatotoxic compounds. Driven by this shortcoming as well as by ethical constraints, increasing attention has been paid over the past 2 decades to the development of human-based liver-derived *in vitro* models for toxicity testing. At present, however, these systems barely identify about half of all clinical drug-induced liver injury cases (Laverty et al., 2010; Xu et al., 2004). This is due, at least in part, to the lack of optimal biomarkers, and in particular combinations of those, to accurately detect drug-induced liver injury, which in turn results from gaps in the current knowledge about the mechanisms that drive drug-induced liver injury (Vinken, 2018). An equally important reason for this flaw includes the limited capacity of the liver-derived *in vitro* models as such to fully imitate the natural *in vivo* hepatic situation. In case of primary hepatocytes and their adherent cultures, considered as the benchmark *in vitro* system in the area of liver-based *in vitro* modeling, this is associated with dedifferentiation. This deteriorative process both at the morphological and functional level can be delayed by a number of classical approaches that are aimed at restoring the natural hepatocyte micro-environment. Although useful, these classical anti-dedifferentiation strategies are only partly successful, yielding primary hepatocyte cultures that can be used for weeks instead of days. This is because these strategies are targeted towards reducing the consequences of dedifferentiation, without acting on its actual causes (Fraczek, Bolleyn, Vanhaecke, Rogiers, & Vinken, 2013; Godoy et al., 2013; Vinken, Vanhaecke, & Rogiers, 2012). With the advent of omics technologies over the past years, insight into the mechanisms underlying hepatocyte dedifferentiation has greatly increased (Baker et al., 2001; Boess et al., 2003). This has formed the rational basis for novel anti-dedifferentiation methodologies that affect the most upstream regulatory level of dedifferentiation by interfering with (epi)genetic control of liver-specific gene expression (Fraczek et al., 2013). These innovative anti-dedifferentiation methods have proven very efficient, yet are still not sufficient on their own to create *in vitro* systems that may fully replace liver toxicity testing *in vivo*. The future not only lies in combining classical and novel anti-dedifferentiation strategies, but also in getting expertise other than cell biology involved in the toxicology research niche. Such interdisciplinary research efforts are indeed an absolute *conditione sine qua non* to move this field forward. Of specific interest in this context is the area of (bio-)engineering, which has already resulted in a number of advanced liver-based *in vitro* models, namely liver bioreactors and liver chips, by implementing cutting-edge technical features, such as microfluidics and in-built sensors to monitor hepatocyte toxicity in real-time (Kimura, Sakai, & Fujii, 2018; Lauschke, Hendriks, Bell, Andersson, & Ingelman-Sundberg, 2016). Nevertheless, several challenges still lie ahead, including furnishing such state-of-the-art *in vitro* models with microbiota, which have emerged lately as critical goalkeepers in drug-induced liver injury pathogenesis (Possamai et al., 2015; Yip et al., 2018), modeling of idiosyncratic drug-induced liver injury (Ballet, 2015; Kenna, 2017) and investigating the role of extracellular vesicles in drug-induced liver injury (Cho, Song, Akbar, & Baek, 2018). Research in these directions should be strongly encouraged, as it opens the way to reliable animal-free and fully human-based drug-induced liver injury prediction.

Acknowledgments

This work was supported by the grants of the European Research Council, the Center for Alternatives to Animal Testing at Johns Hopkins University, Baltimore, USA, the Fund for Scientific Research—Flanders and the University Hospital of the Willy Gepts Fonds UZ-Brussels.

Conflict of interest

The authors have no conflicts of interest to declare.

References

Abdel-Misih, S. R., & Bloomston, M. (2010). Liver anatomy. *Surgical Clinics of North America, 90*, 643–653.

Alpini, G., Phillips, J. O., Vroman, B., & LaRusso, N. F. (1994). Recent advances in the isolation of liver cells. *Hepatology, 20*, 494–514.

Ansede, J. H., Smith, W. R., Perry, C. H., St Claire, R. L., & Brouwer, K. R. (2010). An *in vitro* assay to assess transporter-based cholestatic hepatotoxicity using sandwich-cultured rat hepatocytes. *Drug Metabolism and Disposition, 38*, 276–280.

Auth, M. K., Woitaschek, D., Beste, M., Schreiter, T., Kim, H. S., Oppermann, E., et al. (2005). Preservation of the synthetic and metabolic capacity of isolated human hepatocytes by coculture with human biliary epithelial cells. *Liver Transplantation, 11*, 410–419.

Bailly-Maitre, B., de Sousa, G., Zucchini, N., Gugenheim, J., Boulukos, K. E., Rahmani, R., et al. (2002). Spontaneous apoptosis in primary cultures of human and rat hepatocytes: Molecular mechanisms and regulation by dexamethasone. *Cell Death and Differentiation, 9*, 945–955.

Baker, T. K., Carfagna, M. A., Gao, H., Dow, E. R., Li, Q., Searfoss, G. H., et al. (2001). Temporal gene expression analysis of monolayer cultured rat hepatocytes. *Chemical Research in Toxicology, 14*, 1218–1231.

Ballet, F. (2015). Preventing drug-induced liver injury: How useful are animal models? *Digestive Diseases, 33*, 477–485.

Banic, B., Nipic, D., Suput, D., & Milisav, I. (2011). DMSO modulates the pathway of apoptosis triggering. *Cellular and Molecular Biology Letters, 16*, 328–341.

Baudoin, R., Corlu, A., Griscom, L., Legallais, C., & Leclerc, E. (2007). Trends in the development of microfluidic cell biochips for *in vitro* hepatotoxicity. *Toxicology In Vitro, 21*, 535–544.

Beigel, J., Fella, K., Kramer, P. J., Kroeger, M., & Hewitt, P. (2008). Genomics and proteomics analysis of cultured primary rat hepatocytes. *Toxicology In Vitro, 22*, 171–181.

Bell, C. C., Danker, A. C. A., Lauschke, V. M., Sison-Young, R., Jenkins, R., Rowe, C., et al. (2018). Comparison of hepatic 2D sandwich cultures and 3D spheroids for long-term toxicity applications: A multicenter study. *Toxicological Sciences, 162*, 655–666.

Bell, C. C., Hendriks, D. F., Moro, S. M., Ellis, E., Walsh, J., Renblom, A., et al. (2016). Characterization of primary human hepatocyte spheroids as a model system for drug-induced liver injury, liver function and disease. *Scientific Reports, 6*, 25187.

Bell, C. C., Lauschke, V. M., Vorrink, S. U., Palmgren, H., Duffin, R., Andersson, T. B., et al. (2017). Transcriptional, functional, and mechanistic comparisons of stem cell-derived hepatocytes, HepaRG cells, and three-dimensional human hepatocyte spheroids as predictive *in vitro* systems for drug-induced liver injury. *Drug Metabolism and Disposition, 45*, 419–429.

Berry, M. N., Grivell, A. R., Grivell, M. B., & Phillips, J. W. (1997). Isolated hepatocytes: Past, present and future. *Cell Biology and Toxicology, 13*, 223–233.

Bhadriraju, K., & Hansen, L. K. (2000). Hepatocyte adhesion, growth and differentiated function on RGD-containing proteins. *Biomaterials, 21*, 267–272.

Bhamidimarri, K. R., & Schiff, E. (2013). Drug-induced cholestasis. *Clinics in Liver Disease, 17*, 519–531.

Bismuth, H. (1982). Surgical anatomy and anatomical surgery of the liver. *World Journal of Surgery, 6*, 3–9.

Björnsson, E., & Olsson, R. (2005). Outcome and prognostic markers in severe drug-induced liver disease. *Hepatology, 42*, 481–489.
Boess, F., Kamber, M., Romer, S., Gasser, R., Muller, D., Albertini, S., et al. (2003). Gene expression in two hepatic cell lines, cultured primary hepatocytes, and liver slices compared to the *in vivo* liver gene expression in rats: Possible implications for toxicogenomics use of *in vitro* systems. *Toxicological Sciences, 73*, 386–402.
Bolleyn, J., Fraczek, J., Vinken, M., Lizarraga, D., Gaj, S., van Delft, J. H., et al. (2011). Effect of trichostatin A on miRNA expression in cultures of primary rat hepatocytes. *Toxicology In Vitro, 25*, 1173–1182.
Braet, F., & Wisse, E. (2002). Structural and functional aspects of liver sinusoidal endothelial cell *fenestrae*: A review. *Comparative Hepatology, 1*, 1.
Bresgen, N., Ohlenschlager, I., Wacht, N., Afazel, S., Ladurner, G., & Eckl, P. M. (2008). Ferritin and FasL (CD95L) mediate density dependent apoptosis in primary rat hepatocytes. *Journal of Cellular Physiology, 217*, 800–808.
Caperna, T. J., Blomberg, L. A., Garrett, W. M., & Talbot, N. C. (2011). Culture of porcine hepatocytes or bile duct epithelial cells by inductive serum-free media. *In Vitro Cellular & Developmental Biology. Animal, 47*, 218–233.
Cereghini, S. (1996). Liver-enriched transcription factors and hepatocyte differentiation. *FASEB Journal, 10*, 267–282.
Chatterjee, S., Richert, L., Augustijns, P., & Annaert, P. (2014). Hepatocyte-based *in vitro* model for assessment of drug-induced cholestasis. *Toxicology and Applied Pharmacology, 274*, 124–136.
Cho, Y. E., Song, B. J., Akbar, M., & Baek, M. C. (2018). Extracellular vesicles as potential biomarkers for alcohol- and drug-induced liver injury and their therapeutic applications. *Pharmacology and Therapeutics, 187*, 180–194.
Corlu, A., Ilyin, G., Cariou, S., Lamy, I., Loyer, P., & Guguen-Guillouzo, C. (1997). The coculture: A system for studying the regulation of liver differentiation/proliferation activity and its control. *Cell Biology and Toxicology, 13*, 235–242.
Corlu, A., Lamy, I., Ilyin, G. P., Fardel, O., Kneip, B., Le Jossic, C., et al. (1998). Hematopoiesis-promoting activity of rat liver biliary epithelial cells: Involvement of a cell surface molecule, liver-regulating protein. *Experimental Hematology, 26*, 382–394.
De Kock, J., Ceelen, L., De Spiegelaere, W., Casteleyn, C., Claes, P., Vanhaecke, T., et al. (2011). Simple and quick method for whole-liver decellularization: A novel *in vitro* three-dimensional bioengineering tool? *Archives of Toxicology, 85*, 607–612.
De Leeuw, A. M., Brouwer, A., & Knook, D. L. (1990). Sinusoidal endothelial cells of the liver: Fine structure and function in relation to age. *Journal of Electron Microscopy Technique, 14*, 218–236.
de Longueville, F., Atienzar, F. A., Marcq, L., Dufrane, S., Evrard, S., Wouters, L., et al. (2003). Use of a low-density microarray for studying gene expression patterns induced by hepatotoxicants on primary cultures of rat hepatocytes. *Toxicological Sciences, 75*, 378–392.
Dich, J., Vind, C., & Grunnet, N. (1988). Long-term culture of hepatocytes: Effect of hormones on enzyme activities and metabolic capacity. *Hepatology, 8*, 39–45.
Dunn, J. C., Tompkins, R. G., & Yarmush, M. L. (1991). Long-term *in vitro* function of adult hepatocytes in a collagen sandwich configuration. *Biotechnology Progress, 7*, 237–245.
Edwards, A. M., Glistak, M. L., Lucas, C. M., & Wilson, P. A. (1984). 7-ethoxycoumarin deethylase activity as a convenient measure of liver drug metabolizing enzymes: Regulation in cultured rat hepatocytes. *Biochemical Pharmacology, 33*, 1537–1546.
El-Ali, J., Sorger, P. K., & Jensen, K. F. (2006). Cells on chips. *Nature, 442*, 403–411.
Elaut, G., Henkens, T., Papeleu, P., Snykers, S., Vinken, M., Vanhaecke, T., et al. (2006). Molecular mechanisms underlying the dedifferentiation process of isolated hepatocytes and their cultures. *Current Drug Metabolism, 7*, 629–660.

Elaut, G., Vanhaecke, T., Heyden, Y. V., & Rogiers, V. (2005). Spontaneous apoptosis, necrosis, energy status, glutathione levels and biotransformation capacities of isolated rat hepatocytes in suspension: Effect of the incubation medium. *Biochemical Pharmacology*, *69*, 1829–1838.

Ethier, C., Raymond, V. A., Musallam, L., Houle, R., & Bilodeau, M. (2003). Anti-apoptotic effect of EGF on mouse hepatocytes associated with downregulation of proapoptotic Bid protein. *American Journal of Physiology. Gastrointestinal and Liver Physiology*, *285*, G298–G308.

Evenou, F., Hamon, M., Fujii, T., Takeuchi, S., & Sakai, Y. (2011). Gas-permeable membranes and co-culture with fibroblasts enable high-density hepatocyte culture as multilayered liver tissues. *Biotechnology Progress*, *27*, 1146–1153.

Farkas, D., Bhat, V. B., Mandapati, S., Wishnok, J. S., & Tannenbaum, S. R. (2005). Characterization of the secreted proteome of rat hepatocytes cultured in collagen sandwiches. *Chemical Research in Toxicology*, *18*, 1132–1139.

Farkas, D., & Tannenbaum, S. R. (2005). Characterization of chemically induced hepatotoxicity in collagen sandwiches of rat hepatocytes. *Toxicological Sciences*, *85*, 927–934.

Fladmark, K. E., Gjertsen, B. T., Doskeland, S. O., & Vintermyr, O. K. (1997). Fas/APO-1 (CD95)-induced apoptosis of primary hepatocytes is inhibited by cAMP. *Biochemical and Biophysical Research Communications*, *232*, 20–25.

Fraczek, J., Bolleyn, J., Vanhaecke, T., Rogiers, V., & Vinken, M. (2013). Primary hepatocyte cultures for pharmaco-toxicological studies: At the busy crossroad of various anti-dedifferentiation strategies. *Archives of Toxicology*, *87*, 577–610.

Fraczek, J. E., Vinken, M., Tourwé, D., Vanhaecke, T., & Rogiers, V. (2011). Synergetic effects of DNA demethylation and histone deacetylase inhibition in primary rat hepatocytes. *Investigational New Drugs*, *30*, 1715–1724.

Friedman, S. L. (2015). Hepatic fibrosis: Emerging therapies. *Digestive Diseases*, *33*, 504–507.

Fu, T., Guo, D., Huang, X., O'Gorman, M. R., Huang, L., Crawford, S. E., et al. (2001). Apoptosis occurs in isolated and banked primary mouse hepatocytes. *Cell Transplantation*, *10*, 59–66.

Garside, H., Stevens, A., Farrow, S., Normand, C., Houle, B., Berry, A., et al. (2004). Glucocorticoid ligands specify different interactions with NF-kappaB by allosteric effects on the glucocorticoid receptor DNA binding domain. *Journal of Biological Chemistry*, *279*, 50050–50059.

Genove, E., Schmitmeier, S., Sala, A., Borros, S., Bader, A., Griffith, L. G., et al. (2009). Functionalized self-assembling peptide hydrogel enhance maintenance of hepatocyte activity *in vitro*. *Journal of Cellular and Molecular Medicine*, *13*, 3387–3397.

Ghodsizadeh, A., Taei, A., Totonchi, M., Seifinejad, A., Gourabi, H., Pournasr, B., et al. (2010). Generation of liver disease-specific induced pluripotent stem cells along with efficient differentiation to functional hepatocyte-like cells. *Stem Cell Reviews*, *6*, 622–632.

Gilot, D., Loyer, P., Corlu, A., Glaise, D., Lagadic-Gossmann, D., Atfi, A., et al. (2002). Liver protection from apoptosis requires both blockage of initiator caspase activities and inhibition of ASK1/JNK pathway *via* glutathione S-transferase regulation. *Journal of Biological Chemistry*, *277*, 49220–49229.

Godoy, P., Hewitt, N. J., Albrecht, U., Andersen, M. E., Ansari, N., Bhattacharya, S., et al. (2013). Recent advances in 2D and 3D *in vitro* systems using primary hepatocytes, alternative hepatocyte sources and non-parenchymal liver cells and their use in investigating mechanisms of hepatotoxicity, cell signaling and ADME. *Archives of Toxicology*, *87*, 1315–1530.

Goldberg, D. S., Forde, K. A., Carbonari, D. M., Lewis, J. D., Leidl, K. B., Reddy, K. R., et al. (2015). Population-representative incidence of drug-induced acute liver failure based on an analysis of an integrated health care system. *Gastroenterology*, *148*, 1353–1361.

Gomez-Quiroz, L. E., Factor, V. M., Kaposi-Novak, P., Coulouarn, C., Conner, E. A., & Thorgeirsson, S. S. (2008). Hepatocyte-specific c-Met deletion disrupts redox homeostasis and sensitizes to Fas-mediated apoptosis. *Journal of Biological Chemistry, 283*, 14581–14589.
Gonzalez, F. J. (2008). Regulation of hepatocyte nuclear factor 4 alpha-mediated transcription. *Drug Metabolism and Pharmacokinetics, 23*, 2–7.
Goral, V. N., Hsieh, Y. C., Petzold, O. N., Clark, J. S., Yuen, P. K., & Faris, R. A. (2010). Perfusion-based microfluidic device for three-dimensional dynamic primary human hepatocyte cell culture in the absence of biological or synthetic matrices or coagulants. *Lab on a Chip, 10*, 3380–3386.
Goral, V. N., & Yuen, P. K. (2011). Microfluidic platforms for hepatocyte cell culture: New technologies and applications. *Annals of Biomedical Engineering, 40*, 1244–1254.
Gossard, A. A., & Talwalkar, J. A. (2014). Cholestatic liver disease. *Medical Clinics of North America, 98*, 73–85.
Guguen-Guillouzo, C., Clement, B., Baffet, G., Beaumont, C., Morel-Chany, E., Glaise, D., et al. (1983). Maintenance and reversibility of active albumin secretion by adult rat hepatocytes co-cultured with another liver epithelial cell type. *Experimental Cell Research, 143*, 47–54.
Guguen-Guillouzo, C., & Guillouzo, A. (1983). Modulation of functional activities in cultured rat hepatocytes. *Molecular and Cellular Biochemistry, 53–54*, 35–56.
Hamilton, G. A., Jolley, S. L., Gilbert, D., Coon, D. J., Barros, S., & LeCluyse, E. L. (2001). Regulation of cell morphology and cytochrome P450 expression in human hepatocytes by extracellular matrix and cell-cell interactions. *Cell and Tissue Research, 306*, 85–99.
Hendriks, D. F., Fredriksson Puigvert, L., Messner, S., Mortiz, W., & Ingelman-Sundberg, M. (2016). Hepatic 3D spheroid models for the detection and study of compounds with cholestatic liability. *Scientific Reports, 6*, 35434.
Henkens, T., Papeleu, P., Elaut, G., Vinken, M., Rogiers, V., & Vanhaecke, T. (2007). Trichostatin A, a critical factor in maintaining the functional differentiation of primary cultured rat hepatocytes. *Toxicology and Applied Pharmacology, 218*, 64–71.
Hiramatsu, K., Matsumoto, Y., Miyazaki, M., Tsubouchi, H., Yamamoto, I., & Gohda, E. (2005). Inhibition of hepatocyte growth factor production in human fibroblasts by ursodeoxycholic acid. *Biological and Pharmaceutical Bulletin, 28*, 619–624.
Hughes, C. S., Postovit, L. M., & Lajoie, G. A. (2010). Matrigel: A complex protein mixture required for optimal growth of cell culture. *Proteomics, 10*, 1886–1890.
Humbert, L., Maubert, M. A., Wolf, C., Duboc, H., Mahé, M., Farabos, D., et al. (2012). Bile acid profiling in human biological samples: Comparison of extraction procedures and application to normal and cholestatic patients. *Journal of Chromatography. B, Analytical Technologies in the Biomedical and Life Sciences, 899*, 135–145.
Hwang-Verslues, W. W., & Sladek, F. M. (2010). HNF4alpha: Role in drug metabolism and potential drug target? *Current Opinion in Pharmacology, 10*, 698–705.
Imagawa, K., Takayama, K., Isoyama, S., Tanikawa, K., Shinkai, M., Harada, K., et al. (2017). Generation of a bile salt export pump deficiency model using patient-specific induced pluripotent stem cell-derived hepatocyte-like cells. *Scientific Reports*, 7, 41806.
Inoue, C., Yamamoto, H., Nakamura, T., Ichihara, A., & Okamoto, H. (1989). Nicotinamide prolongs survival of primary cultured hepatocytes without involving loss of hepatocyte-specific functions. *Journal of Biological Chemistry, 264*, 4747–4750.
Irie, S., & Tavassoli, M. (1991). Transendothelial transport of macromolecules: The concept of tissue-blood barriers. *Cell Biology Reviews, 25*, 317–333.
Ishibashi, H., Nakamura, M., Komori, A., Migita, K., & Shimoda, S. (2009). Liver architecture, cell function, and disease. *Seminars in Immunopathology, 31*, 399–409.
Jungermann, K. (1986). Functional heterogeneity of periportal and perivenous hepatocytes. *Enzyme, 35*, 161–180.

Jungermann, K., & Kietzmann, T. (1996). Zonation of parenchymal and nonparenchymal metabolism in liver. *Annual Review of Nutrition, 16*, 179–203.
Kaestner, K. H. (2010). The FoxA factors in organogenesis and differentiation. *Current Opinion in Genetics and Development, 20*, 527–532.
Kang, L., Chung, B. G., Langer, R., & Khademhosseini, A. (2008). Microfluidics for drug discovery and development: From target selection to product lifecycle management. *Drug Discovery Today, 13*, 1–13.
Kasuya, J., Sudo, R., Mitaka, T., Ikeda, M., & Tanishita, K. (2011). Hepatic stellate cell-mediated three-dimensional hepatocyte and endothelial cell triculture model. *Tissue Engineering Part A, 17*, 361–370.
Kenna, J. G. (2017). Human biology-based drug safety evaluation: Scientific rationale, current status and future challenges. *Expert Opinion on Drug Metabolism & Toxicology, 13*, 567–574.
Khetani, S. R., & Bhatia, S. N. (2008). Microscale culture of human liver cells for drug development. *Nature Biotechnology, 26*, 120–126.
Kim, J. J., Park, B. C., Kido, Y., & Accili, D. (2001). Mitogenic and metabolic effects of type I IGF receptor overexpression in insulin receptor-deficient hepatocytes. *Endocrinology, 142*, 3354–3360.
Kim, Y., & Rajagopalan, P. (2010). 3D hepatic cultures simultaneously maintain primary hepatocyte and liver sinusoidal endothelial cell phenotypes. *PLoS One, 5*, e15456.
Kimura, H., Sakai, Y., & Fujii, T. (2018). Organ/body-on-a-chip based on microfluidic technology for drug discovery. *Drug Metabolism and Pharmacokinetics, 33*, 43–48.
Lang, R., Stern, M. M., Smith, L., Liu, Y., Bharadwaj, S., Liu, G., et al. (2011). Three-dimensional culture of hepatocytes on porcine liver tissue-derived extracellular matrix. *Biomaterials, 32*, 7042–7052.
Lauschke, V. M., Hendriks, D. F., Bell, C. C., Andersson, T. B., & Ingelman-Sundberg, M. (2016). Novel 3D culture systems for studies of human liver function and assessments of the hepatotoxicity of drugs and drug candidates. *Chemical Research in Toxicology, 29*, 1936–1955.
Laverty, H. G., Antoine, D. J., Benson, C., Chaponda, M., Williams, D., & Kevin Park, B. (2010). The potential of cytokines as safety biomarkers for drug-induced liver injury. *European Journal of Clinical Pharmacology, 66*, 961–976.
LeCluyse, E., Bullock, P., & Parkinson, A. (1996). Strategies for restoration and maintenance of normal hepatic structure and function in long term cultures of hepatocytes. *Advanced Drug Delivery Reviews, 22*, 133–186.
Lee, W. M. (2013). Drug-induced acute liver failure. *Clinics in Liver Disease, 17*, 575–586.
Lee, Y. A., Wallace, M. C., & Friedman, S. L. (2015). Pathobiology of liver fibrosis: A translational success story. *Gut, 64*, 830–841.
Leite, S. B., Teixeira, A. P., Miranda, J. P., Tostoes, R. M., Clemente, J. J., Sousa, M. F., et al. (2011). Merging bioreactor technology with 3D hepatocyte-fibroblast culturing approaches: Improved *in vitro* models for toxicological applications. *Toxicology In Vitro, 25*, 825–832.
Lu, J. N., Wang, C. C., & Young, T. H. (2011). The behaviors of long-term cryopreserved human hepatocytes on different biomaterials. *Artificial Organs, 35*, E65–E72.
Malarkey, D. E., Johnson, K., Ryan, L., Boorman, G., & Maronpot, R. R. (2005). New insights into functional aspects of liver morphology. *Toxicologic Pathology, 33*, 27–34.
Matsuno, F., Chowdhury, S., Gotoh, T., Iwase, K., Matsuzaki, H., Takatsuki, K., et al. (1996). Induction of the C/EBP beta gene by dexamethasone and glucagon in primary-cultured rat hepatocytes. *Journal of Biochemistry, 119*, 524–532.
McCuskey, R. S. (2008). The hepatic microvascular system in health and its response to toxicants. *Anatomical Record, 291*, 661–671.

Meier, Y., Cavallaro, M., Roos, M., Pauli-Magnus, C., Folkers, G., Meier, P. J., et al. (2005). Incidence of drug-induced liver injury in medical inpatients. *European Journal of Clinical Pharmacology*, *61*, 135–143.

Mesnil, M., Fraslin, J. M., Piccoli, C., Yamasaki, H., & Guguen-Guillouzo, C. (1987). Cell contact but not junctional communication (dye coupling) with biliary epithelial cells is required for hepatocytes to maintain differentiated functions. *Experimental Cell Research*, *173*, 524–533.

Mizuguchi, T., Mitaka, T., Hirata, K., Oda, H., & Mochizuki, Y. (1998). Alteration of expression of liver-enriched transcription factors in the transition between growth and differentiation of primary cultured rat hepatocytes. *Journal of Cellular Physiology*, *174*, 273–284.

Musallam, L., Ethier, C., Haddad, P. S., & Bilodeau, M. (2001). Role of EGF receptor tyrosine kinase activity in antiapoptotic effect of EGF on mouse hepatocytes. *American Journal of Physiology. Gastrointestinal and Liver Physiology*, *280*, G1360–G1369.

Naiki, T., Nagaki, M., Asano, T., Kimata, T., & Moriwaki, H. (2005). Adenovirus-mediated hepatocyte nuclear factor-4alpha overexpression maintains liver phenotype in cultured rat hepatocytes. *Biochemical and Biophysical Research Communications*, *335*, 496–500.

Nakamura, T., Mura, T., Saito, K., Ohsawa, T., Akiyoshi, H., & Sato, K. (1998). Adenovirus-transferred HNF-3 gamma conserves some liver functions in primary cultured hepatocytes of adult rats. *Biochemical and Biophysical Research Communications*, *253*, 352–357.

Nakatsuka, H., Sokabe, T., Yamamoto, K., Sato, Y., Hatakeyama, K., Kamiya, A., et al. (2006). Shear stress induces hepatocyte PAI-1 gene expression through cooperative Sp1/Ets-1 activation of transcription. *American Journal of Physiology. Gastrointestinal and Liver Physiology*, *29*, G26–G34.

Nguyen, K. D., Sundaram, V., & Ayoub, W. S. (2014). Atypical causes of cholestasis. *World Journal of Gastroenterology*, *20*, 9418–9426.

Noor, F. (2015). A shift in paradigm towards human biology-based systems for cholestatic liver diseases. *Journal of Physiology*, *593*, 5043–5055.

Oorts, M., Baze, A., Bachellier, P., Heyd, B., Zacharias, T., Annaert, P., et al. (2016). Drug-induced cholestasis risk assessment in sandwich-cultured human hepatocytes. *Toxicology In Vitro*, *34*, 179–186.

Oorts, M., Richert, L., & Annaert, P. (2015). Drug-induced cholestasis detection in cryopreserved rat hepatocytes in sandwich culture. *Journal of Pharmacological and Toxicological Methods*, *73*, 63–71.

Paine, A. J., & Andreakos, E. (2004). Activation of signalling pathways during hepatocyte isolation: Relevance to toxicology *in vitro*. *Toxicology In Vitro*, *18*, 187–193.

Papeleu, P., Loyer, P., Vanhaecke, T., Henkens, T., Elaut, G., Guguen-Guillouzo, C., et al. (2004). Proliferation of epidermal growth factor-stimulated hepatocytes in a hormonally defined serum-free medium. *Alternatives to Laboratory Animals*, *32*, 57–64.

Papeleu, P., Vanhaecke, T., Henkens, T., Elaut, G., Vinken, M., Snykers, S., et al. (2006). Isolation of rat hepatocytes. *Methods in Molecular Biology*, *320*, 229–237.

Papeleu, P., Wullaert, A., Elaut, G., Henkens, T., Vinken, M., Laus, G., et al. (2007). Inhibition of NF-kappaB activation by the histone deacetylase inhibitor 4-Me_2N-BAVAH induces an early G1 cell cycle arrest in primary hepatocytes. *Cell Proliferation*, *40*, 640–655.

Parker, G. A., & Picut, C. A. (2005). Liver immunobiology. *Toxicologic Pathology*, *33*, 52–62.

Parmentier, C., Couttet, P., Wolf, A., Zaccharias, T., Heyd, B., Bachellier, P., et al. (2017). Evaluation of transcriptomic signature as a valuable tool to study drug-induced cholestasis in primary human hepatocytes. *Archives of Toxicology*, *91*, 2879–2893.

Possamai, L. A., McPhail, M. J., Khamri, W., Wu, B., Concas, D., Harrison, M., et al. (2015). The role of intestinal microbiota in murine models of acetaminophen-induced hepatotoxicity. *Liver International*, *35*, 764–773.

Pradip, A., Steel, D., Jacobsson, S., Holmgren, G., Ingelman-Sundberg, M., Sartipy, P., et al. (2016). High-content analysis of human pluripotent stem cell-derived hepatocytes reveals drug-induced steatosis and phospholipidosis. *Stem Cells International*, *2016*, 2475631.

Prot, J. M., Videau, O., Brochot, C., Legallais, C., Benech, H., & Leclerc, E. (2011). A cocktail of metabolic probes demonstrates the relevance of primary human hepatocyte cultures in a microfluidic biochip for pharmaceutical drug screening. *International Journal of Pharmaceutics*, *408*, 67–75.

Qiao, L., & Farrell, G. C. (1999). The effects of cell density, attachment substratum and dexamethasone on spontaneous apoptosis of rat hepatocytes in primary culture. *In Vitro Cellular & Developmental Biology. Animal*, *35*, 417–424.

Rajagopalan, P., Shen, C. J., Berthiaume, F., Tilles, A. W., Toner, M., & Yarmush, M. L. (2006). Polyelectrolyte nano-scaffolds for the design of layered cellular architectures. *Tissue Engineering*, *12*, 1553–1563.

Reif, R., Karlsson, J., Günther, G., Beattie, L., Wrangborg, D., Hammad, S., et al. (2015). Bile canalicular dynamics in hepatocyte sandwich cultures. *Archives of Toxicology*, *89*, 1861–1870.

Rodrigues, R. M., De Kock, J., Branson, S., Vinken, M., Meganathan, K., Chaudhari, U., et al. (2014). Human skin-derived stem cells as a novel cell source for *in vitro* hepatotoxicity screening of pharmaceuticals. *Stem Cells and Development*, *23*, 44–55.

Rodriguez-Antona, C., Donato, M. T., Boobis, A., Edwards, R. J., Watts, P. S., Castell, J. V., et al. (2002). Cytochrome P450 expression in human hepatocytes and hepatoma cell lines: Molecular mechanisms that determine lower expression in cultured cells. *Xenobiotica*, *32*, 505–520.

Rutkauskas, S., Gedrimas, V., Pundzius, J., Barauskas, G., & Basevicius, A. (2006). Clinical and anatomical basis for the classification of the structural parts of liver. *Medicina*, *42*, 98–106.

Schulze-Bergkamen, H., Brenner, D., Krueger, A., Suess, D., Fas, S. C., Frey, C. R., et al. (2004). Hepatocyte growth factor induces Mcl-1 in primary human hepatocytes and inhibits CD95-mediated apoptosis *via* Akt. *Hepatology*, *39*, 645–654.

Schutte, M., Fox, B., Baradez, M. O., Devonshire, A., Minguez, J., Bokhari, M., et al. (2011). Rat primary hepatocytes show enhanced performance and sensitivity to acetaminophen during three-dimensional culture on a polystyrene scaffold designed for routine use. *Assay and Drug Development Technologies*, *9*, 475–486.

Seglen, P. O. (1976). Preparation of isolated rat liver cells. *Methods in Cell Biology*, *13*, 29–83.

Shinzawa, K., Watanabe, Y., & Akaike, T. (1995). Primary cultured murine hepatocytes but not hepatoma cells regulate the cell number through density-dependent cell death. *Cell Death and Differentiation*, *2*, 133–140.

Sidhu, J. S., Liu, F., & Omiecinski, C. J. (2004). Phenobarbital responsiveness as a uniquely sensitive indicator of hepatocyte differentiation status: Requirement of dexamethasone and extracellular matrix in establishing the functional integrity of cultured primary rat hepatocytes. *Experimental Cell Research*, *292*, 252–264.

Skett, P. (1994). Problems in using isolated and cultured hepatocytes for xenobiotic metabolism/metabolism-based toxicity testing-solutions? *Toxicology In Vitro*, *8*, 491–504.

Skett, P., & Bayliss, M. (1996). Time for a consistent approach to preparing and culturing hepatocytes? *Xenobiotica*, *26*, 1–7.

Smedsrød, B. (2004). Clearance function of scavenger endothelial cells. *Comparative Hepatology*, *3*(Suppl. 1), S22.

Smedsrød, B., De Bleser, P. J., Braet, F., Lovisetti, P., Vanderkerken, K., Wisse, E., et al. (1994). Cell biology of liver endothelial and Kupffer cells. *Gut*, *35*, 1509–1516.
Su, T., & Waxman, D. J. (2004). Impact of dimethyl sulfoxide on expression of nuclear receptors and drug-inducible cytochromes P450 in primary rat hepatocytes. *Archives of Biochemistry and Biophysics*, *424*, 226–234.
Tagliacozzi, D., Mozzi, A. F., Casetta, B., Bertucci, P., Bernardini, S., Di Ilio, C., et al. (2003). Quantitative analysis of bile acids in human plasma by liquid chromatography-electrospray tandem mass spectrometry: A simple and rapid one-step method. *Clinical Chemistry and Laboratory Medicine*, *41*, 1633–1641.
Takemura, A., Izaki, A., Sekine, S., & Ito, K. (2016). Inhibition of bile canalicular network formation in rat sandwich cultured hepatocytes by drugs associated with risk of severe liver injury. *Toxicology In Vitro*, *35*, 121–130.
Tanaka, Y., Sato, K., Yamato, M., Okano, T., & Kitamori, T. (2006). Cell culture and life support system for microbioreactor and bioassay. *Journal of Chromatography A*, *1111*, 233–237.
Trautwein, C., Friedman, S. L., Schuppan, D., & Pinzani, M. (2015). Hepatic fibrosis: Concept to treatment. *Journal of Hepatology*, *62*, S15–S24.
Tuschl, G., Hrach, J., Walter, Y., Hewitt, P. G., & Mueller, S. O. (2009). Serum-free collagen sandwich cultures of adult rat hepatocytes maintain liver-like properties long term: A valuable model for *in vitro* toxicity and drug-drug interaction studies. *Chemico-Biological Interactions*, *181*, 124–137.
Tuschl, G., & Mueller, S. O. (2006). Effects of cell culture conditions on primary rat hepatocytes: Cell morphology and differential gene expression. *Toxicology*, *218*, 205–215.
Van den Hof, W. F., Ruiz-Aracama, A., Van Summeren, A., Jennen, D. G., Gaj, S., Coonen, M. L., et al. (2015). Integrating multiple omics to unravel mechanisms of cyclosporin A induced hepatotoxicity *in vitro*. *Toxicology In Vitro*, *29*, 489–501.
Vanhaecke, T., Henkens, T., Kass, G. E., & Rogiers, V. (2004). Effect of the histone deacetylase inhibitor trichostatin A on spontaneous apoptosis in various types of adult rat hepatocyte cultures. *Biochemical Pharmacology*, *68*, 753–760.
Vinci, B., Duret, C., Klieber, S., Gerbal-Chaloin, S., Sa-Cunha, A., Laporte, S., et al. (2011). Modular bioreactor for primary human hepatocyte culture: Medium flow stimulates expression and activity of detoxification genes. *Biotechnology Journal*, *6*, 554–564.
Vinken, M. (2016). Regulation of connexin signaling by the epigenetic machinery. *Biochimica et Biophysica Acta (BBA)—Gene Regulatory Mechanisms*, *1859*, 262–268.
Vinken, M. (2018). *In vitro* prediction of drug-induced cholestatic liver injury: A challenge for the toxicologist. *Archives of Toxicology*, *92*, 1909–1912.
Vinken, M., Landesmann, B., Goumenou, M., Vinken, S., Shah, I., Jaeschke, H., et al. (2013). Development of an adverse outcome pathway from drug-mediated bile salt export pump inhibition to cholestatic liver injury. *Toxicological Sciences*, *136*, 97–106.
Vinken, M., Papeleu, P., Snykers, S., De Rop, E., Henkens, T., Chipman, J. K., et al. (2006). Involvement of cell junctions in hepatocyte culture functionality. *Critical Reviews in Toxicology*, *36*, 299–318.
Vinken, M., Vanhaecke, T., & Rogiers, V. (2012). Primary hepatocyte cultures as tools in drug development: *Quo vadis*? *Toxicology In Vitro*, *26*, 541–544.
Vorrink, S. U., Ullah, S., Schmidt, S., Nandania, J., Velagapudi, V., Beck, O., et al. (2017). Endogenous and xenobiotic metabolic stability of primary human hepatocytes in long-term 3D spheroid cultures revealed by a combination of targeted and untargeted metabolomics. *FASEB Journal*, *31*, 2696–2708.
Vorrink, S. U., Zhou, Y., Ingelman-Sundberg, M., & Lauschke, V. M. (2018). Prediction of drug-induced hepatotoxicity using long-term stable primary hepatic 3D spheroid cultures in chemically defined conditions. *Toxicological Sciences*, *163*, 655–665.

Weibel, E. R., Stäubli, W., Gnägi, H. R., & Hess, F. A. (1969). Correlated morphometric and biochemical studies on the liver cell: I. Morphometric model, stereologic methods, and normal morphometric data for rat liver. *Journal of Cell Biology*, *42*, 68–91.

Williams, C. M., Mehta, G., Peyton, S. R., Zeiger, A. S., Van Vliet, K. J., & Griffith, L. G. (2011). Autocrine-controlled formation and function of tissue-like aggregates by primary hepatocytes in micropatterned hydrogel arrays. *Tissue Engineering Part A*, *17*, 1055–1068.

Xu, J. J., Diaz, D., & O'Brien, P. J. (2004). Applications of cytotoxicity assays and pre-lethal mechanistic assays for assessment of human hepatotoxicity potential. *Chemico-Biological Interactions*, *150*, 115–128.

Yip, L. Y., Aw, C. C., Lee, S. H., Hong, Y. S., Ku, H. C., Xu, W. H., et al. (2018). The liver-gut microbiota axis modulates hepatotoxicity of tacrine in the rat. *Hepatology*, 7, 282–295.

CHAPTER TWO

Cell death in drug-induced liver injury

Andrea Iorga[a,b], Lily Dara[a,b,*]
[a]Division of Gastrointestinal and Liver Diseases, Department of Medicine, Keck School of Medicine, University of Southern California, Los Angeles, CA, United States
[b]Research Center for Liver Disease, Keck School of Medicine, University of Southern California, Los Angeles, CA, United States
*Corresponding author: e-mail address: lily.dara@usc.edu

Contents

Abstract

Drug-induced liver injury (DILI) is an important cause of liver toxicity which can have varying clinical presentations, the most severe of which being acute liver failure. Hepatocyte death as a cause of drug toxicity is a feature of DILI. There are multiple cell death subroutines; some, like apoptosis, necroptosis, autophagy, and necrosis have been extensively studied, while others such as pyroptosis and ferroptosis have been more recently described. The mode of cell death in DILI depends on the culprit drug, as it largely dictates the mechanism and extent of injury. The main cell death subroutines in DILI are apoptosis and necrosis, with mitochondrial involvement being pivotal for the execution of both. A few drugs such as acetaminophen (APAP) can cause direct, dose-dependent toxicity, while the majority of drugs cause idiosyncratic DILI (IDILI). IDILI is an unpredictable form of liver injury that is not dose dependent, occurs in individuals with a genetic predisposition, and presents with variable latency. APAP-induced programmed necrosis has been extensively studied. However, the mechanisms and pathogenesis of cell death from drugs causing IDILI are harder to elucidate due to the complex and multifactorial nature of the disease. Cell death in IDILI is likely death receptor-mediated apoptosis and the result of an activated innate and adaptive

Advances in Pharmacology, Volume 85
ISSN 1054-3589
https://doi.org/10.1016/bs.apha.2019.01.006
© 2019 Elsevier Inc.
All rights reserved.

immune system, compounded by other host factors such as genetics, gender, age, and capacity for immune tolerance. This chapter will review the different modes of cell death, namely apoptosis, necrosis, necroptosis, autophagy, pyroptosis, and ferroptosis and their pertinence to DILI.

Abbreviations

AIF	apoptosis-inducing factor
AIM2	absent in melanoma-2
ALF	acute liver failure
ALP	alkaline phosphatase
ALT	alanine aminotransferase
AMPK	AMP-activated protein kinase
APAF1	apoptotic peptidase activating factor 1
APAP	acetaminophen
ASC	apoptosis-associated speck-like protein containing a CARD
ASK1	apoptosis signal regulating kinase 1
ATG	autophagy
BSO	buthionine sulfoximine
cFLIP	FLICE inhibitory protein
CASP	caspase
CD95	cluster of differentiation-95, also known as the FAS receptor
cIAP1/2	cellular inhibitor of apoptosis 1/2
CoA	coenzyme A
CTLA-4	cytotoxic T-lymphocyte-associated protein 4, also known as CD152
CYLD	cylandromatosis
CYP	cytochrome P450
DAMP	danger-associated molecular patterns
DD	death domain
DILI	drug-induced liver injury
DISC	death-inducing signaling complex
DR	death receptor
DRP1	dynamin-related protein 1
ER	endoplasmic reticulum
ETC	electron transport chain
FADD	FAS-associated protein with death domain
FAS	also known as APO-1
FASL	FAS ligand
FAT1	FAT atypical cadherin 1
Fer-1	ferrostatin-1
FIP200	FAK family kinase-interacting protein of 200 kDa
FLICE	Fas-associating protein with death domain-like interleukin-1 beta-converting enzyme
GCL	glutamate-cysteine ligase
GPX4	glutathione peroxidase 4
GSDMD	Gasdermin D

GSH	glutathione
GSK3β	glycogen synthase kinase 3 beta
GSS	glutathione synthetase
GWAS	genome-wide association studies
HLA	human leukocyte antigen
HMGB1	high mobility group box -1
IAP	inhibitor of apoptosis
IDILI	idiosyncratic drug-induced liver injury
IKK	IkB kinase
IL	interleukin
JNK	c Jun N-terminal kinase
KC	Kupffer cells
LC3	microtubule-associated protein 1A/1B-light chain 3
LOX	lipoxygenases
LPS	lipopolysaccharides
LSEC	liver sinusoidal endothelial cells
LUBAC	linear ubiquitination assembly complex
MAPK	mitogen-activated protein kinase family
MHC	major histocompatibility complex
MKK4	mitogen-activated protein kinase 4
MLK3	mixed lineage kinase 3
MLKL	pseudokinase mixed lineage domain like
MOMP	mitochondrial outer membrane permeabilization
MPT	mitochondrial permeability transition
mTORC1	mTOR complex1
NAC	*N*-acetyl cysteine
NAPQI	*N*-acetyl-p-benzoquinone imine
NASH	nonalcoholic steatohepatitis
NEMO	NF-κB essential modifier
NF-κB	nuclear factor kappa-light-chain-enhancer of activated B cells
NK	natural killer
NLRP3	NACHT, LRR, and PYD domains-containing protein 3, also known as NALP3
NPC	non-parenchymal cells
NRF2	nuclear factor 2
PD1	programmed cell death-1
PIS	phosphatidylinositol synthase
PKCα	protein kinase C alpha
POLG	polymerase γ
PRR	pattern recognition receptors
PtdIns3K	phosphoinositide 3-kinase
PTPN13	protein tyrosine phosphatase, non-receptor type 13
PUFA	polyunsaturated fatty acids
PUMA	p53 upregulated modulator of apoptosis
PUMAi	PUMA inhibitor
RHIM	RIP homology interaction motif

RIPK1/3	receptor interacting protein kinase-1/3
RNS	reactive nitrogen species
ROS	reactive oxygen species
sFASL	soluble FAS ligand
SH3BP5	also known as Sab
SOD	superoxide dismutase
TAB2/3	TGF-beta-activated kinase 1/MAP 3K7-binding protein 2/3
TAK1	transforming growth factor-b-activated kinase 1
TGFβ	transforming growth factor beta
TNFR	TNF receptor
TRADD	TNFR-associated death domain
TRAF2/5	TNF receptor-associated factors 2/5
TRAIL-L	TRAIL ligand
TRAIL-R	tumor necrosis factor-related apoptosis-inducing receptor, also known as APO-2
TLR	Toll-like receptor
TUNEL	deoxynucleotidyl transferase dUTP nick end labeling
ULK1	UNC-51 like kinase-1
ULN	upper limit of normal
VPA	valproic acid
XIAP	X-chromosome linked inhibitor of apoptosis protein
ZBP1/DAI	Z-DNA binding protein 1

1. Introduction

Drug-induced liver injury (DILI) is an important cause of liver injury, presenting with various manifestations, the most serious of which being acute liver failure (ALF) following drug intake. DILI is defined as liver injury with alanine aminotransferase (ALT) more than 3–5 times the upper limit of normal (ULN) or an alkaline phosphatase (ALP) more than twice the ULN with or without elevated bilirubin (Motamedi & Kaplowitz, 2017). Clinical representations of DILI can vary and include cholestatic liver injury, acute hepatitis with or without jaundice, nodular regenerative hyperplasia, sinusoidal obstruction syndrome, or subclinical injury detected during routine blood tests (Yuan & Kaplowitz, 2013). Whatever the cause or manifestation of injury, DILI results in cellular stress leading to hepatocyte death. The subsequent inflammatory and regenerative responses play a critical role in the outcome. DILI can occur in two different ways: direct, intrinsic and dose dependent, as seen with mitochondrial toxins such as acetaminophen (APAP) or certain chemotherapeutic drugs, or idiosyncratic, which is not dose-dependent and predictable and occurs in a select population due to individual susceptibility (Dara, Liu, & Kaplowitz, 2016a). Our understanding of the pathogenesis of idiosyncratic DILI (IDILI) has greatly advanced in recent years due to the contribution of large-scale genetic studies. IDILI is by definition an unpredictable injury, which is not strictly dose-dependent and usually occurs after a respectively long latency and only in a small percentage of exposed individuals (Bell & Chalasani, 2009). Latency between the initiation of drug therapy and the onset of liver disease usually provides an indication as to the pathogenesis of the disease. Early onset (within days) is usually indicative of a direct effect of a drug or its hapten, which is characteristic of predictable reactions (such as the case of APAP toxicity, the most widely studied drug), while unpredictable reactions manifest as overt or symptomatic disease with intermediate (weeks) or long (months) latency (Dara & Kaplowitz, 2017a, 2017b). Hepatotoxicity to drugs such as sulindac (Tarazi, Harter, Zimmerman, Ishak, & Eaton, 1993), phenytoin (Shear & Spielberg, 1988), and amoxicillin-clavulanic acid (Shear & Spielberg, 1988) are typical examples of intermediate latency, while drugs associated with long latency include isoniazid (Thompson et al., 1995) and troglitazone (Murphy et al., 2000). IDILI can even manifest after the discontinuation of a drug. In many instances of direct DILI, cell death is due to intrinsic hepatocyte stressors, reactive oxygen species (ROS), drug-protein adducts causing endoplasmic reticulum (ER), and mitochondrial stress leading to necrosis or apoptosis. However, cell death in IDILI as we will proceed to discuss in this chapter is likely the result of an aberrantly activated innate and adaptive immune system, and therefore is likely to be through death receptor (DR)-mediated apoptosis (Iorga, Dara, & Kaplowitz, 2017).

2. Modes of cell death

2.1 Apoptosis

Apoptosis, Greek for falling leaves, is programmed cell death which occurs both as a physiologic process (e.g., during development) as well as during pathologic processes such as certain infections. Apoptosis can be initiated either extrinsically, due to perturbations in the extracellular environment and activated by transmembrane receptors such as pattern recognition receptors (PRRs) or death receptors (DR), or intrinsically, activated by the release of mitochondrial stress factors (Dara & Kaplowitz, 2017a, 2017b). Extrinsic apoptosis usually occurs when DRs such as tumor necrosis factor (TNF), FAS (also known as CD95 or APO-1), or Trail (also known as APO-2) bind their ligands initiating downstream events (Fig. 1A). In the first phase of

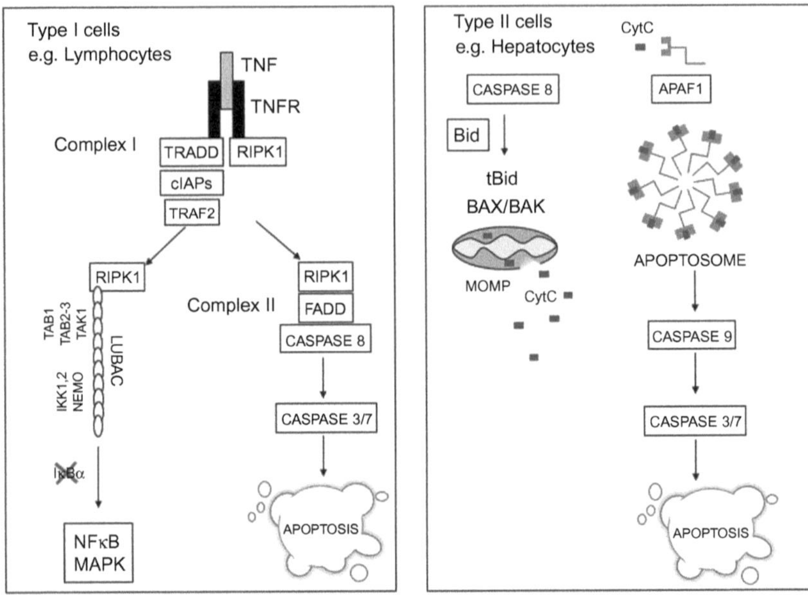

Fig. 1 Mechanism of extrinsic apoptosis in type 1 v.s. type 2 cells. (A) Apoptosis via TNF signaling in type 1 cells. After TNFR is activated by binding TNF, it oligomerizes and recruits TRADD, RIPK1, cIAP1 and 2, and TRAF2 to form complex 1 (also known as DISC). In complex 1 RIPK1 is polyubiquitinated by the cIAPs to form a scaffolding protein for the sequential recruitment of LUBAC, TAB1-TAB2/3-TAK1, and IKK1-IKK2-NEMO. TAK1 phosphorylation of the IKK complex leads to degradation of IκBα and NF-κB activation and transcription of inflammatory/pro-survival genes. For death induction, RIPK1 is deubiquitinated and released from complex 1 to form complex 2, where it associates with FADD and CASP 8 to induce apoptosis by the activation of executioner CASP 3 and CASP 7. In type 1 cells, such as lymphocytes, CASP 8 activation is sufficient for the activation of the downstream executioner caspases. (B). In type 2 cells, such as hepatocytes, the extrinsic apoptotic pathway further requires the involvement of CASP 8 to cleave Bid into tBid to further amplify the apoptotic signal. tBid translocates to the mitochondria where it activates Bax and Bak and leads to MOMP and subsequent release of cytochrome *c*. Cytochrome *c* releases APAF1 from its monomeric autoinhibitory conformation to oligomerize and form the apoptosome, which drives CASP 9-mediated CASP 3 and CASP 7-induced apoptosis.

apoptosis, DR ligation leads to the activation of initiator caspases (caspase 2, 8, 9, and 10), which in turn activate the execution phase by cleaving the effector caspases (caspase 3, 6, and 7), resulting in pyknosis (chromatin condensation), proteolysis and karyorrhexis (nuclear fragmentation) (Galluzzi et al., 2018). DRs share many downstream signaling pathways, a built-in redundancy due to the fact that DRs are critical for tissue hemostasis and regulation of cell death (Guicciardi & Gores, 2009). Apoptosis is the predominant mode of cell death in many forms of liver diseases. For example, apoptotic bodies are a feature of nonalcoholic steatohepatitis (NASH), while councilman bodies are a feature of hepatitis B. Additionally, hepatocytes abundantly express these DRs and while they robustly upregulate nuclear factor kappa-light-chain-enhancer of activated B cells (NF-κB) upon DR ligation, once an insult is large enough or persistent enough in duration (such as in chronic diseases) they die an apoptotic form of cell death.

DR activation leads to the formation of the death-inducing signaling complex (DISC), or complex 1, a dynamic multiprotein complex at the intracellular tail of the transmembrane receptor (Fig. 1A). TNFR activation by its ligand TNF is one of the most widely studied and best described signaling cascades. TNF-induced complex 1 operates as a molecular platform in regulating caspase 8 (CASP 8) activity and downstream functions. Other proteins usually found associating in complex 1 are receptor interacting protein kinase-1 (RIPK1), cellular inhibitor of apoptosis 1 and 2 (cIAP1 and 2), and TNF receptor-associated factors 2 or 5 (TRAF2 or TRAF5) and the adaptor TNFR-associated death domain (TRADD). TNFR activation can have diverse outcomes depending on the post-translational modification status of RIPK1, which has a direct impact on the assembly of pro-survival v.s. pro-death signaling complexes (Gerlach et al., 2011; O'Donnell, Legarda-Addison, Skountzos, Yeh, & Ting, 2007). Once TRADD and RIPK1 are recruited to complex 1 via their death domains, RIPK1 is polyubiquitinated by cIAP1 and 2 and the linear ubiquitination assembly complex (LUBAC) composed of HOIL, HOIP, and Sharpin (Ea, Deng, Xia, Pineda, & Chen, 2006; Haas et al., 2009; Li, Kobayashi, Blonska, You, & Lin, 2006; Peltzer, Darding, & Walczak, 2016; Varfolomeev et al., 2008). Polyubiquitinated RIPK1 promotes inflammation and cell survival by acting as a scaffolding protein for the sequential recruitment of TGF-beta-activated kinase 1/MAP3K7-binding protein 2 and 3 (TAB2 and TAB3) and transforming growth factor-β-activated kinase 1 (TAK1). This induces the activation of IκB kinase (IKK) and NEMO (NF-κB essential modifier), all of which drive the activation of the NF-κB pathway and the mitogen-activated protein kinase (MAPK) cascade (Brenner, Blaser, & Mak, 2015). Activation of the NF-κB pathway results in the transcription of pro-survival and inflammatory genes and prevention of cell death. For death induction, RIPK1 is deubiquitinated by the lysine 63 deubiquitinase cylandromatosis (CYLD), thus releasing it from complex 1 to form complex 2, where it associates with FAS-associated protein with death domain (FADD) and CASP 8 in the cytosol to induce apoptosis (Sun, 2010). Initiator and executioner caspases are present in their catalytically inactive form in the cytosol. Once the apoptotic pathway is engaged, the executioner caspases, caspase 3 and 7 (CASP 3 and CASP 7) are cleaved by the initiator caspases to induce cell death. In many cells, including hepatocytes, formation of complex 2 and apoptosis is blocked by NF-κB target genes such as FAS-associating protein with death domain-like interleukin-1 beta-converting enzyme inhibitory protein (cFLIP) (Irmler et al., 1997; Karin & Lin, 2002; Micheau & Tschopp, 2003). Therefore, interference with NF-κB signaling (transcriptional or translational inhibition) or depletion of glutathione (GSH) is necessary for apoptosis to occur via TNF (Han, Hanawa, Saberi, & Kaplowitz, 2006a; Lou & Kaplowitz, 2007; Matsumaru, Ji, & Kaplowitz, 2003). In type 1 cells, such as lymphocytes, CASP 8 activation is sufficient for the activation of the downstream executioner caspases. However, in type 2 cells, such as hepatocytes, the extrinsic apoptotic pathway further requires the involvement of CASP 8 to cleave Bid into tBid (Fig. 1B). To further amplify the apoptosis signal, tBid translocates to mitochondria, where together with Bim, it activates Bcl-2 proapoptotic proteins Bax and Bak and leads to mitochondrial outer membrane permeabilization (MOMP) and subsequent release of intermitochondrial membrane proteins and cytochrome *c* (Kaufmann et al., 2009; Yin et al., 1999). Cytochrome *c* release in turn activates the apoptosome by releasing apoptotic peptidase activating factor 1 (APAF1) from its autoinhibitory conformation. Once APAF1, which normally exists in a monomeric form, is released, it oligomerizes to form a wheel-like structure called the apoptosome, which promotes self-activation of CASP 9 that in turn cleaves the executioner caspases resulting in cell death (Fig. 1B) (Acehan et al., 2002; Bratton & Salvesen, 2010).

One of the most potent stimuli of hepatocyte death is FAS ligand (Ogasawara et al., 1993). The FAS receptor is a membrane-bound death receptor which is ubiquitously and highly expressed in the liver. FAS ligand (FASL) is mostly expressed on the surface of activated T cells, but also by non-parenchymal cells such as Kupffer cells (KCs, the liver resident macrophages). Additionally, a soluble form of FASL (sFASL) also exists (Malhi, Guicciardi, & Gores, 2010; Strasser, Jost, & Nagata, 2009). FAS receptor activation leads to the formation of complex 1 which consists of: FAS-associated protein with death domain (FADD), CASP 8, and cFLIP. In humans, in addition to CASP 8, FAS activates another initiator enzyme, caspase 10 (CASP 10), which is not present in mice (Strasser et al., 2009). CASP 8 self-cleaves, is released from complex 1 into the cytosol where it cleaves downstream effector caspases thus eventually leading to membrane blebbing, DNA degradation, and apoptosis. Interestingly, CASP 10 can negatively regulate CASP 8 activation by causing the dissociation of CASP 8 from complex 1, thus promoting cell survival (Horn et al., 2017). FAT atypical cadherin 1 (FAT1) also seems to mediate a similar anti-apoptotic function by limiting the association of CASP 8 with complex 1 (Kranz & Boutros, 2014). Similar to TNF signaling, further FAS-mediated apoptosis in hepatocytes requires CASP 8-mediated cleavage of Bid which can be blocked by overexpression of Bcl-2 or Bcl-XL (Scaffidi et al., 1999). In type II cells, X-chromosome linked inhibitor of apoptosis protein (XIAP) associates with CASP 3 to prevent CASP 8 signaling (Jost et al., 2009). This association can be unhinged by mitochondria-derived activator of caspases (SMAC/DIABLO), which is released from the mitochondrial intermembrane space (Jost et al., 2009). Therefore, CASP 8 activation is not sufficient to induce cell death in liver cells, and the mitochondrial pathway must be engaged in order for apoptosis to ensue via MOMP.

Tumor necrosis factor-related apoptosis-inducing receptor (TRAIL-R or APO-2) is a member of the TNF death receptor super family capable of apoptosis induction through binding of its ligand. TRAIL is a homotrimeric ligand capable of interacting with five receptors; of these five, two contain a death domain in their intracellular region (DR5 and DR4), two are decoy receptors (DcR1 and DcR2), which compete with DR4 and DR5 for binding to TRAIL, and one is a soluble receptor capable of binding to TRAIL with low affinity (Wang & El-Deiry, 2003). TRAIL-R1 (DR4) and TRAIL-R2 (DR5) are highly expressed in hepatocytes and can induce caspase-mediated apoptosis in isolated human hepatocytes (Volkmann et al., 2007). TRAIL ligand (TRAIL-L) is mostly expressed by immune cells such as KCs, macrophages, natural killer (NK) cells, and T cells (Malhi et al., 2010). TRAIL was first identified in 1995, and subsequent functional studies have shown that TRAIL-L has a potent ability to trigger apoptosis in numerous tumor cells, but not in most normal cells, thus highlighting the potential therapeutic application of TRAIL-L to cancer treatment (Ashkenazi et al., 1999; Schmaltz et al., 2002; Walczak et al., 1999; Wiley et al., 1995). TRAIL mRNA is constitutively expressed in a wide range of tissues, unlike messenger RNA of other TNF family members which is tightly regulated and often transiently expressed. In the liver, NK cells constitutively express TRAIL for tumor surveillance (Takeda et al., 2001). Upon binding of TRAIL to DR4/DR5, intracellular DD trimerization occurs concomitant with the recruitment of FADD to

DISC/complex 1 and CASP 8/CASP 10 (in humans) activation. Similar to other DR signaling, Bid is cleaved to tBid by CASP 8 and translocates to the mitochondria to further promote cytochrome *c* release by interacting with Bax and Bak (Green, 2000). Such as in the case of TNF or FAS, TRAIL-induced apoptosis proceeds through the apoptosome ultimately leading to activation of CASP 3/6/7. Meanwhile, SMAC/DIABLO activation and binding to inhibitor of apoptosis (IAP) proteins prevents these factors from attenuating the newly active caspases. Additionally, TRAIL binding can result in c Jun N-terminal kinase (JNK) activation through RIPK1 dependent (early phase) and independent (late phase) pathways (Zhang et al., 2015). JNK itself can upregulate DR4 and DR5, increasing sensitivity to TRAIL in certain contexts (Fu et al., 2010; Malhi, 2007; Zou et al., 2004; Zou, Yue, Khuri, & Sun, 2008). The livers of cholestatic mice (bile duct ligation model) also upregulate TRAIL expression, and TRAIL deficiency significantly attenuates liver injury from cholestasis (Kahraman et al., 2008; Takeda et al., 2008). In addition, TRAIL has been shown to play a role in FASL-induced apoptosis in the liver through a JNK-dependent mechanism involving activation of proapoptotic Bim (Corazza et al., 2006).

2.1.1 Apoptosis in drug-induced liver injury

Unlike classic direct-acting hepatotoxins (e.g., APAP), the majority of drugs cause idiosyncratic hepatotoxicity. Due to accumulating amount of evidence pointing to the involvement of the immune system in IDILI, cell death in this instance is thought to be DR-mediated apoptosis. Although the pathogenesis of IDILI is multifactorial and complex, several hypotheses have emerged all of which involve activation of the immune system. To be clear, much of what is hypothesized regarding cell death in IDILI is based on the general understanding of the interplay of the immune system and hepatocytes under stress conditions, as mechanistic insight into IDILI-induced cell death is difficult to ascertain, since the injury is by definition unpredictable, making studying and replicating it extremely difficult in the laboratory setting. It has been hypothesized that drugs can activate the adaptive immune system either through haptenization and neoantigen formation or via molecular mimicry of the parent drug (Dara, Liu, et al., 2015). Thus, hepatotoxicity of drugs can be parent drug-dependent or hapten-dependent, or both. As drug metabolism primarily takes place in the liver, their reactive metabolites are hypothesized to then bind to the liver cytochrome P450 (CYP) enzymes, be presented to major histocompatibility complex (MHC) class II molecules as hapten-antigen adducts and trigger an immune response that activates CD 8+ T cells to express FASL and TNF, thus likely inducing DR-mediated cell death. The consequences of immune activation in response to a drug also include sensitization to cytokines or inflammatory mediators produced by non-parenchymal cells (NPCs). It is also possible that the drug adducts or haptens may covalently bind to or alter CYPs leading to sensitization and immune-mediated injury. In the case of certain drugs, it has been suggested that the idiosyncratic immune reaction in response to a drug or metabolite is further influenced both by genetic and/or environmental factors that determine an injury response (Kaplowitz, 2013). For example, younger patients and women with IDILI from drugs such as amoxicillin/clavulanate often have more severe hepatotoxicity with a hepatitis pattern (high ALT and high bilirubin) while older men present with an indolent and cholestatic injury (Lucena et al., 2006, 2009).

Multiple genome-wide association studies (GWAS) have identified strong correlations between certain human leukocyte antigen (HLA) polymorphisms and the occurrence of IDILI. These studies suggest that IDILI occurs due to a genetic predisposition to an adaptive immune response as well as to the presentation and recognition of a drug-related antigen. For example, strong HLA polymorphic associations have been reported to date in patients who harbor the HLA-B*5701 polymorphism with 80-fold increased risk of flucloxacillin hepatotoxicity (Chalasani et al., 2015; Daly et al., 2009; Wuillemin et al., 2013). GWAS studies also revealed strong associations between HLA polymorphisms and IDILI are the increased risk of amoxicillin-clavulanate toxicity in patients with DRB1*1501, DQB1*0602, and HLA-A*02:01 haplotype and ximelagatran in patients with the HLA-DRB1*0701 polymorphism among many others (Dara, Liu, & Kaplowitz, 2017; Hautekeete et al., 1999; Kindmark et al., 2008; Lucena et al., 2011). Despite the known association of certain HLA polymorphisms with IDILI, only a small percentage of the general population with the known genetic polymorphisms exposed to the drug develop IDILI, highlighting the contribution of other factors to this disease process. For a more comprehensive review of the association of HLA polymorphisms and IDILI, see Grove and Aithal (2015) and Urban, Daly, and Aithal (2014).

2.1.2 Immune tolerance and adaptation

The liver is a site of immune privilege. Due to its routine exposure to foreign ingested antigens, the liver has a tremendous capacity for immune tolerance in order to avoid chronic inflammation (Knolle & Gerken, 2000). This dampening of the liver's immune response is multifaceted and implemented by the various NPCs residing in the liver and may be the reason why many patients exposed to potentially hepatotoxic drugs have transient abnormalities of the liver that normalize with continuous exposure. The liver's capacity for immune tolerance is dependent on the autocrine and paracrine effects of cytokines secreted by KCs, liver sinusoidal endothelial cells (LSECs) as well as the constant exposure to lipopolysaccharides (LPS) (Lohse et al., 1996). LSECs and KCs express interleukin 10 (IL-10), prostaglandins, transforming growth factor beta (TGFβ) and TNFα either in response to LPS stimulation or constitutively, which triggers a signaling cascade leading to expansion of regulatory T cells, attenuation of T cell activation and increased liver immune tolerance (Bissell, Wang, Jarnagin, & Roll, 1995; Dara, Liu, et al., 2015; Knolle et al., 1999, 1995, 1998). The process of attaining immune tolerance after exposure to an inciting antigen is known as adaptation, and several recent studies conducted on animal models demonstrated that bypassing the liver's intrinsic immune checkpoints such as programmed cell death-1 (PD1) and cytotoxic T-lymphocyte-associated protein 4 (CTLA-4), overcomes this adaptive capacity. Preventing immune tolerance can therefore result in sustained injury and DILI from drugs such as amodiaquine and halothane that normally would only give transient rise in ALT values in mice (Chakraborty et al., 2015; Mak & Uetrecht, 2015). Therefore, it is intriguing to hypothesize that for IDILI to occur multiple factors need to be present at the same time, for example a susceptible HLA polymorphism and an acquired or genetic predisposition to the loss of immune tolerance (Dara, Liu, et al., 2015). With the wide use of checkpoint inhibitors for cancer chemotherapy, reports of IDILI from these drugs have been increasing and can range from asymptomatic elevations in liver transaminases to ALF (Suzman, Pelosof, Rosenberg, & Avigan, 2018). The use of immune checkpoint inhibitors to target and kill cancer cells by unleashing a cytotoxic T cell response can have the unwanted adverse effect of targeting hepatocytes for T cell-mediated destruction. The mode of cell death in this novel form of DILI is also likely apoptotic as it is a type of autoimmune response.

2.2 Necrosis

Necrosis is a mode of cell death defined by oncosis (cell swelling and plasma membrane rupture) due to loss of membrane potential, increase of cellular free calcium, activation of many proteases and phospolipases, mitochondrial dysfunction, and subsequent ATP depletion. Morphologically, necrotic cells are identified by cell swelling and the uptake of membrane impermeant dyes such as sytox green or propidium iodide, indicating their ruptured outer plasma membrane (Galluzzi et al., 2015). This is in contrast to apoptosis which morphologically results in cell shrinkage, blebbing and nuclear laddering, although secondary necrosis following apoptosis has been clearly described (Vanden Berghe et al., 2010). The rupture of the plasma membrane results in the release of cellular content into the extracellular milieu, including cytotoxic and pro-inflammatory factors such danger-associated molecular patterns (DAMPs) (Galluzzi et al., 2015). Therefore, necrosis is potentially a much more inflammatory cell death subroutine than apoptosis, although apoptosis, which was previously thought to be a quiescent form of cell death, can also result in an inflammatory response under certain conditions (Newton & Manning, 2016). As ATP depletion due to the loss of mitochondrial oxidative phosphorylation is a trademark of necrosis, much attention has been given to understanding mitochondrial dysfunction and the mitochondrial permeability transition (MPT) in necrosis. Both the adenine nucleotide transporter and the voltage-dependent anion channel have been implicated in MPT, but knockout of either of these genes does not prevent MPT and subsequent cell death (Rasola & Bernardi, 2007). However, knockout or pharmacological inhibition of cyclophilin D (using cyclosporine A), which resides in the mitochondrial matrix and regulates the permeability transition pore opening, is protective against necrosis by inhibiting the MPT (Connern & Halestrap, 1994). Necrosis was initially considered to be an unregulated and incidental form of cell death until more recent evidence revealed that genetic manipulation or pharmacological intervention can interfere with this mode of cell death as well. Therefore, certain types of necrosis are considered "regulated". The best described pathway of regulated necrosis was originally described by Vercammen and colleagues who found that although apoptosis was initiated in L929 cells by TNFR stimulation with its ligand TNF, both ATP depletion or caspase inhibition caused a shift in the cell death subroutine from apoptosis to necrosis (Vercammen et al., 1998). This specific form of cell death which was mainly (although not exclusively) activated via DR signaling and occurred exclusively in the presence of caspase inhibition was termed necroptosis. Over the past 2 decades, many of the molecular mechanisms and signaling pathways which lead to this type of cell death have been discovered and will be discussed below.

2.2.1 Necroptosis

Necroptosis is a regulated modality of necrosis initiated by DRs, PRRs such as Toll-like receptor (TLR), or intracellular sensors such as Z-DNA binding protein 1 (ZBP1/DAI) that occurs in the presence of caspase inhibition (+/− cIAP inhibition in some cells), and requires the involvement of RIPK1, RIPK3, and pseudokinase mixed lineage domain like (MLKL) (Degterev et al., 2008, 2005; Murphy & Vince, 2015; Newton & Manning, 2016; Sun et al., 2012). Necroptosis was first described in cultured cells stimulated with TNF or FASL in the presence of the pan-caspase inhibitor Z-VAD-FMK (Holler et al., 2000; Vercammen et al., 1998). During necroptosis following DR ligand binding and formation of complex 1, which includes TRADD, RIPK1, TRAF2, and E3 ubiquitin ligases, cIAP1 and 2 are recruited to the DR complex promoting ubiquitination of RIPK1. In certain cell types when caspases and cIAPs are inhibited, deubiquitinated RIPK1 does not enter complex 2 to induce apoptosis but instead binds to RIPK3 through their shared RIP homology interaction motif (RHIM). RIPK3 subsequently recruits MLKL and forms the necrosome complex. RIPK3 phospho-activates MLKL leading to its translocation to the plasma membrane where it forms a tetramer to induce pore opening and cell lysis (Fig. 2) (Murphy et al., 2013; Sun et al., 2012). As described in the apoptosis section, cIAP-driven ubiquitination of RIPK1 at the DR complex favors NF-κB signaling, which is pro-inflammatory and pro-survival by enhancing cFLIP transcription. Transcriptional upregulation of cFLIP

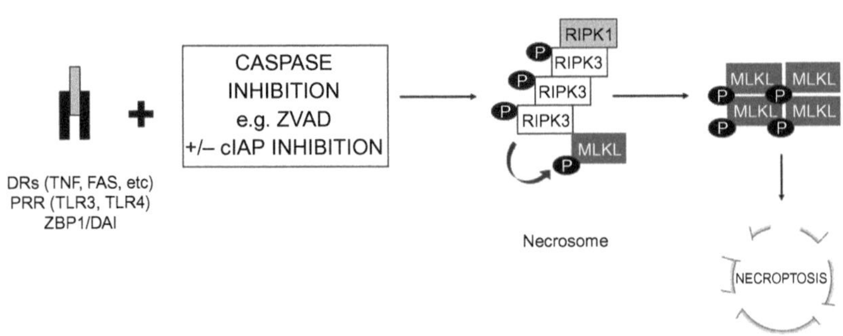

Fig. 2 Mechanism of necroptosis. Necroptosis can be activated through DRs (such as TNF, FAS, etc.), PRRs (TLR3 and 4), or the intracellular pathogen sensor ZBP1/DAI. When these receptors are engaged in the presence of pan-caspase inhibitors to block apoptosis, necroptosis occurs. RIPK1 associates with RIPK3 which in turn recruits MLKL forming the necrosome. RIPK3 phospho-activates MLKL which translocates to the plasma membrane where it forms a tetramer to induce pore opening and oncolysis.

and other NF-κB target genes effectively inhibit DR-induced, CASP 8-mediated apoptosis, which is the default cell death subroutine in most instances. However, if RIPK1 in not ubiquitinated, or if the kinase is deubiquitinated by CYLD, it can initiate the necroptotic cell death cascade upon caspase inhibition (O'Donnell et al., 2007, 2011). In this regard, necroptotic signaling is suppressed by CASP 8-mediated cleavage of RIPK1, RIPK3, and/or CYLD (O'Donnell et al., 2011). Therefore, inhibition of CASP 8 is essential for necroptosis to ensue, questioning the physiological relevance of necroptosis in the pathophysiology of diseases where caspases are intact (Dara, Liu, & Kaplowitz, 2016c). The kinase activity of RIPK1 is dispensable for its pro-survival role, as mice lacking RIPK1 kinase activity are viable and healthy. However, its kinase activity is necessary for necroptosis (and apoptosis) and although the RIPK1 substrate remains unclear, small-molecule inhibitors of RIPK1, the necrostatins, efficiently block necroptosis (Degterev et al., 2008, 2005; Takahashi et al., 2012). Necroptosis also requires the kinase activity of RIPK3, which is required for the activation of the executioner MLKL (Fig. 2). While many cell types such as L929 fibrosarcoma cells, Jurkat T cells, HT29 cells, MEFs, and keratinocytes can undergo necroptosis when apoptosis is inhibited, this cell death subroutine is not universally observed (Degterev, Zhou, Maki, & Yuan, 2014). For example, many epithelial cell lines such as HeLA cells, Hek293, and MCF7 are resistant to necroptosis (Degterev et al., 2014). It is thought that the level of RIPK3 expression correlates with the ability to undergo necroptosis (He et al., 2009). The observation that necroptosis is not a universal phenomenon is highly relevant in DILI and in particular in hepatocyte death, as RIPK3 is undetectable in liver cells under basal conditions and its induction has been controversial (Dara, 2018; Dara et al., 2015; Kasof, Prosser, Liu, Lorenzi, & Gomes, 2000; Sun et al., 1999). However, NPCs do express RIPK3, and MLKL is expressed by all liver cell types. Given that under basal conditions hepatocytes express MLKL but do not express RIPK3, the possibility still remains that MLKL may be activated by a yet unknown kinase. Although RIPK3 is the only known activator of MLKL to date, there have been reports of RIPK3-independent MLKL activation in the Concavalin A (Con A) model of inflammatory hepatocyte death (Gunther et al., 2016). An additional consideration regarding necroptosis in liver injury is that ZVAD and caspase inhibition rescues hepatocytes from apoptotic insults such as TNF/galactosamine or α-galactoceramide (Dara et al., 2016c; Suda et al., 2016). Therefore, in liver cells the switch to a necrotic form of cell death is not seen with inhibition of apoptosis. The role of RIPK1, RIPK3, and MLKL has been studied in DILI and in particular in APAP-induced liver injury, which is a necrotic form of cell death.

2.2.2 Acetaminophen and hepatocyte necrosis

APAP hepatotoxicity from suicidal and accidental overdose is the most common cause of DILI and ALF in the United States (Larson et al., 2005). APAP-induced DILI is commonly used to study hepatocyte necrosis. APAP overdose induces predictable, dose-dependent liver injury. APAP is mainly metabolized into glucuronide and sulfate conjugates, with a small fraction converted by the CYP family (mainly CYP2E1 and CYP1A2) into the highly reactive and toxic metabolite *N*-acetyl-p-benzoquinone imine (NAPQI). NAPQI is inactivated by its preferential conjugation with reduced GSH in the hepatocyte and is subsequently excreted in the bile or urine as a nontoxic conjugate. However, if a large dose of APAP is ingested and GSH storage is depleted, the excess electrophilic metabolite covalently binds to cysteine moieties and protein thiols, altering function, inducing oxidative, and organelle stress and ultimately leading to hepatocyte death (Mitchell, Jollow, Potter, Gillette, & Brodie, 1973). Glutathione replacement by administration of *N*-acetyl cysteine (NAC) prevents liver injury and organ failure if given in a timely manner (8 h post-overdose in humans and 1.5–2 h in mice) (Peterson & Rumack, 1977). GSH availability is dependent on the availability of cysteine in the blood, which is the rate-limiting substrate for glutathione resynthesis (Han, Hanawa, Saberi, & Kaplowitz, 2006b). When NAPQI oxidizes protein thiol groups, it acts as an inter-protein crosslinker, forming disulfide bridges or mixed disulfides. The uncoupling of CYP2E1 and mitochondria results in the accumulation of superoxide and oxidative stress. This not only includes the classical iron-mediated oxidative stress (Fenton reaction) but also involves nitric oxide. Nitric oxide reacts with superoxide to form peroxynitrite, an oxidizing and a nitrating agent detoxified by GSH (Gibson, Pumford, Samokyszyn, & Hinson, 1996; Hinson, Roberts, & James, 2010). The resultant oxidative and nitrosative stress from NAPQI and the generation of NAPQI-protein adducts is not limited to the cytosolic compartments. In fact, NAPQI-protein adducts bind to and cause considerable damage to mitochondria and mitochondrial proteins, depleting mitochondrial GSH stores, and resulting in mitochondrial stress which eventually triggers the MPT and collapse of the membrane potential. These events lead to the release of endonuclease G

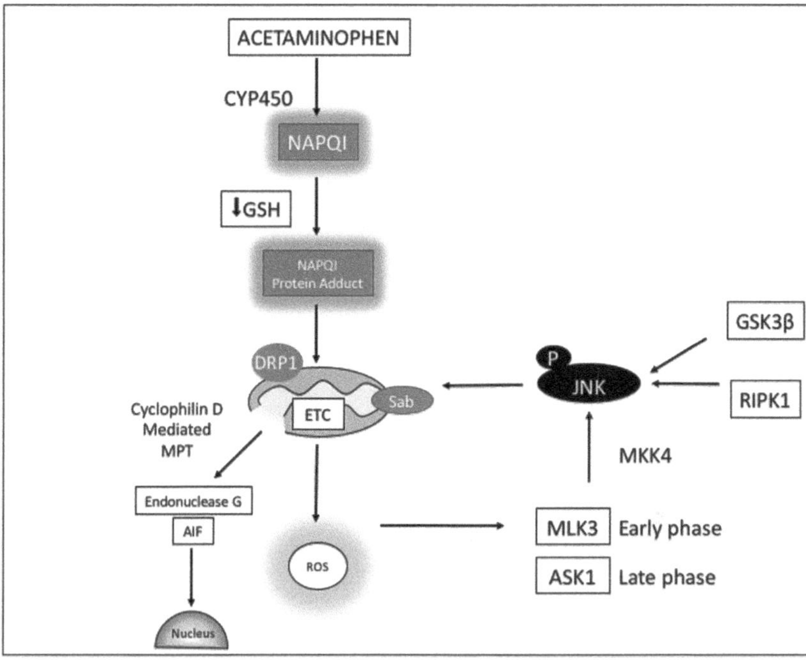

Fig. 3 Mechanism of acetaminophen-induced hepatocyte necrosis. Acetaminophen is converted into its reactive metabolite NAPQI by the CYP450 enzymes (mainly CYP2E1). NAPQI is inactivated by its preferential conjugation with GSH in the cytosol. However, when GSH storage is depleted, reactive NAPQI covalently binds to cysteine moieties and protein thiols to form NAPQI adducts, depleting mitochondrial GSH stores, and resulting in mitochondrial stress and release of ROS. The accumulation of ROS also results in the activation of MLK3 in the early phase of injury and ASK1 in the late phase of injury. Both MLK3 and ASK1 phosphorylate MKK4, which phospho-activates JNK. GSK3β and RIPK1 have been shown to be upstream of pJNK as well. PJNK binds and phosphorylates Sab at the mitochondrial membrane causing the inhibition of the ETC, further release of ROS, which eventually triggers cyclophilin D-mediated MPT and collapse of the membrane potential. These events lead to the release of endonuclease G and AIF, their nuclear translocation, and subsequent DNA fragmentation in the nucleus.

and apoptosis-inducing factor (AIF) and their nuclear translocation, and subsequent DNA fragmentation in the nucleus leading to cellular necrosis (Fig. 3) (Jaeschke, 2015; Jaeschke & Ramachandran, 2018; Kon, Kim, Jaeschke, & Lemasters, 2004). Oxidative stress initiates the cellular stress response but is insufficient to induce MPT and cell death. The role of the MAPKs in sustaining ROS and amplifying stress signals leading to MPT has been well studied in the APAP model (Gunawan et al., 2006; Hanawa et al., 2008; Nakagawa et al., 2008; Saito, Lemasters, & Jaeschke, 2010; Sharma, Gadang, & Jaeschke, 2012). The initial ROS generated by NAPQI results in the activation of the MAPKs. In the early phase of injury mixed lineage kinase 3 (MLK3) is activated, while the redox sensitive protein apoptosis signal regulating kinase 1 (ASK1) is activated in the later phases of injury. Both ASK1 and MLK3 phosphorylate mitogen-activated protein kinase 4 (MKK4), which leads to the phosphor-activation of JNK 1/2 and the translocation of pJNK to mitochondria. The magnitude and duration of pJNK activation correlates with hepatocyte death from APAP (Win et al., 2018). At the mitochondria, pJNK binds to and phosphorylates an outer membrane protein called SH3BP5 or Sab (Chambers & LoGrasso, 2011; Wiltshire, Matsushita, Tsukada, Gillespie, & May, 2002). Sab has been shown to subsequently dephosphorylate the active form of Src (Win, Than, Min, Aghajan, & Kaplowitz, 2016). This inactivation of mitochondrial Src inhibits the electron transport chain (ETC) and increases ROS production, thus creating a sustained activation loop between ASK1 and pJNK leading to cell death (Matsumaru et al., 2003; Win, Than, Han, Petrovic, & Kaplowitz, 2011). The binding of pJNK to Sab is necessary for the downstream effects of JNK on mitochondria, therefore, preventing JNK from binding Sab abrogates hepatocyte death in more than just the APAP DILI model, but also in the ER stress apoptosis model induced by TNF (plus D-galactosamine) and palmitic acid (Win et al., 2018). In addition to JNK and other MAPKs, other kinases and signaling molecules have been implicated in hepatocyte death following APAP overdose. Many of these proteins act upstream of pJNK activation, as it has been shown that interfering with their signaling protects by inhibiting or limiting pJNK activation. Inhibition, knockdown or knockout of RIPK1, glycogen synthase kinase 3 beta (GSK3β), protein kinase C alpha (PKCα), the mitochondrial fission regulator, dynamin-related protein 1 (DRP1), and most recently p53 upregulated modulator of apoptosis (PUMA), have all been shown to attenuate APAP-induced cell death (Chen et al., 2018; Dara, Johnson, et al., 2015; Ramachandran et al., 2013; Saberi et al., 2014; Shinohara et al., 2010). RIPK1 participation in APAP-induced liver injury has been observed by many investigators with inhibitor and knockdown experiments (Dara et al., 2016c). However, one group has argued against the importance of RIPK1 in APAP toxicity with embryonic liver parenchymal cell knockout of the protein (Schneider, Gautheron, Tacke, Vucur, & Luedde, 2015). Since RIPK1 global knockouts are embryonic lethal and the protein is multifunctional and necessary for survival of the embryo, such early embryonic knockouts may result in unforeseen compensatory changes that could explain the contradicting results (Dara & Kaplowitz, 2016). Nevertheless, most investigators that have studied RIPK1 in APAP have found an association with cell death. Given the central role of the kinase in necroptosis, a logical avenue of research has been to determine if the regulated necrosis in APAP is indeed necroptotic cell death. Since the next described protein in necroptosis is RIPK3, the role of RIPK3 was examined in APAP, however, its involvement proved to be controversial. While some investigators observed protection from RIPK3 knockdown or global knockout 6h or 12h after APAP (Deutsch et al., 2015; Ramachandran et al., 2013), we found no difference in liver injury at early or late time points (24h) in RIPK3 KO compared to WT controls (Dara, Johnson, et al., 2015). Importantly, although others had reported increased RIPK3 in the liver, we were unable to detect hepatocyte expression of RIPK3 by immunoblotting or qPCR, with or without APAP (Dara, Johnson, et al., 2015; Dara et al., 2016c). In contrast, liver NPCs and immune cells express high levels of RIPK3 leading to the possibility that the increase in RIPK3 observed in whole liver lysates comes from a source other than hepatocytes. Since the arbiter of necroptosis is the pseudokinase MLKL, in order to determine whether necroptosis was involved in APAP-induced hepatocyte cell death or if RIPK1 was acting through a necroptosis-independent pathway, we treated global MLKL knockout mice with APAP and found no protection compared to substrain matched controls (Dara, Johnson, et al., 2015; Dara, Liu, & Kaplowitz, 2016b). The lack of involvement of MLKL in the APAP cell death pathway was later confirmed by others (Gunther et al., 2016). Therefore, the preponderance of the evidence suggests that APAP does not mediate necroptosis while there is likely a necroptosis-independent role for RIPK1 (and by some accounts RIPK3).

In addition to examining the necroptotic cell death subroutine in APAP, many studies have explored the contribution of apoptotic cell death in APAP hepatotoxicity (Jaeschke, Duan, Akakpo, Farhood, & Ramachandran, 2018; Li et al., 2013; Song, Fu, Xia, Su, & Song, 2014; Wang et al., 2017). Most of the studies attributing apoptosis as the cell death subroutine in APAP are based on immunoblots of cleaved caspases or the non-specific stain and deoxynucleotidyl transferase dUTP nick end labeling (TUNEL), which identifies DNA fragmentation and is falsely positive with a distinctly cytosolic pattern in APAP (Jaeschke, Cover, & Bajt, 2006; Jaeschke, Williams, & Farhood, 2011). However, unlike models of apoptotic cell death, caspase inhibition does not protect against APAP and the observed DNA fragmentation in APAP has been shown to be the result of mitochondrial endonuclease G translocation to the nucleus following MPT (Bajt, Cover, Lemasters, & Jaeschke, 2006). Furthermore, inhibiting MPT by pharmacologic blockade or knockout of cyclophillin D protects against APAP confirming the necrotic cell death subroutine (LoGuidice & Boelsterli, 2011; Ramachandran, Lebofsky, Baines, Lemasters, & Jaeschke, 2011). Interestingly, even PUMA, a member of the BL2 family has been recently implicated as participating in APAP-induced hepatocyte death. However, in this context PUMA is not functioning as a mediator of apoptosis (Chen et al., 2018). PUMA deficiency strongly suppressed APAP-induced liver injury. However, PUMA induction requires RIPK1/JNK in the liver and PMH, as pre-treatment with RIPK1 or JNK inhibitors prior to APAP abrogated the induction of PUMA protein and mRNA levels post-APAP. Pharmacological intervention with the PUMA small-molecule inhibitor (PUMAi) 2 h post-APAP also attenuated liver injury (Chen et al., 2018). Thus, in this case, the data suggest that PUMA-induced hepatocyte necrosis downstream of pJNK. In addition to necrosis, autophagy and mitophagy are a consequence and feature of APAP DILI, as removal of dead organelle and clearance of dead hepatocytes is necessary to dampen ROS, reactive nitrogen species (RNS), and DAMPs. The role of autophagy in APAP DILI will be discussed below.

2.2.3 *Mitochondria, cell death, and DILI*

Mitochondria are vital organelles to the hepatocyte. They play a very important role in the execution of apoptosis, necrosis, and APAP-induced regulated necrosis but they do not contribute to necroptotic cell death (Tait et al., 2013). Therefore, it is not surprising that many drugs that are hepatotoxic directly target the mitochondria. The role of the mitochondria in generating ROS when stressed or damaged is central to cell death from drugs and toxic metabolites. Mice which partially lack the manganese superoxide dismutase (MnSOD) gene, an enzyme that catalyzes the partitioning of the superoxide radical into molecular oxygen or hydrogen peroxide, have increased liver injury post-APAP, highlighting the importance of mitochondrial oxidant stress in the progression of injury (Agarwal et al., 2011; Fujimoto et al., 2009; Ramachandran, Lebofsky, Weinman, & Jaeschke, 2011). Mito-tempo is a recently reported SOD mimetic which dismutates superoxide, and has the ability to accumulate several hundred-fold within the mitochondria, thus being a very efficient superoxide scavenger. Mito-tempo has been shown to protect against oxidative injury in various liver injury models and just recently it has been shown to protect against APAP hepatotoxicity as well (Dikalova et al., 2010; Du, Farhood, & Jaeschke, 2017; Trnka, Blaikie, Smith, & Murphy, 2008; Wang et al., 2014). Nitrosative stress and generation of nitrotyrosine adducts especially in mitochondria is an additional stress signal leading to the downstream signaling events, stress response, and cell death in APAP (Cover et al., 2005) DILI. Tamoxifen, amiodarone, tetracycline, and antiretrovirals are examples of drugs that target mitochondria thus resulting in steatosis, injury, and even ALF (Fromenty & Pessayre, 1995; Lemasters et al., 1998; Lewis et al., 1989; Silva et al., 1997). Hepatotoxicity from mitochondria-targeting agents can occur in a few different ways. Some drugs such as nucleoside analogs and reverse transcriptase inhibitors used in HIV treatment can interfere with mitochondrial DNA synthesis. Examples include fialuridine, zidovudine, and didanosine (Bissuel et al., 1994). Fialuridine-treated patients were noted to exhibit elevated liver enzymes, pancreatitis, lactic acidosis, and even death after a long latency, all clinical features of mitochondrial toxicity (McKenzie et al., 1995). Valproic acid (VPA) is a mood stabilizer and anticonvulsant which causes DILI and kills liver cells by targeting mitochondria in several ways. VPA binds coenzyme A (CoA) to form valproyl-CoA moieties, thus interfering with natural fatty acyl-CoA oxidation, as well as pyruvate dehydrogenase which requires CoA (Ponchaut, van Hoof, & Veitch, 1992; Silva et al., 1997). VPA is converted into a highly electrophilic metabolite 2,4-iene VPA in the mitochondria, where it can uncouple respiration by interfering with the ETC thus causing mitochondrial toxicity resulting in microvesicular steatosis and Reye's syndrome similar to aspirin (Kassahun, Farrell, & Abbott, 1991; Levy et al., 1990). VPA toxicity has been associated with amino acid substitutions which decrease the activity of mitochondrial DNA polymerase γ (POLG). Alpers-Huttenlocher syndrome is a rare disorder belonging to a group of conditions called the POLG-related disorders, characterized by recurrent seizures, ataxia, neuropathy, psychomotor regression, and liver disease. VPA toxicity occurs in nearly one-third of Alpers-Huttenlocher patients due to their POLG mutations (Naviaux & Nguyen, 2004). VPA-induced mitochondrial toxicity and DILI even occur in patients with heterozygous mutations in POLG (Stewart et al., 2010). It is possible that the mutations in POLG affect mitochondrial DNA synthesis thus sensitizing patients to VPA toxicity, but this remains to be validated. It is however unclear if VPA causes direct toxicity to the mitochondria or if there is an immune activation mechanism (Dara & Kaplowitz, 2017a, 2017b). Amiodarone and tamoxifen are widely used medications with the potential for inducing mitochondrial toxicity. Amiodarone, an anti-arrythmic, has been shown in animal models and in vitro to increase hydrogen peroxide formation and to inhibit mitochondrial complex I activity, resulting in uncoupling of oxidative phosphorylation (Serviddio et al., 2011). Importantly, amiodarone inhibits mitochondrial beta oxidation, which explains the classic clinical presentation of microvesicular steatohepatitis seen with amiodarone toxicity (Fromenty et al., 1990). A similar mechanim of toxicity from tamoxifen has also been reported. Tamoxifen interferes with mitochondrial respiration, increases tyrosine nitration and lipid peroxidation of mitochodnrial proteins, ultimately leading to apoptotic cell death and cytochrome *c* release (Nazarewicz et al., 2007). Tamoxifen induces its hepatotoxicity partly by downregulating MnSOD activity, thereby increasing ROS generation (Razandi, Pedram, Jordan, Fuqua, & Levin, 2013). There are many more examples of DILI drugs that are mitochondrial toxins, which can be reviewed here (Pessayre, Mansouri, Berson, & Fromenty, 2010).

2.3 Autophagy in DILI

Autophagy is the cellular degradation pathway through which damaged organelles and other cellular content is recycled (Xie & Klionsky, 2007). This occurs through the formation of the autophagosome, a double membrane vesicle originating from the ER or cell membrane, which then fuses with the lysosome to deliver its contents for hydrolase degradation. Autophagy can be induced by starvation, stressors such as oxidative stress, as well as pathogen infection. It is a critical mechanism for cell survival, as failure to get rid of intracellular wastes by autophagy disrupts cellular homeostasis and leads to inflammation and death. Autophagy is controlled by over 30 autophagy (ATG) genes, and in line with its pro-survival role, knockout of ATG genes in most instances accelerates cell death rather than prevents it (Galluzzi et al., 2012). However, there are certain instances in which the molecular machinery for autophagy ultimately leads to cellular demise and regulated cell death (Galluzzi et al., 2018). The most studied is its interaction with apoptotic cell death, however, other forms of regulated cell death have also been linked to autophagy (Marino, Niso-Santano, Baehrecke, & Kroemer, 2014). For example, ferroptosis (discussed below) can be promoted by the autophagic degradation of ferritin in a process termed ferritinophagy, necroptosis can occur with the autophagic degradation of cIAP1 and cIAP2, and FAS-driven apoptosis is enhanced by autophagic degradation of protein tyrosine phosphatase, non-receptor type 13 (PTPN13) (Gao et al., 2016; Goodall et al., 2016; Gump et al., 2014; He et al., 2014; Hou et al., 2016; Marino et al., 2014).

The UNC-51 like kinase-1 (ULK) complex consisting of ULK1, FAK family kinase-interacting protein of 200 kDa (FIP200), ATG 13 and ATG 101 initiates autophagy, translocates to an ER subdomain enriched in

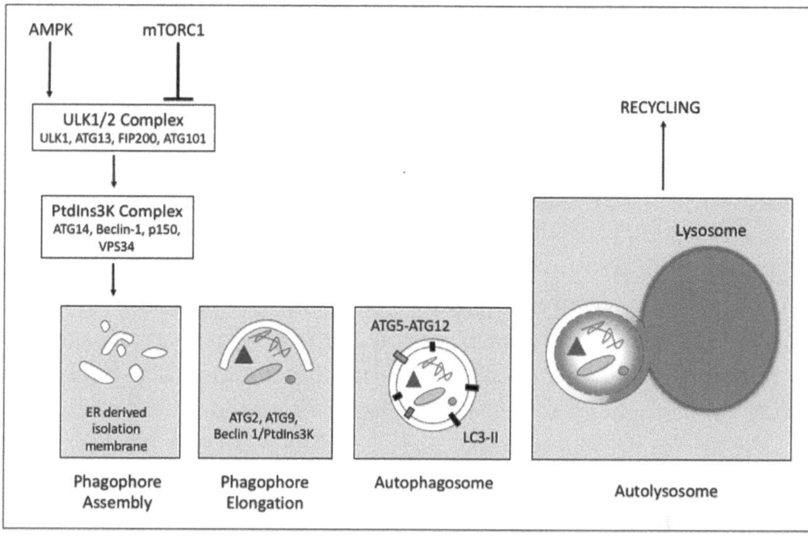

Fig. 4 Mechanism of autophagy. mTORC1 inhibits autophagy when nutrients are readily available by directly phoshorylating ULK1/2 and inhibiting its activity. However, in conditions of low ATP, AMPK is activated, and it phosphorylates ULK1/2 at different sites than mTORC1 to promote autophagy. Once activated, the ULK complex further phosphorylates Beclin1, part of the PtdIns3K complex, which also includes ATG14, p150, and VPS34. PtdIns3K signals for phagophore formation by recruiting ATG18 (not depicted) and further helps in phagophore elongation by membrane addition. ATG2 and ATG9 also contribute to the early steps of elongation. ATG3, ATG4, and ATG7 are necessary for the processing of nascent LC3 by conjugating it to phosphatidylethanolamine to form LC3-II. The expanding membrane then closes around its cargo to form an autophagosome which is achieved by ATG5-ATG12 and LC3-II. The autophagosome then travels along microtubules until it fuses with lysosomes to form autolysosomes leading to digestion and recycling of cellular contents.

phosphatidylinositol synthase (PIS), and induces the recruitment of other downstream factors such as ATG 14 and ATG 9A leading to the elongation of the phagophore membrane (Fig. 4) (Nishimura & Mizushima, 2017). The activity of the ULK complex is regulated by the energy-sensing mTOR complex 1 kinase (mTORC1), and the AMP-activated protein kinase (AMPK) that phosphorylates ATG 13 preventing it from interacting with the ULK complex. mTORC1 is a pivotal enzyme in regulating autophagy and integrating growth factor, metabolic, and energy signaling. mTORC1 inhibits autophagy when nutrients are readily available by directly phoshorylating ULK1/2 and inhibiting its activity. However, in conditions of low ATP, AMPK is activated, and it phosphorylates ULK1/2 at different sites than mTORC1 to promote autophagy (Glick, Barth, & Macleod, 2010).

Once activated, the ULK complex further phosphorylates Beclin1, which is part of the multiprotein autophagy promoting class III complex phosphoinositide 3-kinase (PtdIns3K). PtdIns3K signals for phagophore formation and elongation by membrane addition, which are achieved by two ubiquitin-like conjugation systems, ATG 12 and LC3 (Fig. 4) (Chao, Wang, Jaeschke, & Ding, 2018). The expanding membrane then closes around its cargo to form the autophagosome and travels along microtubules until it fuses with lysosomes to form autolysosomes (Chao et al., 2018).

As hepatocytes require a larger number of organelles such as mitochondria, ER, Golgi, and lysosomes in order to perform their synthetic and secretory functions while maintaining cellular homeostasis, they have a high capacity for autophagy to recycle damaged organelles and proteins. The ER is the site for protein assembly and one of the main sites for drug metabolism in the liver; therefore, ER stress induced by reactive and toxic metabolites or drugs is an important autophagy stimulus and regulator of cell death (Baehrecke, 2005). Consistent with the protective and pro-survival role of autophagy, knockout of ATG 5 and ATG 7 in mouse liver leads to the development of an abnormal and swollen hepatic lobule due to the inability of these mice to clear ubiquitinated proteins and aberrant molecules (Amir et al., 2013; Ding, 2014; Komatsu et al., 2005). Moreover, global ATG 5 and ATG 7 knockouts die shortly after birth, while liver-specific knockout sensitizes mice to liver injury and cell death and compensatory nuclear factor 2 (NRF2) accumulation and activation leading to improved oxidative stress defenses (Ding, 2014; Ni et al., 2012). D-Galactosamine/LPS or D-galactosamine/TNF challenge of hepatocyte-specific ATG 7 knockout mice leads to worsened liver injury and apoptotic cell death by CASP 8 activation and tBid cleavage (Amir et al., 2013).

Autophagy and mitophagy (autophagy of mitochondria) have been studied in APAP-induced hepatotoxicity (Chao et al., 2018). Treatment of transgenic GFP-LC3 with APAP results in the accumulation of LC3 positive autophagosomes in the peri-central areas of the hepatic lobule (Ni, Bockus, Boggess, Jaeschke, & Ding, 2012). Activation of autophagy transcriptionally or pharmacologically has been shown to be protective against liver toxicity induced by APAP, while inhibition of autophagy using chloroquine, leupeptin, or genetic manipulation worsened APAP-induced cell death (Ni, Bockus, et al., 2012; Sydor et al., 2017). Since APAP toxicity results in mitochondrial damage and the generation of oxidative stress, it seems that autophagy and mitophagy in particular are necessary cellular mechanisms to limit cell death and MPT by the clearance of damaged mitochondria, as well as APAP-protein adducts (Chao et al., 2018). The molecular mechanisms of autophagy are complex and beyond the scope of this chapter. For a detailed review, please refer to Chao et al. (2018), Glick et al. (2010), and Marino et al. (2014).

2.4 Pyroptosis

Pyroptosis ("pyro" Greek for fire and "ptosis," falling) is a highly inflammatory mode of regulated cell death which has evolved as a way of removing intracellular pathogens and has a distinct morphology which depends on the formation of plasma membrane pores resulting in cell explosion. Thus, pyroptosis is related to innate immunity activation, but is different from other forms of cell death in that it manifests with a very specific molecular signature. Pyroptosis was originally thought to have evolved as a means of removing invading intracellular pathogens from the body by activating caspase 1 (CASP 1), but more recent findings have demonstrated that other caspases such CASP 4, CASP 5, CASP 12 in humans (CASP 11 in mice) and even CASP 8 can participate in pyroptosis (Aglietti & Dueber, 2017; Orning et al., 2018). Once activated, these inflammatory caspases then cleave Gasdermin D (GSDMD), releasing it from its autoinhibitory conformation. Activated GSDMD then translocates to the plasma membrane where it binds membrane phospholipids (cardiolopin, phosphatidylinositol phosphates, and phosphatidylserine) and initiates pore formation resulting in loss of membrane integrity, cytosolic swelling, and release of cellular contents leading to cell death (Fig. 5) (Aglietti & Dueber, 2017; Kayagaki et al., 2015; Shi et al., 2015). The resultant chromatin condensation and cellular swelling are morphologically different in pyroptosis than that observed in apoptosis (Jorgensen & Miao, 2015). Most recently, pyroptosis has been divided in to two modes: canonical, in which the inflammasome sensors such as NLRP3 (oligomerized NOD-like receptor family, pyrin domain-containing-3) or AIM2 (absent in melanoma-2) are activated by pathogens and recruit CASP 1 via the inflammasome adapter protein apoptosis-associated speck-like protein containing a CARD (ASC) to cleave GSDMD into its active form to drive pyroptosis after sensing a pathogenic signal; or non-canonical, in which cytosolic LPS activates CASP 4, 5, and 11 which then cleave GSDMD (Fig. 5) (Man & Kanneganti, 2015; Sagulenko et al., 2013). Pyroptosis results in the release of cytosolic contents such as ATP, high mobility group box-1 (HMGB-1), and IL-1α, and is subsequently accompanied by processing of inflammatory cytokines such as IL-1β and IL-18

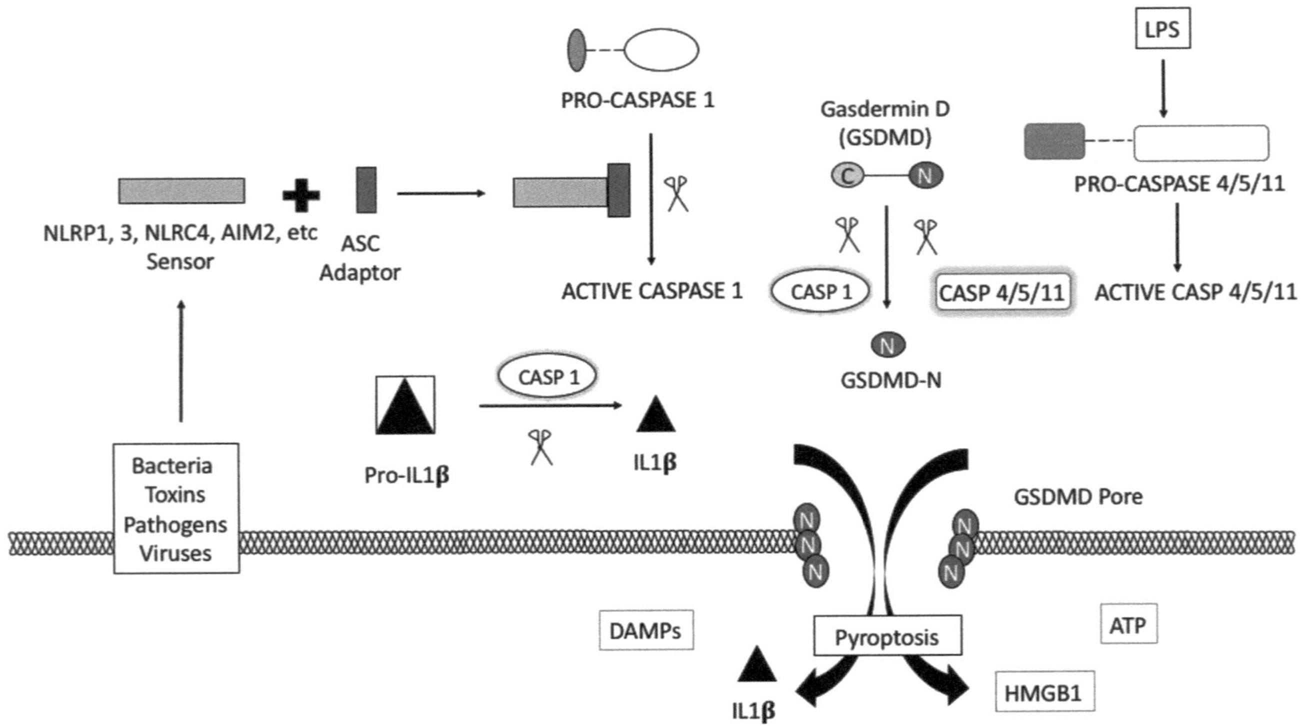

Fig. 5 Mechanism of pyroptosis. There are two pyroptotic pathways. In the canonical pathway, upon detection of pathogens, the inflammasome (NLRP1, NLRP3, NLRC4, AIM2) recruits CASP 1 via ASC and activates it by cleavage. CASP 1 cleaves IL-1β as well as GSDMD. The N-terminal cleavage product, GSDMD-N, mediates the lytic and highly inflammatory cell death subroutine by formation of the GSDMD pore and extracellular release of activated IL-1β. In addition to IL-1β, DAMPs such as HMGB1 and ATP are also released from the pore. GDSMD is a substrate for other caspases as well. In the non-canonical pathway, CASP 4, 5, and 11 are activated directly by LPS. These caspases in turn cleave GSDMD to form the pore and drive pyroptosis.

which elicit an immune response (Aglietti & Dueber, 2017; Franchi, Eigenbrod, Munoz-Planillo, & Nunez, 2009).

Most recently, in addition to pathogen removal, pyroptosis has been implicated in other disease processes such as alcoholic liver disease and LPS-induced septic shock (Khanova et al., 2018; Shao, Yeretssian, Doiron, Hussain, & Saleh, 2007). For example, CASP 11 deletion protected mice against pyroptosis-dependent endotoxic shock following systemic LPS administration (Aachoui, Sagulenko, Miao, & Stacey, 2013). The role of pyroptosis and in particular the inflammasome which is the sensor bio-activating CASP 1 in the pathway has been studied in the APAP model of DILI. Using aspirin to inhibit the inflammasome or mice deficient in the inflammasome components NLRP3 (NALP3), ASC, and CASP 1, as well as TLR9, the role of the inflammasome in APAP-induced liver injury has been studied (Imaeda et al., 2009). The original reports in the NLRP3 −/−, ASC −/−, CASP 1 −/− mice were strongly suggestive of the involvement of the inflammasome (Imaeda et al., 2009); however, subsequent studies by others have found no role for this pathway in APAP toxicity (Williams et al., 2011). In fact, the degree of necrosis, the release of DAMPs, and the recruitment of neutrophils to the site of injury were unaltered in mice lacking inflammasome components compared to controls after APAP (Williams et al., 2011). The role of the innate immunity and neutrophils in particular in aggravating injury and cell death following APAP-induced hepatocyte necrosis has been largely controversial, and therefore it is not surprising that pyroptosis does not contribute significantly to APAP DILI (Woolbright & Jaeschke, 2017). However, in order to conclusively determine whether pyroptotic cell death plays a role in APAP DILI, the participation of GSDMD, the mediator of cell death in pyroptosis, should be studied.

2.5 Ferroptosis

Ferroptosis is a form of regulated cell death initiated by an intracellular milieu of severe lipid peroxidation that relies on ROS generation and iron availability (Dixon, 2017; Dixon et al., 2012;Stockwell et al., 2017; Yang & Stockwell, 2016). Ferroptosis is characterized by an increase of iron-catalyzed H_2O_2-dependent ROS (Fenton chemistry) and occurs independently of caspases, CYPs, necroptosis, apoptosis, the autophagy machinery, and the pyroptosis cascade. However, it does have some subcellular components reminiscent of necrosis, such as mitochondrial alterations and shrinkage, aberrant cristae and MPT, and could be associated with a release of DAMPs (Dixon et al., 2012; Kim et al., 2016; Vanden Berghe, Linkermann, Jouan-Lanhouet, Walczak, & Vandenabeele, 2014). Ferroptosis was first described when the small-molecule inhibitor erastin was administered to RAS-mutant cell lines, severely depleting GSH and inducing a non-necroptotic, non-apoptotic form of cell death that was iron dependent (Dixon et al., 2012). GSH is synthesized in two steps by the ATP-dependent cytosolic enzymes glutamate-cysteine ligase (GCL) and glutathione synthetase (GSS), cysteine availability is the rate-limiting step in GSH synthesis. Cystine enters the cell via the cystine/glutamate antiporter (system x_c^-) where it is reduced to cysteine and used to synthesize GSH (Fig. 6). Certain agents such

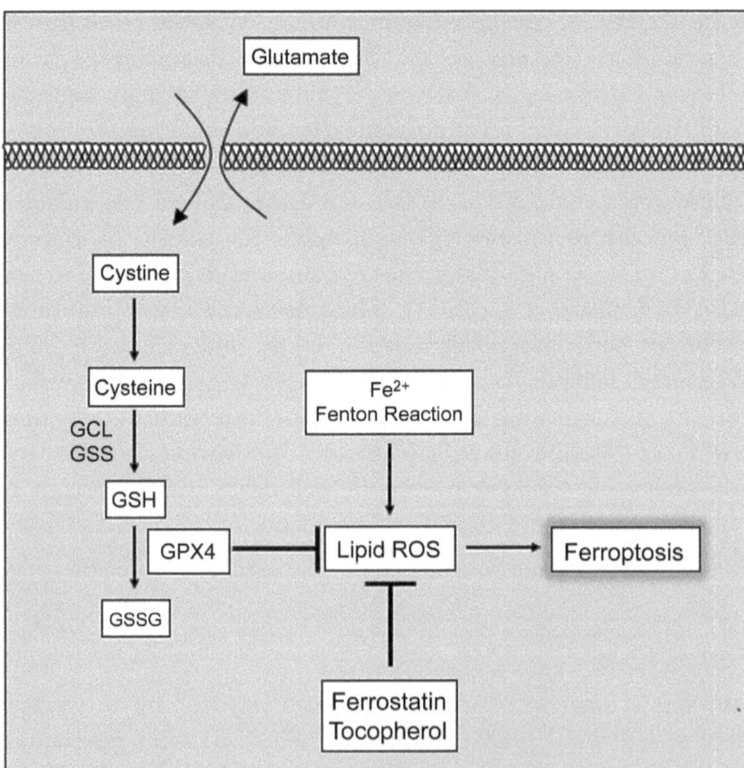

Fig. 6 Mechanism of ferroptosis. Cystine enters the cell via the cystine/glutamate antiporter (system x_c^-) where it is reduced to cysteine and synthesized to GSH in two steps by the ATP-dependent cytosolic enzymes GCL and GSS. GSH is then reduced by GPX4 to glutathione disulfide (GSSG). GPX4 inhibits lipid peroxidation. In the absence of GPX4, lipid peroxidation and accumulation of peroxides occurs, which leads to ferroptosis. Ferroptosis is inhibited by free radical scavengers such as Ferrostatin or Tocopherol.

as buthionine sulfoximine (BSO) can induce ferroptosis by inhibiting GCL and thus depleting GSH (Stockwell et al., 2017; Yang & Stockwell, 2016). Further molecular elucidation of ferroptosis has revealed that GSH depletion by erastin and subsequent glutathione peroxidase 4 (GPX4) inactivation was necessary for cell death to occur, as ferroptotic cell death could be prevented by GSH or NAC supplementation (Yang et al., 2014). The reduced GSH-dependent enzyme GPX4 has emerged as the main endogenous inhibitor of ferroptosis due to its ability to limit lipid peroxidation by catalyzing lipid alcohols from hydroperoxides (Fig. 6) (Yang et al., 2014). Deletion of GPX4 results in accumulation of peroxides and subsequent ferroptotic cell death, which can be inhibited by the ferroptosis inhibitor ferrostatin-1 (Fer-1) or other iron chelators, liproxstatin, and lipophilic antioxidants (Dixon et al., 2012; Friedmann Angeli et al., 2014). Inducible GPX4 knockout mice lose body weight and die within 2 weeks, while global knockout mice die within 48h of birth (Yoo et al., 2012). Transgenic overexpression of human GPX4 in mice greatly reduced buthylhydroperoxide and diquant-induced liver damage and lipid peroxidation as well as reduced CASP 3 activation and cytochrome *c* release from the mitochondria (Ran et al., 2004). Interestingly, the mode of cell death in this model was reported to be apoptosis, pointing to the complexity and interplay of these cell death subroutines (Ran et al., 2004). Non-heme iron-containing proteins including lipoxygenases (LOXs) can mediate ferroptotic peroxidation of free polyunsaturated fatty acids (PUFAs), and genetic mutation of LOXs also protects against erastin-induced ferroptosis (Kagan et al., 2017; Kuhn, Banthiya, & van Leyen, 2015). Based on this evidence, ferroptosis-inducing agents have been classified into two classes: class I agents involve GSH depletion, while class II agents trigger ferroptosis through inhibition of GPX4 (Cao & Dixon, 2016).

Ferroptosis is a relatively novel form of cell death and its role in liver cell pathobiology has not been fully investigated. However, since GSH depletion is an important feature of APAP DILI and hepatotoxicity some have speculated that ferroptosis may account for cell death in this model. Fer-1, a free radical scavenger which dampens the accumulation of lipid hydroperoxides, was shown to protect primary mouse hepatocytes from APAP treatment in vitro (Lorincz, Jemnitz, Kardon, Mandl, & Szarka, 2015). It is important to note that lipid peroxidation has been reported in APAP toxicity but its contribution to APAP-induced hepatocyte necrosis has been controversial. Tocopherol treatment, which blocks lipid peroxidation, had no effect on APAP-induced cell death (Knight, Fariss, Farhood, & Jaeschke, 2003). Although Fer-1 is noted to have greater potency than tocopherol in blocking ferroptosis (Zilka et al., 2017), Fer-1 may play a role as a promiscuous free radical scavenger dampening ROS post-APAP and thereby interfering with sustained pJNK activation. Further studies using GPX4 knockout mice are needed to further investigate the contribution of ferroptosis to cell death in APAP toxicity.

3. Conclusions

Cell death is a dominant feature of hepatotoxicity due to drugs. Despite the many subroutines of cell death which have been recently described, apoptosis and necrosis remain the most relevant in the context of DILI with the culprit drug or toxin largely dictating the mechanism and extent of cell death. DILI can be direct, intrinsic and dose dependent, as we have discussed in the case of APAP, or idiosyncratic (IDILI). While there is not much direct evidence for the subroutine of cell death in IDILI, since liver injury in this instance is immune-mediated and death receptor-driven, apoptosis is likely involved. Idiosyncratic hepatotoxicity is one of the most common reasons for failure of drugs in clinical trials or their withdrawal from the market. The pathogenesis of IDILI is multifactorial, made even more complex by host factors such as age, gender, concomitant diseases and medications, epigenetics, infections, diet, microbiome, activities of CYPs, drug transporters, and detoxifying enzymes (Dara et al., 2017). Recent technological advancements have also helped elucidate the role of genetic polymorphisms in predisposing certain individuals to IDILI (Daly & Day, 2009).

Mitochondria are critical organelles in the liver and their involvement is pivotal for the execution of MPT-driven necrosis (such as in APAP) and hepatocyte apoptosis, but not necroptosis. Given their role in liver homeostasis, it is not surprising that many hepatotoxic drugs directly target the mitochondria. APAP-induced DILI is the best studied animal model of hepatotoxicity. APAP is metabolized to a toxic moiety, NAPQI, which is highly electrophilic and covalently binds proteins, depletes GSH, damages mitochondria, generates ROS, and ultimately results in necrotic cell death of hepatocytes (Dara & Kaplowitz, 2017a, 2017b; McGill et al., 2012). APAP-induced cell death involves the activation of the GSK3β, RIPK1, and the MAPK pathways, culminating in a feedback loop of sustained JNK activation, leading to MPT, the mitochondrial release of endonuclease G and AIF, and cell death. There is no significant caspase activation in

APAP, and the mode of cell death is clearly necrotic. However, since cell death in this model can be abrogated by genetic manipulation or pharmacologic inhibition, it is considered a form of regulated necrosis (Dara et al., 2016c). Necroptosis is a form of regulated cell death which occurs when caspases are inhibited following an apoptotic stimulus in certain cell types. This form of cell death has been largely ruled out as contributing to APAP toxicity as MLKL knockout mice do not seem to be protected (Dara, 2018). However, the RIPK proteins have been suggested to participate in APAP DILI independent of necroptosis. Autophagy, a homeostatic process which promotes the orderly destruction and recycling of cellular components, has been considered a cell death subroutine when excessively activated (Baehrecke, 2005). In the context of APAP DILI, autophagy and mitophagy seem to be mainly protective (Chao et al., 2018). Other more recently discovered forms of cell death have also been studied in DILI models. Ferroptosis is an iron-dependent form of cell death involving lipid peroxidation and GSH depletion and is mediated by GPX4. Pyroptosis is inflammasome-mediated activation of caspases 1 and 11 that leads to Gasdermin-D-induced plasma membrane rupture. However, not enough is known about the importance and participation of ferroptosis and pyroptosis in acute liver injury from DILI to draw firm conclusions.

Acknowledgment

This work was supported by NIH grant K08DK109141 to L.D.

Conflict of interest

We have no conflict of interest or disclosures.

References

Aachoui, Y., Sagulenko, V., Miao, E. A., & Stacey, K. J. (2013). Inflammasome-mediated pyroptotic and apoptotic cell death, and defense against infection. *Current Opinion in Microbiology*, *16*(3), 319–326. https://doi.org/10.1016/j.mib.2013.04.004.

Acehan, D., Jiang, X., Morgan, D. G., Heuser, J. E., Wang, X., & Akey, C. W. (2002). Three-dimensional structure of the apoptosome: Implications for assembly, procaspase-9 binding, and activation. *Molecular Cell*, *9*(2), 423–432. S1097276502004422 [pii].

Agarwal, R., MacMillan-Crow, L. A., Rafferty, T. M., Saba, H., Roberts, D. W., Fifer, E. K., et al. (2011). Acetaminophen-induced hepatotoxicity in mice occurs with inhibition of activity and nitration of mitochondrial manganese superoxide dismutase. *The Journal of Pharmacology and Experimental Therapeutics*, *337*(1), 110–116. https://doi.org/10.1124/jpet.110.176321.

Aglietti, R. A., & Dueber, E. C. (2017). Recent insights into the molecular mechanisms underlying pyroptosis and gasdermin family functions. *Trends in Immunology*, *38*(4), 261–271. https://doi.org/10.1016/j.it.2017.01.003.

Amir, M., Zhao, E., Fontana, L., Rosenberg, H., Tanaka, K., Gao, G., et al. (2013). Inhibition of hepatocyte autophagy increases tumor necrosis factor-dependent liver injury by promoting caspase-8 activation. *Cell Death and Differentiation*, *20*(7), 878–887. https://doi.org/10.1038/cdd.2013.21.

Ashkenazi, A., Pai, R. C., Fong, S., Leung, S., Lawrence, D. A., Marsters, S. A., et al. (1999). Safety and antitumor activity of recombinant soluble Apo2 ligand. *The Journal of Clinical Investigation*, *104*(2), 155–162. https://doi.org/10.1172/JCI6926.

Baehrecke, E. H. (2005). Autophagy: Dual roles in life and death? *Nature Reviews. Molecular Cell Biology*, *6*(6), 505–510. https://doi.org/10.1038/nrm1666.

Bajt, M. L., Cover, C., Lemasters, J. J., & Jaeschke, H. (2006). Nuclear translocation of endonuclease G and apoptosis-inducing factor during acetaminophen-induced liver cell injury. *Toxicological Sciences*, *94*(1), 217–225. kfl077 [pii]. https://doi.org/10.1093/toxsci/kfl077.

Bell, L. N., & Chalasani, N. (2009). Epidemiology of idiosyncratic drug-induced liver injury. *Seminars in Liver Disease*, *29*(4), 337–347. https://doi.org/10.1055/s-0029-1240002.

Bissell, D. M., Wang, S. S., Jarnagin, W. R., & Roll, F. J. (1995). Cell-specific expression of transforming growth factor-beta in rat liver. Evidence for autocrine regulation of hepatocyte proliferation. *The Journal of Clinical Investigation*, *96*(1), 447–455. https://doi.org/10.1172/JCI118055.

Bissuel, F., Bruneel, F., Habersetzer, F., Chassard, D., Cotte, L., Chevallier, M., et al. (1994). Fulminant hepatitis with severe lactate acidosis in HIV-infected patients on didanosine therapy. *Journal of Internal Medicine*, *235*(4), 367–371.

Bratton, S. B., & Salvesen, G. S. (2010). Regulation of the Apaf-1-caspase-9 apoptosome. Journal of Cell Science, 123(Pt 19), 3209–3214. doi:https://doi.org/10.1242/jcs.073643

Brenner, D., Blaser, H., & Mak, T. W. (2015). Regulation of tumour necrosis factor signalling: Live or let die. *Nature Reviews. Immunology*, *15*(6), 362–374. https://doi.org/10.1038/nri3834.

Cao, J. Y., & Dixon, S. J. (2016). Mechanisms of ferroptosis. *Cellular and Molecular Life Sciences*, *73*(11 – 12), 2195–2209. https://doi.org/10.1007/s00018-016-2194-1.

Chakraborty, M., Fullerton, A. M., Semple, K., Chea, L. S., Proctor, W. R., Bourdi, M., et al. (2015). Drug-induced allergic hepatitis develops in mice when myeloid-derived suppressor cells are depleted prior to halothane treatment. *Hepatology*, *62*(2), 546–557. https://doi.org/10.1002/hep.27764.

Chalasani, N., Bonkovsky, H. L., Fontana, R., Lee, W., Stolz, A., Talwalkar, J., et al. (2015). Features and outcomes of 899 patients with drug-induced liver injury: The DILIN prospective study. *Gastroenterology*, *148*(7), 1340–1352. e1347. https://doi.org/10.1053/j.gastro.2015.03.006.

Chambers, J. W., & LoGrasso, P. V. (2011). Mitochondrial c-Jun N-terminal kinase (JNK) signaling initiates physiological changes resulting in amplification of reactive oxygen species generation. *The Journal of Biological Chemistry*, *286*(18), 16052–16062. https://doi.org/10.1074/jbc.M111.223602.

Chao, X., Wang, H., Jaeschke, H., & Ding, W. X. (2018). Role and mechanisms of autophagy in acetaminophen-induced liver injury. *Liver International*, *38*(8), 1363–1374. https://doi.org/10.1111/liv.13866.

Chen, D., Ni, H. M., Wang, L., Ma, X., Yu, J., Ding, W. X., et al. (2018). PUMA induction mediates acetaminophen-induced necrosis and liver injury. *Hepatology*. https://doi.org/10.1002/hep.30422 [Epub ahead of print].

Connern, C. P., & Halestrap, A. P. (1994). Recruitment of mitochondrial cyclophilin to the mitochondrial inner membrane under conditions of oxidative stress that enhance the opening of a calcium-sensitive non-specific channel. *The Biochemical Journal*, *302*(Pt 2), 321–324.

Corazza, N., Jakob, S., Schaer, C., Frese, S., Keogh, A., Stroka, D., et al. (2006). TRAIL receptor-mediated JNK activation and Bim phosphorylation critically regulate Fas-mediated liver damage and lethality. *The Journal of Clinical Investigation, 116*(9), 2493–2499. https://doi.org/10.1172/JCI27726.

Cover, C., Mansouri, A., Knight, T. R., Bajt, M. L., Lemasters, J. J., Pessayre, D., et al. (2005). Peroxynitrite-induced mitochondrial and endonuclease-mediated nuclear DNA damage in acetaminophen hepatotoxicity. *The Journal of Pharmacology and Experimental Therapeutics, 315*(2), 879–887. https://doi.org/10.1124/jpet.105.088898.

Daly, A. K., & Day, C. P. (2009). Genetic association studies in drug-induced liver injury. *Seminars in Liver Disease, 29*(4), 400–411. https://doi.org/10.1055/s-0029-1240009.

Daly, A. K., Donaldson, P. T., Bhatnagar, P., Shen, Y., Pe'er, I., Floratos, A., et al. (2009). HLA-B*5701 genotype is a major determinant of drug-induced liver injury due to flucloxacillin. *Nature Genetics, 41*(7), 816–819. https://doi.org/10.1038/ng.379.

Dara, L. (2018). The receptor interacting protein kinases in the liver. *Seminars in Liver Disease, 38*(1), 73–86. https://doi.org/10.1055/s-0038-1629924.

Dara, L., Johnson, H., Suda, J., Win, S., Gaarde, W., Han, D., et al. (2015). Receptor interacting protein kinase 1 mediates murine acetaminophen toxicity independent of the necrosome and not through necroptosis. *Hepatology, 62*(6), 1847–1857. https://doi.org/10.1002/hep.27939. Dec.

Dara, L., & Kaplowitz, N. (2016). Reply. *Hepatology, 64*(1), 308–309. https://doi.org/10.1002/hep.28221.

Dara, L., & Kaplowitz, N. (2017a). Cell death in drug induced liver injury. In W.-X. Ding & X.-M. Yin (Eds.), *Cellular injury in liver diseases* (pp. 1–29). Springer International Publishing AG.

Dara, L., & Kaplowitz, N. (2017b). Cell death in drug-induced liver injury. In W.-X. Yin & X.-M. Ding (Eds.), *Cell death in biology and diseases* (pp. 1–35). Cham, Switzerland: Springer International Publishing AG.

Dara, L., Liu, X. Z., & Kaplowitz, N. (2017). Pathogenesis if idiosyncratic drug induced liver injury. In P. Muriel (Ed.), *Liver pathophysiology, therapies and antioxidants*. Cambridge: Elsevier.

Dara, L., Liu, Z. X., & Kaplowitz, N. (2016a). Mechanisms of adaptation and progression in idiosyncratic drug induced liver injury, clinical implications. *Liver International, 36*(2), 158–165. https://doi.org/10.1111/liv.12988.

Dara, L., Liu, Z. X., & Kaplowitz, N. (2016b). A murder mystery in the liver: Who done it and how? *The Journal of Clinical Investigation, 126*(11), 4068–4071. https://doi.org/10.1172/JCI90830.

Dara, L., Liu, Z. X., & Kaplowitz, N. (2016c). Questions and controversies: The role of necroptosis in liver disease. *Cell Death & Disease, 2*, 16089. https://doi.org/10.1038/cddiscovery.2016.89.

Degterev, A., Hitomi, J., Germscheid, M., Ch'en, I. L., Korkina, O., Teng, X., et al. (2008). Identification of RIP1 kinase as a specific cellular target of necrostatins. *Nature Chemical Biology, 4*(5), 313–321. https://doi.org/10.1038/nchembio.83.

Degterev, A., Huang, Z., Boyce, M., Li, Y., Jagtap, P., Mizushima, N., et al. (2005). Chemical inhibitor of nonapoptotic cell death with therapeutic potential for ischemic brain injury. *Nature Chemical Biology, 1*(2), 112–119. https://doi.org/10.1038/nchembio711.

Degterev, A., Zhou, W., Maki, J. L., & Yuan, J. (2014). Assays for necroptosis and activity of RIP kinases. *Methods in Enzymology, 545*, 1–33. https://doi.org/10.1016/B978-0-12-801430-1.00001-9.

Deutsch, M., Graffeo, C. S., Rokosh, R., Pansari, M., Ochi, A., Levie, E. M., et al. (2015). Divergent effects of RIP1 or RIP3 blockade in murine models of acute liver injury. *Cell Death & Disease, 6*, e1759. https://doi.org/10.1038/cddis.2015.126.

Dikalova, A. E., Bikineyeva, A. T., Budzyn, K., Nazarewicz, R. R., McCann, L., Lewis, W., et al. (2010). Therapeutic targeting of mitochondrial superoxide in hypertension. *Circulation Research*, *107*(1), 106–116. https://doi.org/10.1161/CIRCRESAHA.109.214601.

Ding, W. X. (2014). Induction of autophagy, a promising approach for treating liver injury. *Hepatology*, *59*(1), 340–343. https://doi.org/10.1002/hep.26572.

Dixon, S. J. (2017). Ferroptosis: Bug or feature? *Immunological Reviews*, *277*(1), 150–157. https://doi.org/10.1111/imr.12533.

Dixon, S. J., Lemberg, K. M., Lamprecht, M. R., Skouta, R., Zaitsev, E. M., Gleason, C. E., et al. (2012). Ferroptosis: An iron-dependent form of nonapoptotic cell death. *Cell*, *149*(5), 1060–1072. https://doi.org/10.1016/j.cell.2012.03.042.

Du, K., Farhood, A., & Jaeschke, H. (2017). Mitochondria-targeted antioxidant Mito-Tempo protects against acetaminophen hepatotoxicity. *Archives of Toxicology*, *91*(2), 761–773. https://doi.org/10.1007/s00204-016-1692-0.

Ea, C. K., Deng, L., Xia, Z. P., Pineda, G., & Chen, Z. J. (2006). Activation of IKK by TNFalpha requires site-specific ubiquitination of RIP1 and polyubiquitin binding by NEMO. *Molecular Cell*, *22*(2), 245–257. https://doi.org/10.1016/j.molcel.2006.03.026.

Franchi, L., Eigenbrod, T., Munoz-Planillo, R., & Nunez, G. (2009). The inflammasome: A caspase-1-activation platform that regulates immune responses and disease pathogenesis. *Nature Immunology*, *10*(3), 241–247. https://doi.org/10.1038/ni.1703.

Friedmann Angeli, J. P., Schneider, M., Proneth, B., Tyurina, Y. Y., Tyurin, V. A., Hammond, V. J., et al. (2014). Inactivation of the ferroptosis regulator Gpx4 triggers acute renal failure in mice. *Nature Cell Biology*, *16*(12), 1180–1191. https://doi.org/10.1038/ncb3064.

Fromenty, B., Fisch, C., Labbe, G., Degott, C., Deschamps, D., Berson, A., et al. (1990). Amiodarone inhibits the mitochondrial beta-oxidation of fatty acids and produces microvesicular steatosis of the liver in mice. *The Journal of Pharmacology and Experimental Therapeutics*, *255*(3), 1371–1376.

Fromenty, B., & Pessayre, D. (1995). Inhibition of mitochondrial beta-oxidation as a mechanism of hepatotoxicity. *Pharmacology & Therapeutics*, *67*(1), 101–154.

Fu, L., Lin, Y. D., Elrod, H. A., Yue, P., Oh, Y., Li, B., et al. (2010). C-Jun NH2-terminal kinase-dependent upregulation of DR5 mediates cooperative induction of apoptosis by perifosine and TRAIL. *Molecular Cancer*, *9*, 315. https://doi.org/10.1186/1476-4598-9-315.

Fujimoto, K., Kumagai, K., Ito, K., Arakawa, S., Ando, Y., Oda, S., et al. (2009). Sensitivity of liver injury in heterozygous Sod2 knockout mice treated with troglitazone or acetaminophen. *Toxicologic Pathology*, *37*(2), 193–200. 37/2/193 [pii]. https://doi.org/10.1177/0192623308329282.

Galluzzi, L., Bravo-San Pedro, J. M., Vitale, I., Aaronson, S. A., Abrams, J. M., Adam, D., et al. (2015). Essential versus accessory aspects of cell death: Recommendations of the NCCD 2015. *Cell Death and Differentiation*, *22*(1), 58–73. https://doi.org/10.1038/cdd.2014.137.

Galluzzi, L., Vitale, I., Aaronson, S. A., Abrams, J. M., Adam, D., Agostinis, P., et al. (2018). Molecular mechanisms of cell death: Recommendations of the nomenclature committee on cell death 2018. *Cell Death and Differentiation*, *25*(3), 486–541. https://doi.org/10.1038/s41418-017-0012-4.

Galluzzi, L., Vitale, I., Abrams, J. M., Alnemri, E. S., Baehrecke, E. H., Blagosklonny, M. V., et al. (2012). Molecular definitions of cell death subroutines: Recommendations of the nomenclature committee on cell death 2012. *Cell Death and Differentiation*, *19*(1), 107–120. https://doi.org/10.1038/cdd.2011.96.

Gao, M., Monian, P., Pan, Q., Zhang, W., Xiang, J., & Jiang, X. (2016). Ferroptosis is an autophagic cell death process. *Cell Research*, *26*(9), 1021–1032. https://doi.org/10.1038/cr.2016.95.

Gerlach, B., Cordier, S. M., Schmukle, A. C., Emmerich, C. H., Rieser, E., Haas, T. L., et al. (2011). Linear ubiquitination prevents inflammation and regulates immune signalling. *Nature*, *471*(7340), 591–596. https://doi.org/10.1038/nature09816.

Gibson, J. D., Pumford, N. R., Samokyszyn, V. M., & Hinson, J. A. (1996). Mechanism of acetaminophen-induced hepatotoxicity: Covalent binding versus oxidative stress. *Chemical Research in Toxicology*, *9*(3), 580–585. https://doi.org/10.1021/tx950153d.

Glick, D., Barth, S., & Macleod, K. F. (2010). Autophagy: Cellular and molecular mechanisms. *The Journal of Pathology*, *221*(1), 3–12. https://doi.org/10.1002/path.2697.

Goodall, M. L., Fitzwalter, B. E., Zahedi, S., Wu, M., Rodriguez, D., Mulcahy-Levy, J. M., et al. (2016). The autophagy machinery controls cell death switching between apoptosis and necroptosis. *Developmental Cell*, *37*(4), 337–349. https://doi.org/10.1016/j.devcel.2016.04.018.

Green, D. R. (2000). Apoptotic pathways: Paper wraps stone blunts scissors. *Cell*, *102*(1), 1–4.

Grove, J. I., & Aithal, G. P. (2015). Human leukocyte antigen genetic risk factors of drug-induced liver toxicology. *Expert Opinion on Drug Metabolism & Toxicology*, *11*(3), 395–409. https://doi.org/10.1517/17425255.2015.992414.

Guicciardi, M. E., & Gores, G. J. (2009). Life and death by death receptors. *The FASEB Journal*, *23*(6), 1625–1637. https://doi.org/10.1096/fj.08-111005.

Gump, J. M., Staskiewicz, L., Morgan, M. J., Bamberg, A., Riches, D. W., & Thorburn, A. (2014). Autophagy variation within a cell population determines cell fate through selective degradation of Fap-1. *Nature Cell Biology*, *16*(1), 47–54. https://doi.org/10.1038/ncb2886.

Gunawan, B. K., Liu, Z. X., Han, D., Hanawa, N., Gaarde, W. A., & Kaplowitz, N. (2006). C-Jun N-terminal kinase plays a major role in murine acetaminophen hepatotoxicity. *Gastroenterology*, *131*(1), 165–178. S0016-5085(06)00712-8 [pii]. https://doi.org/10.1053/j.gastro.2006.03.045.

Gunther, C., He, G. W., Kremer, A. E., Murphy, J. M., Petrie, E. J., Amann, K., et al. (2016). The pseudokinase MLKL mediates programmed hepatocellular necrosis independently of RIPK3 during hepatitis. *The Journal of Clinical Investigation*, *126*(11), 4346–4360. https://doi.org/10.1172/JCI87545.

Haas, T. L., Emmerich, C. H., Gerlach, B., Schmukle, A. C., Cordier, S. M., Rieser, E., et al. (2009). Recruitment of the linear ubiquitin chain assembly complex stabilizes the TNF-R1 signaling complex and is required for TNF-mediated gene induction. *Molecular Cell*, *36*(5), 831–844. https://doi.org/10.1016/j.molcel.2009.10.013.

Han, D., Hanawa, N., Saberi, B., & Kaplowitz, N. (2006a). Hydrogen peroxide and redox modulation sensitize primary mouse hepatocytes to TNF-induced apoptosis. *Free Radical Biology & Medicine*, *41*(4), 627–639. S0891-5849(06)00294-2 [pii]. https://doi.org/10.1016/j.freeradbiomed.2006.05.002.

Han, D., Hanawa, N., Saberi, B., & Kaplowitz, N. (2006b). Mechanisms of liver injury. III. Role of glutathione redox status in liver injury. *American Journal of Physiology. Gastrointestinal and Liver Physiology*, *291*(1), G1–G7. 00001.2006 [pii]. https://doi.org/10.1152/ajpgi.00001.2006.

Hanawa, N., Shinohara, M., Saberi, B., Gaarde, W. A., Han, D., & Kaplowitz, N. (2008). Role of JNK translocation to mitochondria leading to inhibition of mitochondria bioenergetics in acetaminophen-induced liver injury. *The Journal of Biological Chemistry*, *283*(20), 13565–13577. M708916200 [pii]. https://doi.org/10.1074/jbc.M708916200.

Hautekeete, M. L., Horsmans, Y., Van Waeyenberge, C., Demanet, C., Henrion, J., Verbist, L., et al. (1999). HLA association of amoxicillin-clavulanate–induced hepatitis. *Gastroenterology, 117*(5), 1181–1186.

He, S., Wang, L., Miao, L., Wang, T., Du, F., Zhao, L., et al. (2009). Receptor interacting protein kinase-3 determines cellular necrotic response to TNF-alpha. *Cell, 137*(6), 1100–1111. S0092-8674(09)00578-9 [pii]. https://doi.org/10.1016/j.cell.2009.05.021.

He, W., Wang, Q., Srinivasan, B., Xu, J., Padilla, M. T., Li, Z., et al. (2014). A JNK-mediated autophagy pathway that triggers c-IAP degradation and necroptosis for anticancer chemotherapy. *Oncogene, 33*(23), 3004–3013. https://doi.org/10.1038/onc.2013.256.

Hinson, J. A., Roberts, D. W., & James, L. P. (2010). Mechanisms of acetaminophen-induced liver necrosis. *Handbook of Experimental Pharmacology, 196*, 369–405. https://doi.org/10.1007/978-3-642-00663-0_12.

Holler, N., Zaru, R., Micheau, O., Thome, M., Attinger, A., Valitutti, S., et al. (2000). Fas triggers an alternative, caspase-8-independent cell death pathway using the kinase RIP as effector molecule. *Nature Immunology, 1*(6), 489–495. https://doi.org/10.1038/82732.

Horn, S., Hughes, M. A., Schilling, R., Sticht, C., Tenev, T., Ploesser, M., et al. (2017). Caspase-10 negatively regulates caspase-8-mediated cell death, switching the response to CD95L in favor of NF-kappaB activation and cell survival. *Cell Reports, 19*(4), 785–797. https://doi.org/10.1016/j.celrep.2017.04.010.

Hou, W., Xie, Y., Song, X., Sun, X., Lotze, M. T., Zeh, H. J., 3rd, et al. (2016). Autophagy promotes ferroptosis by degradation of ferritin. *Autophagy, 12*(8), 1425–1428. https://doi.org/10.1080/15548627.2016.1187366.

Imaeda, A. B., Watanabe, A., Sohail, M. A., Mahmood, S., Mohamadnejad, M., Sutterwala, F. S., et al. (2009). Acetaminophen-induced hepatotoxicity in mice is dependent on Tlr9 and the Nalp3 inflammasome. *The Journal of Clinical Investigation, 119*(2), 305–314. https://doi.org/10.1172/JCI35958.

Iorga, A., Dara, L., & Kaplowitz, N. (2017). Drug-induced liver injury: Cascade of events leading to cell death, apoptosis or necrosis. *International Journal of Molecular Sciences, 18*(5). https://doi.org/10.3390/ijms18051018.

Irmler, M., Thome, M., Hahne, M., Schneider, P., Hofmann, K., Steiner, V., et al. (1997). Inhibition of death receptor signals by cellular FLIP. *Nature, 388*(6638), 190–195. https://doi.org/10.1038/40657.

Jaeschke, H. (2015). Acetaminophen: Dose-dependent drug hepatotoxicity and acute liver failure in patients. *Digestive Diseases, 33*(4), 464–471. https://doi.org/10.1159/000374090.

Jaeschke, H., Cover, C., & Bajt, M. L. (2006). Role of caspases in acetaminophen-induced liver injury. *Life Sciences, 78*(15), 1670–1676. https://doi.org/10.1016/j.lfs.2005.07.003.

Jaeschke, H., Duan, L., Akakpo, J. Y., Farhood, A., & Ramachandran, A. (2018). The role of apoptosis in acetaminophen hepatotoxicity. *Food and Chemical Toxicology, 118*, 709–718. https://doi.org/10.1016/j.fct.2018.06.025.

Jaeschke, H., & Ramachandran, A. (2018). Oxidant stress and lipid peroxidation in acetaminophen hepatotoxicity. *Reactive Oxygen Species, 5*(15), 145–158.

Jaeschke, H., Williams, C. D., & Farhood, A. (2011). No evidence for caspase-dependent apoptosis in acetaminophen hepatotoxicity. *Hepatology, 53*(2), 718–719. https://doi.org/10.1002/hep.23940.

Jorgensen, I., & Miao, E. A. (2015). Pyroptotic cell death defends against intracellular pathogens. *Immunological Reviews, 265*(1), 130–142. https://doi.org/10.1111/imr.12287.

Jost, P. J., Grabow, S., Gray, D., McKenzie, M. D., Nachbur, U., Huang, D. C., et al. (2009). XIAP discriminates between type I and type II FAS-induced apoptosis. *Nature, 460*(7258), 1035–1039. https://doi.org/10.1038/nature08229.

Kagan, V. E., Mao, G., Qu, F., Angeli, J. P., Doll, S., Croix, C. S., et al. (2017). Oxidized arachidonic and adrenic PEs navigate cells to ferroptosis. *Nature Chemical Biology, 13*(1), 81–90. https://doi.org/10.1038/nchembio.2238.

Kahraman, A., Barreyro, F. J., Bronk, S. F., Werneburg, N. W., Mott, J. L., Akazawa, Y., et al. (2008). TRAIL mediates liver injury by the innate immune system in the bile duct-ligated mouse. *Hepatology*, *47*(4), 1317–1330. https://doi.org/10.1002/hep.22136.

Kaplowitz, N. (2013). Drug-induced liver injury. Introduction and overview. In N. Kaplowitz & L. D. DeLeve (Eds.), *Drug-induced liver injury* (3rd ed., pp. 3–13). Elsevier.

Karin, M., & Lin, A. (2002). NF-kappaB at the crossroads of life and death. *Nature Immunology*, *3*(3), 221–227. https://doi.org/10.1038/ni0302-221.

Kasof, G. M., Prosser, J. C., Liu, D., Lorenzi, M. V., & Gomes, B. C. (2000). The RIP-like kinase, RIP3, induces apoptosis and NF-kappaB nuclear translocation and localizes to mitochondria. *FEBS Letters*, *473*(3), 285–291.

Kassahun, K., Farrell, K., & Abbott, F. (1991). Identification and characterization of the glutathione and N-acetylcysteine conjugates of (E)-2-propyl-2,4-pentadienoic acid, a toxic metabolite of valproic acid, in rats and humans. *Drug Metabolism and Disposition*, *19*(2), 525–535.

Kaufmann, T., Jost, P. J., Pellegrini, M., Puthalakath, H., Gugasyan, R., Gerondakis, S., et al. (2009). Fatal hepatitis mediated by tumor necrosis factor TNFalpha requires caspase-8 and involves the BH3-only proteins bid and Bim. *Immunity*, *30*(1), 56–66. S1074-7613(08)00543-8 [pii]. https://doi.org/10.1016/j.immuni.2008.10.017.

Kayagaki, N., Stowe, I. B., Lee, B. L., O'Rourke, K., Anderson, K., Warming, S., et al. (2015). Caspase-11 cleaves gasdermin D for non-canonical inflammasome signalling. *Nature*, *526*(7575), 666–671. https://doi.org/10.1038/nature15541.

Khanova, E., Wu, R., Wang, W., Yan, R., Chen, Y., French, S. W., et al. (2018). Pyroptosis by caspase11/4-gasdermin-D pathway in alcoholic hepatitis in mice and patients. *Hepatology*, *67*(5), 1737–1753. https://doi.org/10.1002/hep.29645.

Kim, S. E., Zhang, L., Ma, K., Riegman, M., Chen, F., Ingold, I., et al. (2016). Ultrasmall nanoparticles induce ferroptosis in nutrient-deprived cancer cells and suppress tumour growth. *Nature Nanotechnology*, *11*(11), 977–985. https://doi.org/10.1038/nnano.2016.164.

Kindmark, A., Jawaid, A., Harbron, C. G., Barratt, B. J., Bengtsson, O. F., Andersson, T. B., et al. (2008). Genome-wide pharmacogenetic investigation of a hepatic adverse event without clinical signs of immunopathology suggests an underlying immune pathogenesis. *The Pharmacogenomics Journal*, *8*(3), 186–195. https://doi.org/10.1038/sj.tpj.6500458.

Knight, T. R., Fariss, M. W., Farhood, A., & Jaeschke, H. (2003). Role of lipid peroxidation as a mechanism of liver injury after acetaminophen overdose in mice. *Toxicological Sciences*, *76*(1), 229–236. https://doi.org/10.1093/toxsci/kfg220.

Knolle, P. A., & Gerken, G. (2000). Local control of the immune response in the liver. *Immunological Reviews*, *174*, 21–34.

Knolle, P. A., Germann, T., Treichel, U., Uhrig, A., Schmitt, E., Hegenbarth, S., et al. (1999). Endotoxin down-regulates T cell activation by antigen-presenting liver sinusoidal endothelial cells. *Journal of Immunology*, *162*(3), 1401–1407.

Knolle, P., Schlaak, J., Uhrig, A., Kempf, P., Meyer zum Buschenfelde, K. H., & Gerken, G. (1995). Human Kupffer cells secrete IL-10 in response to lipopolysaccharide (LPS) challenge. *Journal of Hepatology*, *22*(2), 226–229.

Knolle, P. A., Uhrig, A., Protzer, U., Trippler, M., Duchmann, R., Meyer zum Buschenfelde, K. H., et al. (1998). Interleukin-10 expression is autoregulated at the transcriptional level in human and murine Kupffer cells. *Hepatology*, *27*(1), 93–99. https://doi.org/10.1002/hep.510270116.

Komatsu, M., Waguri, S., Ueno, T., Iwata, J., Murata, S., Tanida, I., et al. (2005). Impairment of starvation-induced and constitutive autophagy in Atg7-deficient mice. *The Journal of Cell Biology*, *169*(3), 425–434. jcb.200412022 [pii]. https://doi.org/10.1083/jcb.200412022.

Kon, K., Kim, J. S., Jaeschke, H., & Lemasters, J. J. (2004). Mitochondrial permeability transition in acetaminophen-induced necrosis and apoptosis of cultured mouse hepatocytes. *Hepatology*, *40*(5), 1170–1179. https://doi.org/10.1002/hep.20437.

Kranz, D., & Boutros, M. (2014). A synthetic lethal screen identifies FAT1 as an antagonist of caspase-8 in extrinsic apoptosis. *The EMBO Journal, 33*(3), 181–197. https://doi.org/10.1002/embj.201385686.

Kuhn, H., Banthiya, S., & van Leyen, K. (2015). Mammalian lipoxygenases and their biological relevance. *Biochimica et Biophysica Acta, 1851*(4), 308–330. https://doi.org/10.1016/j.bbalip.2014.10.002.

Larson, A. M., Polson, J., Fontana, R. J., Davern, T. J., Lalani, E., Hynan, L. S., et al. (2005). Acetaminophen-induced acute liver failure: Results of a United States multicenter, prospective study. *Hepatology, 42*(6), 1364–1372. https://doi.org/10.1002/hep.20948.

Lemasters, J. J., Nieminen, A. L., Qian, T., Trost, L. C., Elmore, S. P., Nishimura, Y., et al. (1998). The mitochondrial permeability transition in cell death: A common mechanism in necrosis, apoptosis and autophagy. *Biochimica et Biophysica Acta, 1366*(1–2), 177–196.

Levy, R. H., Rettenmeier, A. W., Anderson, G. D., Wilensky, A. J., Friel, P. N., Baillie, T. A., et al. (1990). Effects of polytherapy with phenytoin, carbamazepine, and stiripentol on formation of 4-ene-valproate, a hepatotoxic metabolite of valproic acid. *Clinical Pharmacology and Therapeutics, 48*(3), 225–235.

Lewis, J. H., Ranard, R. C., Caruso, A., Jackson, L. K., Mullick, F., Ishak, K. G., et al. (1989). Amiodarone hepatotoxicity: Prevalence and clinicopathologic correlations among 104 patients. *Hepatology, 9*(5), 679–685.

Li, G., Chen, J. B., Wang, C., Xu, Z., Nie, H., Qin, X. Y., et al. (2013). Curcumin protects against acetaminophen-induced apoptosis in hepatic injury. *World Journal of Gastroenterology, 19*(42), 7440–7446. https://doi.org/10.3748/wjg.v19.i42.7440.

Li, H., Kobayashi, M., Blonska, M., You, Y., & Lin, X. (2006). Ubiquitination of RIP is required for tumor necrosis factor alpha-induced NF-kappaB activation. *The Journal of Biological Chemistry, 281*(19), 13636–13643. https://doi.org/10.1074/jbc.M600620200.

LoGuidice, A., & Boelsterli, U. A. (2011). Acetaminophen overdose-induced liver injury in mice is mediated by peroxynitrite independently of the cyclophilin D-regulated permeability transition. *Hepatology, 54*(3), 969–978. https://doi.org/10.1002/hep.24464.

Lohse, A. W., Knolle, P. A., Bilo, K., Uhrig, A., Waldmann, C., Ibe, M., et al. (1996). Antigen-presenting function and B7 expression of murine sinusoidal endothelial cells and Kupffer cells. *Gastroenterology, 110*(4), 1175–1181.

Lorincz, T., Jemnitz, K., Kardon, T., Mandl, J., & Szarka, A. (2015). Ferroptosis is involved in acetaminophen induced cell death. *Pathology Oncology Research, 21*(4), 1115–1121. https://doi.org/10.1007/s12253-015-9946-3.

Lou, H., & Kaplowitz, N. (2007). Glutathione depletion down-regulates tumor necrosis factor alpha-induced NF-kappaB activity via IkappaB kinase-dependent and -independent mechanisms. *The Journal of Biological Chemistry, 282*(40), 29470–29481. https://doi.org/10.1074/jbc.M706145200.

Lucena, M. I., Andrade, R. J., Fernandez, M. C., Pachkoria, K., Pelaez, G., Duran, J. A., et al. (2006). Determinants of the clinical expression of amoxicillin-clavulanate hepatotoxicity: A prospective series from Spain. *Hepatology, 44*(4), 850–856. https://doi.org/10.1002/hep.21324.

Lucena, M. I., Andrade, R. J., Kaplowitz, N., Garcia-Cortes, M., Fernandez, M. C., Romero-Gomez, M., et al. (2009). Phenotypic characterization of idiosyncratic drug-induced liver injury: The influence of age and sex. *Hepatology, 49*(6), 2001–2009. https://doi.org/10.1002/hep.22895.

Lucena, M. I., Molokhia, M., Shen, Y., Urban, T. J., Aithal, G. P., Andrade, R. J., et al. (2011). Susceptibility to amoxicillin-clavulanate-induced liver injury is influenced by multiple HLA class I and II alleles. *Gastroenterology, 141*(1), 338–347. https://doi.org/10.1053/j.gastro.2011.04.001.

Mak, A., & Uetrecht, J. (2015). The combination of anti-CTLA-4 and PD1 −/− mice unmasks the potential of isoniazid and Nevirapine to cause liver injury. *Chemical Research in Toxicology*. https://doi.org/10.1021/acs.chemrestox.5b00305.
Malhi, H. (2007). TRAILs and tribulation. *Hepatology*, *46*(5), 1320–1322. https://doi.org/10.1002/hep.21913.
Malhi, H., Guicciardi, M. E., & Gores, G. J. (2010). Hepatocyte death: A clear and present danger. *Physiological Reviews*, *90*(3), 1165–1194. 90/3/1165 [pii]. https://doi.org/10.1152/physrev.00061.2009.
Man, S. M., & Kanneganti, T. D. (2015). Gasdermin D: The long-awaited executioner of pyroptosis. *Cell Research*, *25*(11), 1183–1184. https://doi.org/10.1038/cr.2015.124.
Marino, G., Niso-Santano, M., Baehrecke, E. H., & Kroemer, G. (2014). Self-consumption: The interplay of autophagy and apoptosis. *Nature Reviews. Molecular Cell Biology*, *15*(2), 81–94. https://doi.org/10.1038/nrm3735.
Matsumaru, K., Ji, C., & Kaplowitz, N. (2003). Mechanisms for sensitization to TNF-induced apoptosis by acute glutathione depletion in murine hepatocytes. *Hepatology*, *37*(6), 1425–1434. https://doi.org/10.1053/jhep.2003.50230.
McGill, M. R., Sharpe, M. R., Williams, C. D., Taha, M., Curry, S. C., & Jaeschke, H. (2012). The mechanism underlying acetaminophen-induced hepatotoxicity in humans and mice involves mitochondrial damage and nuclear DNA fragmentation. *The Journal of Clinical Investigation*, *122*(4), 1574–1583. https://doi.org/10.1172/JCI59755.
McKenzie, R., Fried, M. W., Sallie, R., Conjeevaram, H., Di Bisceglie, A. M., Park, Y., et al. (1995). Hepatic failure and lactic acidosis due to fialuridine (FIAU), an investigational nucleoside analogue for chronic hepatitis B. *The New England Journal of Medicine*, *333*(17), 1099–1105. https://doi.org/10.1056/NEJM199510263331702.
Micheau, O., & Tschopp, J. (2003). Induction of TNF receptor I-mediated apoptosis via two sequential signaling complexes. *Cell*, *114*(2), 181–190. S009286740300521X [pii].
Mitchell, J. R., Jollow, D. J., Potter, W. Z., Gillette, J. R., & Brodie, B. B. (1973). Acetaminophen-induced hepatic necrosis. IV. Protective role of glutathione. *The Journal of Pharmacology and Experimental Therapeutics*, *187*(1), 211–217.
Motamedi, N. D. L., & Kaplowitz, N. (2017). Clinical considerations of drug-induced hepatotoxicity. In C. MacQueen (Ed.), *Comprehensive toxicology* (3rd ed., pp. 369–381). Elsevier Science.
Murphy, J. M., Czabotar, P. E., Hildebrand, J. M., Lucet, I. S., Zhang, J. G., Alvarez-Diaz, S., et al. (2013). The pseudokinase MLKL mediates necroptosis via a molecular switch mechanism. *Immunity*, *39*(3), 443–453. https://doi.org/10.1016/j.immuni.2013.06.018.
Murphy, E. J., Davern, T. J., Shakil, A. O., Shick, L., Masharani, U., Chow, H., et al. (2000). Troglitazone-induced fulminant hepatic failure. Acute Liver Failure Study Group. *Acute Liver Failure Study Group*, *45*(3), 549–553.
Murphy, J. M., & Vince, J. E. (2015). Post-translational control of RIPK3 and MLKL mediated necroptotic cell death. *F1000Res*, 4. https://doi.org/10.12688/f1000research.7046.1.
Nakagawa, H., Maeda, S., Hikiba, Y., Ohmae, T., Shibata, W., Yanai, A., et al. (2008). Deletion of apoptosis signal-regulating kinase 1 attenuates acetaminophen-induced liver injury by inhibiting c-Jun N-terminal kinase activation. *Gastroenterology*, *135*(4), 1311–1321. https://doi.org/10.1053/j.gastro.2008.07.006.
Naviaux, R. K., & Nguyen, K. V. (2004). POLG mutations associated with Alpers' syndrome and mitochondrial DNA depletion. *Annals of Neurology*, *55*(5), 706–712. https://doi.org/10.1002/ana.20079.
Nazarewicz, R. R., Zenebe, W. J., Parihar, A., Larson, S. K., Alidema, E., Choi, J., et al. (2007). Tamoxifen induces oxidative stress and mitochondrial apoptosis via stimulating mitochondrial nitric oxide synthase. *Cancer Research*, *67*(3), 1282–1290. https://doi.org/10.1158/0008-5472.CAN-06-3099.

Newton, K., & Manning, G. (2016). Necroptosis and inflammation. *Annual Review of Biochemistry*, *85*, 743–763. https://doi.org/10.1146/annurev-biochem-060815-014830.
Ni, H. M., Bockus, A., Boggess, N., Jaeschke, H., & Ding, W. X. (2012). Activation of autophagy protects against acetaminophen-induced hepatotoxicity. *Hepatology*, *55*(1), 222–232. https://doi.org/10.1002/hep.24690.
Ni, H. M., Boggess, N., McGill, M. R., Lebofsky, M., Borude, P., Apte, U., et al. (2012). Liver-specific loss of Atg5 causes persistent activation of Nrf2 and protects against acetaminophen-induced liver injury. *Toxicological Sciences*, *127*(2), 438–450. https://doi.org/10.1093/toxsci/kfs133.
Nishimura, T., & Mizushima, N. (2017). The ULK complex initiates autophagosome formation at phosphatidylinositol synthase-enriched ER subdomains. *Autophagy*, *13*(10), 1795–1796. https://doi.org/10.1080/15548627.2017.1358344.
O'Donnell, M. A., Legarda-Addison, D., Skountzos, P., Yeh, W. C., & Ting, A. T. (2007). Ubiquitination of RIP1 regulates an NF-kappaB-independent cell-death switch in TNF signaling. *Current Biology*, *17*(5), 418–424. https://doi.org/10.1016/j.cub.2007.01.027.
O'Donnell, M. A., Perez-Jimenez, E., Oberst, A., Ng, A., Massoumi, R., Xavier, R., et al. (2011). Caspase 8 inhibits programmed necrosis by processing CYLD. *Nature Cell Biology*, *13*(12), 1437–1442. https://doi.org/10.1038/ncb2362.
Ogasawara, J., Watanabe-Fukunaga, R., Adachi, M., Matsuzawa, A., Kasugai, T., Kitamura, Y., et al. (1993). Lethal effect of the anti-Fas antibody in mice. *Nature*, *364*(6440), 806–809. https://doi.org/10.1038/364806a0.
Orning, P., Weng, D., Starheim, K., Ratner, D., Best, Z., Lee, B., et al. (2018). Pathogen blockade of TAK1 triggers caspase-8-dependent cleavage of gasdermin D and cell death. *Science*, *362*(6418), 1064–1069. https://doi.org/10.1126/science.aau2818.
Peltzer, N., Darding, M., & Walczak, H. (2016). Holding RIPK1 on the ubiquitin leash in TNFR1 signaling. *Trends in Cell Biology*, *26*(6), 445–461. https://doi.org/10.1016/j.tcb.2016.01.006.
Pessayre, D., Mansouri, A., Berson, A., & Fromenty, B. (2010). Mitochondrial involvement in drug-induced liver injury. *Handbook of Experimental Pharmacology*, *196*, 311–365. https://doi.org/10.1007/978-3-642-00663-0_11.
Peterson, R. G., & Rumack, B. H. (1977). Treating acute acetaminophen poisoning with acetylcysteine. *JAMA*, *237*(22), 2406–2407.
Ponchaut, S., van Hoof, F., & Veitch, K. (1992). In vitro effects of valproate and valproate metabolites on mitochondrial oxidations. Relevance of CoA sequestration to the observed inhibitions. *Biochemical Pharmacology*, *43*(11), 2435–2442.
Ramachandran, A., Lebofsky, M., Baines, C. P., Lemasters, J. J., & Jaeschke, H. (2011). Cyclophilin D deficiency protects against acetaminophen-induced oxidant stress and liver injury. *Free Radical Research*, *45*(2), 156–164. https://doi.org/10.3109/10715762.2010.520319.
Ramachandran, A., Lebofsky, M., Weinman, S. A., & Jaeschke, H. (2011). The impact of partial manganese superoxide dismutase (SOD2)-deficiency on mitochondrial oxidant stress, DNA fragmentation and liver injury during acetaminophen hepatotoxicity. *Toxicology and Applied Pharmacology*, *251*(3), 226–233. https://doi.org/10.1016/j.taap.2011.01.004.
Ramachandran, A., McGill, M. R., Xie, Y., Ni, H. M., Ding, W. X., & Jaeschke, H. (2013). The receptor interacting protein kinase 3 is a critical early mediator of acetaminophen-induced hepatocyte necrosis in mice. *Hepatology*, *58*(6), 2099–2108. https://doi.org/10.1002/hep.26547.
Ran, Q., Liang, H., Gu, M., Qi, W., Walter, C. A., Roberts, L. J., 2nd, Van Remmen, H. (2004). Transgenic mice overexpressing glutathione peroxidase 4 are protected against oxidative stress-induced apoptosis. The Journal of Biological Chemistry, 279(53), 55137–55146. https://doi.org/10.1074/jbc.M410387200

Rasola, A., & Bernardi, P. (2007). The mitochondrial permeability transition pore and its involvement in cell death and in disease pathogenesis. *Apoptosis*, *12*(5), 815–833. https://doi.org/10.1007/s10495-007-0723-y.

Razandi, M., Pedram, A., Jordan, V. C., Fuqua, S., & Levin, E. R. (2013). Tamoxifen regulates cell fate through mitochondrial estrogen receptor beta in breast cancer. *Oncogene*, *32*(27), 3274–3285. https://doi.org/10.1038/onc.2012.335.

Saberi, B., Ybanez, M. D., Johnson, H. S., Gaarde, W. A., Han, D., & Kaplowitz, N. (2014). Protein kinase C (PKC) participates in acetaminophen hepatotoxicity through c-Jun-N-terminal kinase (JNK)-dependent and -independent signaling pathways. *Hepatology*, *59*(4), 1543–1554. https://doi.org/10.1002/hep.26625.

Sagulenko, V., Thygesen, S. J., Sester, D. P., Idris, A., Cridland, J. A., Vajjhala, P. R., et al. (2013). AIM2 and NLRP3 inflammasomes activate both apoptotic and pyroptotic death pathways via ASC. *Cell Death and Differentiation*, *20*(9), 1149–1160. https://doi.org/10.1038/cdd.2013.37.

Saito, C., Lemasters, J. J., & Jaeschke, H. (2010). C-Jun N-terminal kinase modulates oxidant stress and peroxynitrite formation independent of inducible nitric oxide synthase in acetaminophen hepatotoxicity. *Toxicology and Applied Pharmacology*, *246*(1–2), 8–17. S0041-008X(10)00142-0 [pii]. https://doi.org/10.1016/j.taap.2010.04.015.

Scaffidi, C., Schmitz, I., Zha, J., Korsmeyer, S. J., Krammer, P. H., & Peter, M. E. (1999). Differential modulation of apoptosis sensitivity in CD95 type I and type II cells. *The Journal of Biological Chemistry*, *274*(32), 22532–22538.

Schmaltz, C., Alpdogan, O., Kappel, B. J., Muriglan, S. J., Rotolo, J. A., Ongchin, J., et al. (2002). T cells require TRAIL for optimal graft-versus-tumor activity. *Nature Medicine*, *8*(12), 1433–1437. https://doi.org/10.1038/nm797.

Schneider, A. T., Gautheron, J., Tacke, F., Vucur, M., & Luedde, T. (2015). Receptor interacting protein Kinase-1 (RIPK1) in hepatocytes does not mediate murine acetaminophen toxicity. *Hepatology*, *64*, 306–308. https://doi.org/10.1002/hep.28225.

Serviddio, G., Bellanti, F., Giudetti, A. M., Gnoni, G. V., Capitanio, N., Tamborra, R., et al. (2011). Mitochondrial oxidative stress and respiratory chain dysfunction account for liver toxicity during amiodarone but not dronedarone administration. *Free Radical Biology & Medicine*, *51*(12), 2234–2242. https://doi.org/10.1016/j.freeradbiomed.2011.09.004.

Shao, W., Yeretssian, G., Doiron, K., Hussain, S. N., & Saleh, M. (2007). The caspase-1 digestome identifies the glycolysis pathway as a target during infection and septic shock. *The Journal of Biological Chemistry*, *282*(50), 36321–36329. https://doi.org/10.1074/jbc.M708182200.

Sharma, M., Gadang, V., & Jaeschke, A. (2012). Critical role for mixed-lineage kinase 3 in acetaminophen-induced hepatotoxicity. *Molecular Pharmacology*, *82*(5), 1001–1007. mol.112.079863 [pii]. https://doi.org/10.1124/mol.112.079863.

Shear, N. H., & Spielberg, S. P. (1988). Anticonvulsant hypersensitivity syndrome. In vitro assessment of risk. *The Journal of Clinical Investigation*, *82*(6), 1826–1832. https://doi.org/10.1172/JCI113798.

Shi, J., Zhao, Y., Wang, K., Shi, X., Wang, Y., Huang, H., et al. (2015). Cleavage of GSDMD by inflammatory caspases determines pyroptotic cell death. *Nature*, *526*(7575), 660–665. https://doi.org/10.1038/nature15514.

Shinohara, M., Ybanez, M. D., Win, S., Than, T. A., Jain, S., Gaarde, W. A., et al. (2010). Silencing glycogen synthase kinase-3beta inhibits acetaminophen hepatotoxicity and attenuates JNK activation and loss of glutamate cysteine ligase and myeloid cell leukemia sequence 1. *The Journal of Biological Chemistry*, *285*(11), 8244–8255. M109.054999 [pii]. https://doi.org/10.1074/jbc.M109.054999.

Silva, M. F., Ruiter, J. P., Illst, L., Jakobs, C., Duran, M., de Almeida, I. T., et al. (1997). Valproate inhibits the mitochondrial pyruvate-driven oxidative phosphorylation in vitro. *Journal of Inherited Metabolic Disease*, *20*(3), 397–400.

Song, E., Fu, J., Xia, X., Su, C., & Song, Y. (2014). Bazhen decoction protects against acetaminophen induced acute liver injury by inhibiting oxidative stress, inflammation and apoptosis in mice. *PLoS One*, *9*(9), e107405. https://doi.org/10.1371/journal.pone.0107405.

Stewart, J. D., Horvath, R., Baruffini, E., Ferrero, I., Bulst, S., Watkins, P. B., et al. (2010). Polymerase gamma gene POLG determines the risk of sodium valproate-induced liver toxicity. *Hepatology*, *52*(5), 1791–1796. https://doi.org/10.1002/hep.23891.

Stockwell, B. R., Friedmann Angeli, J. P., Bayir, H., Bush, A. I., Conrad, M., Dixon, S. J., et al. (2017). Ferroptosis: A regulated cell death Nexus linking metabolism, redox biology, and disease. *Cell*, *171*(2), 273–285. https://doi.org/10.1016/j.cell.2017.09.021.

Strasser, A., Jost, P. J., & Nagata, S. (2009). The many roles of FAS receptor signaling in the immune system. *Immunity*, *30*(2), 180–192. https://doi.org/10.1016/j.immuni.2009.01.001.

Suda, J., Dara, L., Yang, L., Aghajan, M., Song, Y., Kaplowitz, N., et al. (2016). Knockdown of RIPK1 markedly exacerbates murine immune-mediated liver injury through massive apoptosis of hepatocytes, independent of necroptosis and inhibition of NF-kappaB. *Journal of Immunology*, *197*, 3120–3129. https://doi.org/10.4049/jimmunol.1600690.

Sun, S. C. (2010). CYLD: A tumor suppressor deubiquitinase regulating NF-kappaB activation and diverse biological processes. *Cell Death and Differentiation*, *17*(1), 25–34. https://doi.org/10.1038/cdd.2009.43.

Sun, X., Lee, J., Navas, T., Baldwin, D. T., Stewart, T. A., & Dixit, V. M. (1999). RIP3, a novel apoptosis-inducing kinase. *The Journal of Biological Chemistry*, *274*(24), 16871–16875.

Sun, L., Wang, H., Wang, Z., He, S., Chen, S., Liao, D., et al. (2012). Mixed lineage kinase domain-like protein mediates necrosis signaling downstream of RIP3 kinase. *Cell*, *148*(1–2), 213–227. S0092-8674(11)01422-X [pii]. https://doi.org/10.1016/j.cell.2011.11.031.

Suzman, D. L., Pelosof, L., Rosenberg, A., & Avigan, M. I. (2018). Hepatotoxicity of immune checkpoint inhibitors: An evolving picture of risk associated with a vital class of immunotherapy agents. *Liver International*, *38*(6), 976–987. https://doi.org/10.1111/liv.13746.

Sydor, S., Manka, P., Best, J., Jafoui, S., Sowa, J. P., Zoubek, M. E., et al. (2017). Kruppel-like factor 6 is a transcriptional activator of autophagy in acute liver injury. *Scientific Reports*, 7(1), 8119. https://doi.org/10.1038/s41598-017-08680-w.

Tait, S. W., Oberst, A., Quarato, G., Milasta, S., Haller, M., Wang, R., et al. (2013). Widespread mitochondrial depletion via mitophagy does not compromise necroptosis. *Cell Reports*, *5*(4), 878–885. https://doi.org/10.1016/j.celrep.2013.10.034.

Takahashi, N., Duprez, L., Grootjans, S., Cauwels, A., Nerinckx, W., DuHadaway, J. B., et al. (2012). Necrostatin-1 analogues: Critical issues on the specificity, activity and in vivo use in experimental disease models. *Cell Death & Disease, 3,* e437. https://doi.org/10.1038/cddis.2012.176.

Takeda, K., Hayakawa, Y., Smyth, M. J., Kayagaki, N., Yamaguchi, N., Kakuta, S., et al. (2001). Involvement of tumor necrosis factor-related apoptosis-inducing ligand in surveillance of tumor metastasis by liver natural killer cells. *Nature Medicine*, 7(1), 94–100. https://doi.org/10.1038/83416.

Takeda, K., Kojima, Y., Ikejima, K., Harada, K., Yamashina, S., Okumura, K., et al. (2008). Death receptor 5 mediated-apoptosis contributes to cholestatic liver disease. *Proceedings of the National Academy of Sciences of the United States of America*, *105*(31), 10895–10900. https://doi.org/10.1073/pnas.0802702105.

Tarazi, E. M., Harter, J. G., Zimmerman, H. J., Ishak, K. G., & Eaton, R. A. (1993). Sulindac-associated hepatic injury: Analysis of 91 cases reported to the Food and Drug Administration. *Gastroenterology*, *104*(2), 569–574.

Thompson, N. P., Caplin, M. E., Hamilton, M. I., Gillespie, S. H., Clarke, S. W., Burroughs, A. K., et al. (1995). Anti-tuberculosis medication and the liver: Dangers and recommendations in management. *The European Respiratory Journal, 8*(8), 1384–1388.

Trnka, J., Blaikie, F. H., Smith, R. A., & Murphy, M. P. (2008). A mitochondria-targeted nitroxide is reduced to its hydroxylamine by ubiquinol in mitochondria. *Free Radical Biology & Medicine, 44*(7), 1406–1419. https://doi.org/10.1016/j.freeradbiomed.2007.12.036.

Urban, T. J., Daly, A. K., & Aithal, G. P. (2014). Genetic basis of drug-induced liver injury: Present and future. *Seminars in Liver Disease, 34*(2), 123–133. https://doi.org/10.1055/s-0034-1375954.

Vanden Berghe, T., Linkermann, A., Jouan-Lanhouet, S., Walczak, H., & Vandenabeele, P. (2014). Regulated necrosis: The expanding network of non-apoptotic cell death pathways. *Nature Reviews. Molecular Cell Biology, 15*(2), 135–147. https://doi.org/10.1038/nrm3737.

Vanden Berghe, T., Vanlangenakker, N., Parthoens, E., Deckers, W., Devos, M., Festjens, N., et al. (2010). Necroptosis, necrosis and secondary necrosis converge on similar cellular disintegration features. *Cell Death and Differentiation, 17*(6), 922–930. https://doi.org/10.1038/cdd.2009.184.

Varfolomeev, E., Goncharov, T., Fedorova, A. V., Dynek, J. N., Zobel, K., Deshayes, K., et al. (2008). C-IAP1 and c-IAP2 are critical mediators of tumor necrosis factor alpha (TNFalpha)-induced NF-kappaB activation. *The Journal of Biological Chemistry, 283*(36), 24295–24299. https://doi.org/10.1074/jbc.C800128200.

Vercammen, D., Beyaert, R., Denecker, G., Goossens, V., Van Loo, G., Declercq, W., et al. (1998). Inhibition of caspases increases the sensitivity of L929 cells to necrosis mediated by tumor necrosis factor. *The Journal of Experimental Medicine, 187*(9), 1477–1485.

Volkmann, X., Fischer, U., Bahr, M. J., Ott, M., Lehner, F., Macfarlane, M., et al. (2007). Increased hepatotoxicity of tumor necrosis factor-related apoptosis-inducing ligand in diseased human liver. *Hepatology, 46*(5), 1498–1508. https://doi.org/10.1002/hep.21846.

Walczak, H., Miller, R. E., Ariail, K., Gliniak, B., Griffith, T. S., Kubin, M., et al. (1999). Tumoricidal activity of tumor necrosis factor-related apoptosis-inducing ligand in vivo. *Nature Medicine, 5*(2), 157–163. https://doi.org/10.1038/5517.

Wang, S., & El-Deiry, W. S. (2003). TRAIL and apoptosis induction by TNF-family death receptors. *Oncogene, 22*(53), 8628–8633. https://doi.org/10.1038/sj.onc.1207232.

Wang, Z., Hu, J. N., Yan, M. H., Xing, J. J., Liu, W. C., & Li, W. (2017). Caspase-mediated anti-apoptotic effect of Ginsenoside Rg5, a main rare Ginsenoside, on acetaminophen-induced hepatotoxicity in mice. *Journal of Agricultural and Food Chemistry, 65*(42), 9226–9236. https://doi.org/10.1021/acs.jafc.7b03361.

Wang, A., Keita, A. V., Phan, V., McKay, C. M., Schoultz, I., Lee, J., et al. (2014). Targeting mitochondria-derived reactive oxygen species to reduce epithelial barrier dysfunction and colitis. *The American Journal of Pathology, 184*(9), 2516–2527. https://doi.org/10.1016/j.ajpath.2014.05.019.

Wiley, S. R., Schooley, K., Smolak, P. J., Din, W. S., Huang, C. P., Nicholl, J. K., et al. (1995). Identification and characterization of a new member of the TNF family that induces apoptosis. *Immunity, 3*(6), 673–682.

Williams, C. D., Antoine, D. J., Shaw, P. J., Benson, C., Farhood, A., Williams, D. P., et al. (2011). Role of the Nalp3 inflammasome in acetaminophen-induced sterile inflammation and liver injury. *Toxicology and Applied Pharmacology, 252*(3), 289–297. https://doi.org/10.1016/j.taap.2011.03.001.

Wiltshire, C., Matsushita, M., Tsukada, S., Gillespie, D. A., & May, G. H. (2002). A new c-Jun N-terminal kinase (JNK)-interacting protein, Sab (SH3BP5), associates with mitochondria. The Biochemical Journal, 367(Pt 3), 577–585. doi:https://doi.org/10.1042/BJ20020553

Win, S., Than, T. A., Han, D., Petrovic, L. M., & Kaplowitz, N. (2011). C-Jun N-terminal kinase (JNK)-dependent acute liver injury from acetaminophen or tumor necrosis factor (TNF) requires mitochondrial Sab protein expression in mice. *The Journal of Biological Chemistry*, *286*(40), 35071–35078. M111.276089 [pii]. https://doi.org/10.1074/jbc.M111.276089.

Win, S., Than, T. A., Min, R. W., Aghajan, M., & Kaplowitz, N. (2016). C-Jun N-terminal kinase mediates mouse liver injury through a novel Sab (SH3BP5)-dependent pathway leading to inactivation of intramitochondrial Src. *Hepatology*, *63*(6), 1987–2003. https://doi.org/10.1002/hep.28486.

Win, S., Than, T. A., Zhang, J., Oo, C., Min, R. W. M., & Kaplowitz, N. (2018). New insights into the role and mechanism of c-Jun-N-terminal kinase signaling in the pathobiology of liver diseases. *Hepatology*, *67*(5), 2013–2024. https://doi.org/10.1002/hep.29689.

Woolbright, B. L., & Jaeschke, H. (2017). Role of the inflammasome in acetaminophen-induced liver injury and acute liver failure. *Journal of Hepatology*, *66*(4), 836–848. https://doi.org/10.1016/j.jhep.2016.11.017.

Wuillemin, N., Adam, J., Fontana, S., Krahenbuhl, S., Pichler, W. J., & Yerly, D. (2013). HLA haplotype determines hapten or p-i T cell reactivity to flucloxacillin. *Journal of Immunology*, *190*(10), 4956–4964. https://doi.org/10.4049/jimmunol.1202949.

Xie, Z., & Klionsky, D. J. (2007). Autophagosome formation: Core machinery and adaptations. *Nature Cell Biology*, *9*(10), 1102–1109. https://doi.org/10.1038/ncb1007-1102.

Yang, W. S., SriRamaratnam, R., Welsch, M. E., Shimada, K., Skouta, R., Viswanathan, V. S., et al. (2014). Regulation of ferroptotic cancer cell death by GPX4. *Cell*, *156*(1–2), 317–331. https://doi.org/10.1016/j.cell.2013.12.010.

Yang, W. S., & Stockwell, B. R. (2016). Ferroptosis: Death by lipid peroxidation. *Trends in Cell Biology*, *26*(3), 165–176. https://doi.org/10.1016/j.tcb.2015.10.014.

Yin, X. M., Wang, K., Gross, A., Zhao, Y., Zinkel, S., Klocke, B., et al. (1999). Bid-deficient mice are resistant to Fas-induced hepatocellular apoptosis. *Nature*, *400*(6747), 886–891. https://doi.org/10.1038/23730.

Yoo, S. E., Chen, L., Na, R., Liu, Y., Rios, C., Van Remmen, H., et al. (2012). Gpx4 ablation in adult mice results in a lethal phenotype accompanied by neuronal loss in brain. *Free Radical Biology & Medicine*, *52*(9), 1820–1827. https://doi.org/10.1016/j.freeradbiomed.2012.02.043.

Yuan, L., & Kaplowitz, N. (2013). Mechanisms of drug-induced liver injury. *Clinics in Liver Disease*, *17*(4), 507–518. viihttps://doi.org/10.1016/j.cld.2013.07.002.

Zhang, L., Dittmer, M. R., Blackwell, K., Workman, L. M., Hostager, B., & Habelhah, H. (2015). TRAIL activates JNK and NF-kappaB through RIP1-dependent and -independent pathways. *Cellular Signalling*, *27*(2), 306–314. https://doi.org/10.1016/j.cellsig.2014.11.014.

Zilka, O., Shah, R., Li, B., Friedmann Angeli, J. P., Griesser, M., Conrad, M., et al. (2017). On the mechanism of cytoprotection by ferrostatin-1 and liproxstatin-1 and the role of lipid peroxidation in ferroptotic cell death. *ACS Central Science*, *3*(3), 232–243. https://doi.org/10.1021/acscentsci.7b00028.

Zou, W., Liu, X., Yue, P., Zhou, Z., Sporn, M. B., Lotan, R., et al. (2004). C-Jun NH2-terminal kinase-mediated up-regulation of death receptor 5 contributes to induction of apoptosis by the novel synthetic triterpenoid methyl-2-cyano-3,12-dioxooleana-1, 9-dien-28-oate in human lung cancer cells. *Cancer Research*, *64*(20), 7570–7578. https://doi.org/10.1158/0008-5472.CAN-04-1238.

Zou, W., Yue, P., Khuri, F. R., & Sun, S. Y. (2008). Coupling of endoplasmic reticulum stress to CDDO-me-induced up-regulation of death receptor 5 via a CHOP-dependent mechanism involving JNK activation. *Cancer Research*, *68*(18), 7484–7492. https://doi.org/10.1158/0008-5472.CAN-08-1318.

CHAPTER THREE

Drug-induced liver injury in obesity and nonalcoholic fatty liver disease

Julien Allard†, Dounia Le Guillou†, Karima Begriche, Bernard Fromenty*
INSERM, Univ. Rennes, INRA, Institut NUMECAN (Nutrition Metabolisms and Cancer) UMR_A 1341, UMR_S 1241, Rennes, France
*Corresponding author: e-mail address: bernard.fromenty@inserm.fr

Contents

Abstract

Obesity is commonly associated with nonalcoholic fatty liver (NAFL), a benign condition characterized by hepatic lipid accumulation. However, NAFL can progress in some patients to nonalcoholic steatohepatitis (NASH) and then to severe liver lesions including extensive fibrosis, cirrhosis and hepatocellular carcinoma. The entire spectrum of these hepatic lesions is referred to as nonalcoholic fatty liver disease (NAFLD). The

† Equal contributors.

Advances in Pharmacology, Volume 85
ISSN 1054-3589
https://doi.org/10.1016/bs.apha.2019.01.003
© 2019 Elsevier Inc.
All rights reserved.

transition of simple fatty liver to NASH seems to be favored by several genetic and environmental factors. Different experimental and clinical investigations showed or suggested that obesity and NAFLD are able to increase the risk of hepatotoxicity of different drugs. Some of these drugs may cause more severe and/or more frequent acute liver injury in obese individuals whereas others may trigger the transition of simple fatty liver to NASH or may worsen hepatic lipid accumulation, necroinflammation and fibrosis. This review presents the available information regarding drugs that may cause a specific risk in the context of obesity and NAFLD. These drugs, which belong to different pharmacological classes, include acetaminophen, halothane, methotrexate, rosiglitazone and tamoxifen. For some of these drugs, experimental investigations confirmed the clinical observations and unveiled different pathophysiological mechanisms which may explain why these pharmaceuticals are particularly hepatotoxic in obesity and NAFLD. Because obese people often take several drugs for the treatment of different obesity-related diseases, there is an urgent need to identify the main pharmaceuticals that may cause acute liver injury on a fatty liver background or that may enhance the risk of severe chronic liver disease.

Abbreviations

ALI acute liver injury
APAP acetaminophen
CYP cytochrome P450
DILI drug-induced liver injury
DNL de novo lipogenesis
ER endoplasmic reticulum
FAO fatty acid oxidation
GSH glutathione
HFD high-fat diet
MCD methionine choline-deficient
MRC mitochondrial respiratory chain
NAFL nonalcoholic fatty liver
NAFLD nonalcoholic fatty liver disease
NAPQI *N*-acetyl-*p*-benzoquinone imine
NASH nonalcoholic steatohepatitis
OXPHOS oxidative phosphorylation
PPAR peroxisome proliferator-activated receptor
ROS reactive oxygen species
T2D type 2 diabetes
VLDL very low-density lipoprotein.
XME xenobiotic-metabolizing enzyme

1. Introduction

More than 350 drugs are able to induce liver injury with different clinical, biochemical and pathological presentations (Björnsson & Hoofnagle, 2016; Massart, Begriche, Moreau, & Fromenty, 2017). For instance, histological features in drug-induced liver injury (DILI) include necrosis, cholestatic hepatitis, steatosis (microvesicular and/or macrovacuolar), inflammatory cell infiltrates and fibrosis (Begriche, Massart, Robin, Borgne-Sanchez, & Fromenty, 2011; Wang et al., 2013). Although severe DILI is a rare event, it can require orthotopic liver transplantation, or lead to the death of the patient (Björnsson & Hoofnagle, 2016; Massart et al., 2017).

Different predisposing factors are known to enhance the risk of DILI such as underlying genetic diseases, polymorphisms in genes coding for xenobiotic metabolizing enzymes (XMEs) and pre-existing liver diseases including alcoholic liver diseases and viral hepatitis (Begriche et al., 2011; Labbe, Pessayre, & Fromenty, 2008). Nonalcoholic fatty liver disease (NAFLD) is another liver disease that is increasingly recognized to favor DILI, at least for some drugs (Bessone, Dirchwolf, Rodil, Razori, & Roma, 2018; Fromenty, 2013; Lammert, Imler, Teal, & Chalasani, 2019; Massart et al., 2017). The main goal of this chapter is to review the available information regarding the drugs that can pose a potential risk in patients with NAFLD. Beforehand, some major features of NAFLD pathophysiology will be briefly recalled. Indeed, such information could be important to understand why some drugs can be particularly hepatotoxic in this pathological context. As we recently wrote a review on the same topic (Massart et al., 2017), the present article has been rewritten in order to avoid major duplications of the information and to provide novel data regarding several drugs such as androgenic steroids, benzbromarone and troglitazone. Numerous news references of articles published on the subject have also been added. In addition, a new paragraph entitled "experimental models of NAFLD" has been included since this might be useful for readers who are not familiar with these models and want to have some important information regarding their respective advantages and limitations.

2. Pathophysiology of NAFLD

NAFLD refers to the whole spectrum of hepatic lesions linked to obesity including nonalcoholic fatty liver (NAFL, also referred to as hepatic steatosis), nonalcoholic steatohepatitis (NASH) and cirrhosis. Importantly, most obese patients present simple NAFL but this lesion can progress in the long term to NASH in 10–20% of patients. Besides fatty liver, NASH is characterized by necroinflammation, hepatocyte ballooning and some degree of fibrosis (Denk, Abuja, & Zatloukal, 2019). Different factors such as genetic polymorphisms and exposure to some xenobiotics could explain why NAFL progresses to NASH only in a subset of obese patients (Begriche, Massart, Robin, Bonnet, & Fromenty, 2013; Massart et al., 2017). Besides drugs (discussed in this review), ethanol and environmental contaminants (e.g. benzo[*a*]pyrene, dioxin and polychlorinated biphenyls) could also promote the progression from simple NAFL to NASH (Bucher et al., 2018; Duval et al., 2017; Wahlang et al., 2014).

Insulin resistance in white adipose tissue and skeletal muscle plays a key role in the pathogenesis of NAFL (Begriche et al., 2013; Hardy, Oakley, Anstee, & Day, 2016). Insulin resistance in adipose tissue favors triacylglycerol lipolysis, which leads to the release in the circulation of large amounts of non-esterified fatty acids entering the liver in a concentration-dependent manner. In addition, fatty acids are synthesized more actively in liver because insulin resistance-associated hyperinsulinemia favors hepatic de novo lipogenesis (DNL) via the activation of sterol regulatory element-binding protein 1c (SREBP1c) and peroxisome proliferator-activated receptor-γ (PPARγ). Insulin resistance in muscle impairs glucose intake and glycogen synthesis, thus favoring glucose utilization for hepatic DNL.

The pathogenesis of NAFL progression to NASH is complex and remains incompletely understood. Different events could be involved such as overproduction of reactive oxygen species (ROS), reduced ROS detoxification, endoplasmic reticulum (ER) stress and mitochondrial dysfunction (Begriche et al., 2013; Hardy et al., 2016). Hence, any xenobiotics able to induce one or several of these deleterious events might be able to favor NAFL evolution to NASH (Bucher et al., 2018; Massart et al., 2017). Other important factors include increased production of pro-inflammatory and profibrogenic cytokines by non-parenchymal liver cells (Begriche et al., 2013; Hardy et al., 2016). Importantly, ROS overproduction during NAFL could mainly occur within mitochondria, in particular at the level of different complexes of the mitochondrial respiratory chain (MRC) and some enzymes of the fatty acid oxidation (FAO) pathway (Begriche et al., 2013; Satapati et al., 2015).

Another substantial source of ROS in NAFL seems to be cytochrome P450 2E1 (CYP2E1), a XME able to generate superoxide anion during its catalytic cycle (Abdelmegeed et al., 2017; Aubert, Begriche, Knockaert, Robin, & Fromenty, 2011). CYP2E1 catalyzes the biotransformation of different xenobiotics (e.g. carbon tetrachloride, ethanol and acetaminophen) and endogenous derivatives such as acetone and some fatty acids (Aubert et al., 2011; Seth et al., 2017). Notably, CYP2E1 is an enzyme located not only within the ER but also within mitochondria (Hartman, Miller, & Meyer, 2017; Knockaert, Fromenty, & Robin, 2011).

Numerous experimental and clinical studies have reported higher hepatic CYP2E1 expression and/or activity in NAFLD, and more broadly in obesity (Aubert et al., 2011; Gade et al., 2018; Massart et al., 2017; Sadler et al., 2018; van Rongen et al., 2016). Moreover, a role of higher CYP2E1 activity in the pathogenesis of NAFLD is supported by different experimental investigations (Abdelmegeed et al., 2017; Aubert et al., 2011; Seth et al., 2017). Interestingly, induction of CYP2E1 could not only favor oxidative stress but also lipid accumulation (Abdelmegeed et al., 2017; Chen, Zhang, Zhao, Xie, & Zeng, 2014), possibly via a ROS-mediated reduction of PPARα activity (Lu, Zhuge, Wang, Bai, & Cederbaum, 2008; Zeng, Zhang, Song, Zhao, & Xie, 2014). The mechanism whereby CYP2E1 activity is increased in obesity and NAFLD is still unknown, even though some studies suggested a role of the accumulation of some fatty acids such as stearic acid (Aubert et al., 2011; Michaut et al., 2016).

3. Experimental models of NAFLD

Numerous experimental models of obesity and NAFLD can be useful in order to study the pathophysiology of NAFLD, or xenobiotic-induced hepatotoxicity in this metabolic condition. Readers are invited to peruse excellent recent reviews in order to have a comprehensive outlook on these different in vitro and in vivo models (Denk et al., 2019; Haczeyni et al., 2018; Kanuri & Bergheim, 2013; Santhekadur, Kumar, & Sanyal, 2018). However, important remarks should be done regarding some of these models:

(1) Different types of energy-rich diets can be used in order to induce obesity and NAFLD. However, the extent of steatosis, necroinflammation and fibrosis can greatly vary between diets. Rodent species and strain also greatly influence liver pathology including the extent of steatosis.

(2) Although genetic animal models such as ob/ob and db/db mice can be useful (Aubert et al., 2012; Garcia-Ruiz et al., 2007; Massart et al., 2012), these models tally with morbid obesity and thus do not represent the common clinical situation. Experimenters should also bear in mind that leptin deficiency in ob/ob mice limits the development of liver fibrosis, even after xenobiotic exposure (Cao et al., 2018; Trak-Smayra et al., 2011).

Hence, ob/ob mice are not appropriate in order to determine whether xenobiotics (or other pathogenic factors) are able to aggravate liver fibrosis.

(3) Mice fed a methionine choline-deficient (MCD) diet develop hepatic pathological features that are comparable to human NASH (Li, Toth, & Cherrington, 2018; Takahashi, Soejima, & Fukusato, 2012). However, it should be underlined that the MCD model, unlike high-fat diet (HFD) models, does not reflect the metabolic context of obesity because the MCD diet induces cachexia (i.e. significant loss of body weight) and lower glycemia (Jha et al., 2014; Kanuri & Bergheim, 2013).

(4) Different in vitro models of NAFL have been developed in order to study the pathophysiological consequences related to hepatocellular fat accumulation, including XME expression and drug-induced cytotoxicity (Kanuri & Bergheim, 2013; Luo, Rana, & Will, 2012). However, most of these studies used human hepatoma cell lines (e.g. HuH7, HepG2) that do not have the full repertoire of XMEs, or rodent hepatocytes that do not have the same profile of drug metabolism than human hepatocytes. Moreover, most studies were carried out in cells incubated with fatty acids for a short duration of time (from a few hours to 2 or 3 days), which does not allow prolonged xenobiotic exposure. Recently, we set up a cellular model of NAFL by using differentiated HepaRG cells incubated with stearic acid for 7 days (Michaut et al., 2016) or with a mixture of stearic and oleic acids for 14 days (Bucher, Le Guillou, et al., 2018; Bucher, Tête, et al., 2018; Le Guillou et al., 2018). Importantly, CYP2E1 activity was increased in these HepaRG-based models of NAFL, thus reproducing what has been consistently observed in clinical studies, as previously mentioned. More generally, it should be underscored that the HepaRG cell line expresses a large repertoire of XMEs including CYPs and glutathione *S*-transferases (Aninat et al., 2006; Anthérieu, Chesné, Li, Guguen-Guillouzo, & Guillouzo, 2012). In addition, mitochondrial function in differentiated HepaRG cells is close to primary human hepatocytes and significantly superior compared to HepG2 and HuH7 cells (Le Guillou et al., 2018; Peyta et al., 2016).

4. Drug-induced hepatotoxicity in obesity and NAFLD

Different clinical and experimental investigations suggested or showed that some drugs might be particularly hepatotoxic in NAFLD and obesity. Actually, three pathophysiological settings seem to exist (Table 1): (1) Some drugs may cause more severe and/or more frequent acute liver injury (ALI) in obese patients as compared to healthy patients. (2) Other drugs may cause

Table 1 Drugs that may pose a specific risk in obesity and NAFLD.

Drugs that may cause more severe (and/or more frequent) acute liver injury	Drugs that may favor the transition of pre-existing fatty liver to NASH, fibrosis or cirrhosis	Drugs that may worsen pre-existing fatty liver or NASH
Acetaminophen (C, E)[a]	Androgenic steroids (E)	Androgenic steroids (E)
Fosipronil (C)	Benzbromarone (E)	Benzbromarone (C, E)
Halothane (C)	Corticosteroids (E)	Corticosteroids (E)
Isoflurane (C)	Irinotecan (C)	Irinotecan (E)
Losartan (C)	Methotrexate (C)	Methotrexate (C, E)
Omeprazole (C)	Tamoxifen (C)	NRTIs[b] (C)
Piperacillin/tazobactam (C)		Pentoxifylline (E)
Sorafenib (C)		Phenobarbital (E)
Telithromycin (C)		Rosiglitazone (C, E)
Ticlopidine (C)		Tamoxifen (C)
Troglitazone (E)		Tetracycline (E)

[a]Letters C and E indicate the existence of one or several clinical or experimental studies, respectively.
[b]NRTIs, nucleoside reverse transcriptase inhibitors.

chronic liver injury (e.g. steatohepatitis, fibrosis and cirrhosis) more frequently in obese patients; hence, because obesity is consistently associated with NAFL, these drugs might favor its transition to NASH and cirrhosis. (3) Some drugs may worsen pre-existing obesity-related NAFL or NASH, with for instance an exacerbation of lipid deposition or necroinflammation, respectively. It is noteworthy that the two latter situations could be difficult to ascertain in clinical practice, for at least three reasons: (1) The usual causality assessment methods used to identify DILI (including the RUCAM score) are not suitable in the context of drug-associated chronic liver injury (Aithal et al., 2011). (2) The bona fide diagnosis of drug-induced NAFLD progression or worsening requires a strict follow-up of patients, either with serial liver biopsies or with sequential non-invasive methods such as serum (or plasma) biomarkers, ultrasonography or transient elastography. (3) In addition to drugs, unidentified confounding factors such as genetic polymorphisms and environmental contaminants might participate to NAFLD progression or worsening. Hence, for drugs suspected to favor the transition of pre-existing fatty liver to NASH and cirrhosis, or to worsen fatty liver (or

NASH), further experimental investigations in obese rodents could be useful to confirm or not their potential detrimental effects in NAFLD. Finally, it appears that drugs able to trigger the transition of fatty liver to NASH or cirrhosis could also be able to worsen fatty liver, or NASH (Table 1). This could be due to their mechanisms of toxicity, as discussed below.

The mechanisms whereby some drugs could be more hepatotoxic in NAFLD are still poorly understood. Nonetheless, pathophysiological mechanisms have been proposed for several drugs, as mentioned below. Fig. 1 summarizes the different possible mechanisms that can explain how drugs can pose a specific risk in the context of obesity and NAFLD. More severe and/or more frequent acute liver injury seems to be explained by the increased generation of toxic reactive metabolites, in particular by CYPs. Reduced mitochondrial FAO, increased DNL and/or impaired very low-density lipoprotein (VLDL) export can explain why some drugs are able to worsen fatty liver. Finally, drug-induced oxidative stress can explain NASH worsening or faster transition of fatty liver to NASH. In addition, oxidative stress might also worsen fatty liver (Fig. 1), possibly by favoring DNL (Lee, Homma, Kurahashi, Kang, & Fujii, 2015; Sekiya, Hiraishi,

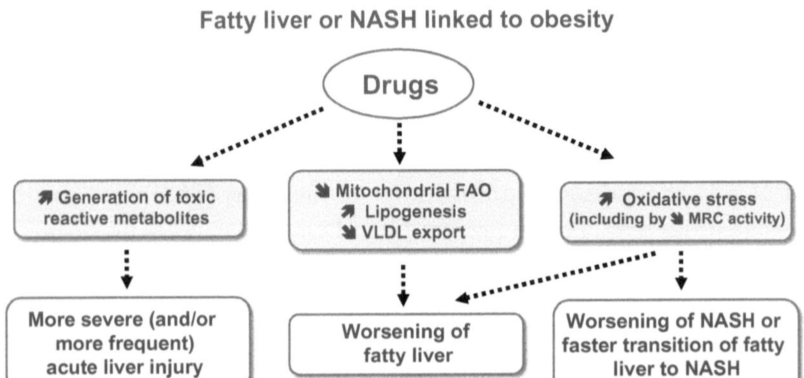

Fig. 1 Mechanisms whereby some drugs could be more toxic in the context of obesity and NAFLD. More severe (and/or more frequent) drug-induced acute liver injury can occur because of higher generation of one or several toxic reactive metabolite(s). Hepatic triglyceride accumulation can be greater with some drugs (thus leading to the worsening fatty liver) via different mechanisms, including impairment of mitochondrial fatty acid oxidation (FAO), activation of de novo lipogenesis and/or reduction of very low-density lipoprotein (VLDL) secretion. A few drugs could also worsen NASH or promote a more rapid transition from fatty liver to NASH by favoring oxidative stress, for instance by impairing the activity of the mitochondrial respiratory chain (MRC) activity. Oxidative stress might also worsen fatty liver by favoring de novo lipogenesis.

Touyama, & Sakamoto, 2008) and/or reducing FAO via a reduction of PPARα activity (Lu et al., 2008; Zeng et al., 2014).

In the following sections, only some drugs will be particularly discussed due to the existence of several clinical reports and/or experimental investigations regarding their deleterious effects in NAFLD. Other drugs will be more rapidly mentioned because no novel data are available since the publication of our recent review on the same topic (Massart et al., 2017).

4.1 Acetaminophen

The painkiller acetaminophen (APAP, also known as paracetamol), is mainly metabolized in the liver into the harmless sulfate and glucuronide conjugates. However, a small amount of APAP is oxidized to the highly toxic metabolite *N*-acetyl-*p*-benzoquinone imine (NAPQI) by several CYPs. In human, CYP2E1, CYP3A4 and CYP1A2 seem to be the main CYPs involved in NAPQI generation (Chowdhary et al., 2017; Michaut, Moreau, Robin, & Fromenty, 2014), although the respective contribution of each CYP isoform is still unknown. Whereas NAPQI is usually safely detoxified in liver by reduced glutathione (GSH) when APAP is taken at the maximum recommended dose (i.e. 4 g per day), high levels of NAPQI after an acute overdose consistently induce a fall in the GSH stores. This GSH shortage subsequently promotes the covalent binding of free NAPQI to different cellular proteins, in particular at the mitochondrial level (Ramachandran & Jaeschke, 2017). This leads to profound oxidative phosphorylation (OXPHOS) impairment and ATP deficiency, massive hepatocellular necrosis and acute liver failure (Maes, Vinken, & Jaeschke, 2016; Michaut et al., 2014). Besides the context of APAP overdose, it should be underlined that therapeutic dose of APAP can induce mild to moderate hepatic cytolysis (Michaut et al., 2014; van Rongen et al., 2016).

Different clinical studies suggest that APAP-induced hepatotoxicity at therapeutic dosage or after an overdose, could be more frequent and more severe in obese patients with NAFLD (Massart et al., 2017; Michaut et al., 2014). Regarding therapeutic doses of APAP, a recent study reported a significant increase in plasma transaminases (i.e. ALT and AST) in morbidly obese patients but not in non-obese individuals (van Rongen et al., 2016). In this study, increased levels of transaminases were more than three times the reference values in some obese patients.

Concerning APAP overdose, two large retrospective studies reported that APAP-induced ALI was more frequent in NAFLD patients (Myers & Shaheen, 2009; Nguyen, Sam, & Thuluvath, 2008). A recent study also showed that APAP-induced ALI after acute APAP overdose was more frequent in overweight or obese patients (Chomchai & Chomchai, 2018). In contrast to these studies, the occurrence to APAP-induced ALI was reported to be similar, or even lower, in obese patients compared to non-obese individuals (Radosevich, Patanwala, & Erstad, 2016; Rutherford et al., 2006). However, one of these studies showed that obese patients had significantly poorer outcomes after acute liver failure (Rutherford et al., 2006).

The discrepancies between some of the above-mentioned studies might be due to the variability of hepatic CYP2E1 activity in obese individuals. Indeed, although liver CYP2E1 activity is statistically greater in obesity and NAFLD, this activity is highly variable between obese patients. In particular, whereas some obese patients present very high hepatic CYP2E1 activity, others are in the range of non-obese individuals (Emery et al., 2003; Gade et al., 2018; Lucas et al., 1998; van Rongen et al., 2016; Wang et al., 2003). Hence, a subset of obese (NAFLD) subjects may not be particularly at risk for APAP-induced hepatotoxicity.

Besides CYP2E1, CYP3A4 and CYP1A2 seem to be also involved in the generation of the highly toxic APAP metabolite NAPQI, as already mentioned (Chowdhary et al., 2017; Michaut et al., 2014). However, hepatic CYP3A4 activity is consistently reduced in human obesity and NAFLD (Brill et al., 2012; Jamwal et al., 2018; Woolsey, Mansell, Kim, Tirona, & Beaton, 2015). Clinical data regarding CYP1A2 in obesity and NAFLD are inconsistent with reduced, unchanged or increased hepatic CYP1A2 activity depending of the studies (Brill et al., 2012; Cobbina & Akhlaghi, 2017; Merrell & Cherrington, 2011). Hence, CYP3A4 and CYP1A2 may not be responsible for greater APAP-induced hepatotoxicity in obese patients.

Different experimental investigations have been performed in lean and obese rodents treated with a single toxic dose of APAP (Massart et al., 2017; Michaut et al., 2014). Although different investigations reported greater APAP-induced hepatotoxicity in obese rodents, others showed no difference or even lower APAP hepatotoxicity compared to lean rodents (Kim, Choi, Kim, Lee, & Koo, 2017; Massart et al., 2017; Michaut et al., 2014). The reasons of such discrepancies are unknown, but several hypotheses can be put forward such as differences in animal models, diets and APAP doses, or the lack of high hepatic CYP2E1 activity in some rodent models of obesity (Kim et al., 2017; Michaut et al., 2014). Indeed, our investigations in ob/ob and db/db obese mice clearly indicated that greater APAP hepatotoxicity was correlated with enhanced hepatic CYP2E1 activity (Aubert et al., 2012). In contrast, greater APAP hepatotoxicity was not correlated with the importance of liver fat accumulation since ob/ob mice presented similar APAP hepatotoxicity than lean mice despite massive fatty liver (Aubert et al., 2012). Interestingly, a recent study showed that mice fed a high-cholesterol diet for 4 weeks were more sensitive to liver injury induced by APAP (500 mg/kg), possibly through the Toll-like receptor 9 (TLR9)/inflammasome pathway (Teratani et al., 2017). Unfortunately, hepatic CYP2E1 activity was not determined in this study. Conversely, another recent study carried out in transgenic *fat-1* mice, which endogenously convert n-6 polyunsaturated fatty acids (PUFA) to n-3 PUFA, showed that these mice were partially protected from APAP-induced acute liver injury despite unchanged CYP2E1 expression (Feng et al., 2018). Mechanistic investigations, however, suggested that reduced activation of apoptosis signal-regulating kinase 1 (ASK1) and Jun N-terminal kinase (JNK) could have played a role in such protection (Feng et al., 2018). These last two studies illustrate the major role played by the intrahepatic lipid content on APAP hepatotoxicity. Indeed, the accumulation of some lipid species may modulate key pathways involved in cell survival or death (Garcia-Ruiz et al., 2007; Mota, Banini, Cazanave, & Sanyal, 2016), and/or may favor CYP2E1 induction and NAPQI formation, as discussed below.

Finally, investigations have also been performed in a cellular model of NAFL (Michaut et al., 2016). By using differentiated HepaRG cells incubated 7 days with stearic acid or oleic acid, we found that stearate supplementation was associated with greater APAP-induced cytotoxicity, which was blunted by the CYP2E1 inhibitor chlormethiazole (Michaut et al., 2016). In contrast, oleate supplementation did not modify CYP2E1 activity and did not favor APAP cytotoxicity. This study, along with ongoing investigations in our lab, indicates that not all fatty acids are able to enhance CYP2E1 activity and that fatty acid-induced increase in CYP2E1 activity is leading to greater APAP cytotoxicity. Finally, we also found that supplementation with stearate (but not oleate) was associated with lower CYP3A4 activity (Michaut et al., 2016), which is consistent with different clinical investigations carried out in obese patients with NAFLD (Brill et al., 2012; Jamwal et al., 2018; Woolsey et al., 2015).

In summary, APAP-induced acute hepatotoxicity seems to occur more frequently and to be more severe in obese patients with NAFLD, although all these patients might not be at risk. Obese patients with higher risk of APAP-induced liver injury might be those with greater hepatic CYP2E1 activity but the involvement of other factors (i.e. lower hepatic GSH stores and mitochondrial dysfunction) requires further investigations (Michaut et al., 2014). Conversely, some metabolic factors might protect a subset of obese patients against APAP-induced hepatotoxicity such as lower gastro-intestinal absorption of APAP, higher volume of distribution as well as normal CYP2E1 activity and increased APAP glucuronidation in liver (Michaut et al., 2014).

4.2 Benzbromarone

Benzbromarone, a non-competitive inhibitor of xanthine oxidase, is a potent uricosuric drug used in the treatment of gout. In the 2000s, this drug was withdrawn from the market in different countries after reports of severe (sometimes fatal) hepatotoxicity in some patients (Lee, Graham, Williams, & Day, 2008). Indeed, benzbromarone was reported to induce massive necrosis leading to severe hepatic cytolysis and fulminant liver failure (Biour et al., 2004; Lee et al., 2008). However, despite its hepatotoxicity, benzbromarone is still marketed in several countries such as China and Japan (Sun et al., 2018).

Mechanisms of benzbromarone-induced hepatotoxicity might include mitochondrial dysfunction, increased ROS production and formation of toxic epoxide intermediate(s) responsible for protein covalent binding (Felser et al., 2014; Wang et al., 2017). Interestingly, benzbromarone, which is structurally similar to amiodarone, induces deleterious mitochondrial effects that resemble those brought about by this antiarrhythmic drug with dual effect on OXPHOS (i.e. uncoupling followed by inhibition with high drug concentrations) and impairment of mitochondrial FAO (Felser et al., 2014; Kaufmann et al., 2005).

Recent experimental investigations performed in db/db and HFD mice showed that an 11-week treatment with benzbromarone (25 or 50 mg/kg) was able to aggravate NAFL, while this treatment did not affect the liver of lean mice (Sun et al., 2018). Moreover, increased fat accumulation in treated db/db and HFD mice was associated with higher serum ALT, thus suggesting that benzbromarone favored the transition of fatty liver to NASH (Sun et al., 2018). Although the possible involvement of benzbromarone-induced mitochondrial toxicity in NAFL aggravation was not explored in this study, gene expression analysis in HFD mouse liver showed that benzbromarone treatment increased the mRNA expression of several key enzymes involved in DNL (e.g. ACC1 and SCD1) and triacylglycerol synthesis (e.g. DGAT and GPAT) (Sun et al., 2018). Furthermore, in vitro investigations using reporter assays revealed that benzbromarone was able to activate PPARγ, a nuclear receptor controlling the expression of many lipogenic enzymes (Sun et al., 2018). Interestingly, pathological and biochemical data gathered in 22 hyperuricemic patients treated by benzbromarone suggested that this drug could aggravate NASH in overweight or obese individuals (Sun et al., 2018).

4.3 Corticosteroids and androgenic steroids

Corticosteroids such as cortisone, corticosterone, dexamethasone and prednisone are used in various diseases for their anti-inflammatory and anti-allergic effects. However, one of the main adverse effects of these drugs is the occurrence of metabolic and endocrine disturbances including central (i.e. abdominal) obesity, hyperlipidemia, insulin resistance and type 2 diabetes (T2D) (Rafacho, Ortsäter, Nadal, & Quesada, 2014; Zhou et al., 2016). As a whole, corticosteroids also induce different types of liver lesions including hepatic cytolysis (sometimes severe), steatosis, steatohepatitis and benign liver tumors (Biour et al., 2004; Gutkowski, Chwist, & Hartleb, 2011).

The mechanism of corticosteroid-induced hepatotoxicity is poorly understood. Steatosis may primarily be related to corticosteroid-induced increased adiposity and insulin resistance (Begriche et al., 2011; Woods, Hazlehurst, & Tomlinson, 2015). However, it should be mentioned that corticosteroids might also trigger liver lipid accumulation through direct intrahepatic effects. For instance, it has been shown that corticosteroids are able to disturb mitochondrial FAO, MRC activity and OXPHOS in liver (Lettéron et al., 1997; Massart et al., 2017). Increased DNL and reduced triglyceride secretion also seem to be involved (Amatruda, Danahy, & Chang, 1983; Lettéron et al., 1997; Woods et al., 2015).

In two experimental studies carried out in HFD obese rodents, long-term treatment with corticosteroids (corticosterone or dexamethasone) significantly worsened hepatic steatosis (D'souza et al., 2012; Poggioli et al., 2013). In one of these studies, plasma bilirubin and ALT and liver collagen content were significantly increased in HFD rats treated with corticosterone while no such disturbances were observed in untreated HFD rats (D'souza et al., 2012). Thus, in the context of obesity, corticosteroids might not only exacerbate liver lipid accumulation but might also favor the transition of simple fatty liver to NASH.

Androgenic steroids such as testosterone and dihydrotestosterone (also referred to as androstanolone) are mainly prescribed for male primary or secondary hypogonadism. However, some androgenic steroids such as boldenone and stanozolol can be used non-therapeutically to increase muscle mass, in particular by bodybuilders. As a whole, anabolic-androgenic steroids can induce different types of liver injury including hepatic cytolysis, cholestasis, steatosis and liver cancers (Biour et al., 2004; Niedfeldt, 2018). A recent study performed in lean and HFD obese mice showed that a 12-week treatment with testosterone was able to aggravate NAFL in obese mice, possibly via increased DNL, whereas no hepatic steatosis was observed in lean mice (Santos et al., 2018). Moreover, plasma levels of AST and ALT were increased in testosterone-treated HFD obese mice (but not in untreated HFD mice), thus suggesting a transition of fatty liver to NASH. Interestingly, different parameters of hepatic oxidative stress such as thiobarbituric acid reactive substances (TBARS) and protein carbonyls were specifically enhanced in testosterone-treated obese mice (Santos et al., 2018).

4.4 Halothane and isoflurane

The volatile halogenated general anesthetics halothane and isoflurane can both induce severe hepatotoxicity, although the number of reported cases is much higher with halothane. Consequently, the use of halothane has been largely limited in recent years. In the most severe cases, halothane and isoflurane are able to induce massive hepatic cytolysis that can require orthotopic liver transplantation, or lead to the death of the patients (Brunt, White, Marsh, Holtmann, & Peters, 1991; Massart et al., 2017).

Halothane and isoflurane-induced hepatotoxicity is due to the CYP2E1-mediated generation of electrophilic acyl chloride reactive metabolites able to covalently bind to a large array of hepatocyte proteins (Kharasch, Hankins, & Cox, 1999; Massart et al., 2017). Regarding halothane, covalent binding of the trifluoroacetyl chloride metabolite to key cellular targets is deemed to be involved in liver injury by triggering an immune-mediated reaction but also by inducing glutathione depletion, oxidative stress and mitochondrial dysfunction (Ijiri et al., 2018; Massart et al., 2017). Similar mechanisms of hepatotoxicity have been proposed for isoflurane (Kharasch et al., 1999; Kim et al., 2006).

Both halothane and isoflurane have been reported to induce ALI more frequently in obese individuals (Brunt et al., 1991; Massart et al., 2017; Moult & Sherlock, 1975). Moreover, obesity seems to be associated with

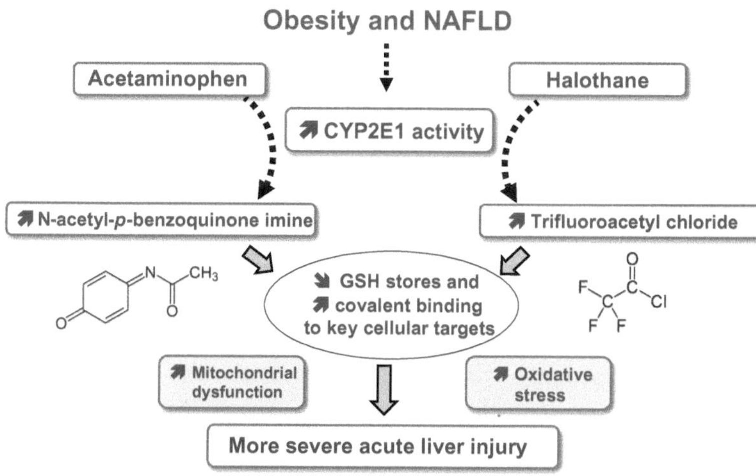

Fig. 2 Increased hepatotoxicity induced by acetaminophen and halothane in obesity and NAFLD. Obesity and NAFLD are associated with higher hepatic cytochrome P450 2E1 (CYP2E1) activity, which is responsible for a greater biotransformation of acetaminophen and halothane to the highly reactive metabolites *N*-acetyl-*p*-benzoquinone imine and trifluoroacetyl chloride, respectively. The higher generation of these toxic reactive metabolites induces a greater reduction of the hepatic glutathione (GSH) stores and more covalent binding to different key cellular targets, in particular at the mitochondrial level. These deleterious events cause more profound mitochondrial dysfunction and oxidative stress, thus favoring the occurrence of more severe acute liver injury.

poor prognosis during halothane and isoflurane-induced hepatitis (Brunt et al., 1991; Moult & Sherlock, 1975). Besides obesity, other factors such as genetic predisposition, female sex and repeated exposures to these halogenated anesthetics could also augment the risk of hepatotoxicity (Brunt et al., 1991; Massart et al., 2017).

Considering the major role of CYP2E1 in the pathogenesis of halogenated anesthetic-induced liver injury, one can assume that the greater risk of liver injury in obese patients treated with halothane or isoflurane might be the consequence of the higher CYP2E1 activity commonly observed in obese individuals (Fig. 2) (Fromenty, 2013; Massart et al., 2017). In keeping with this assumption, plasma levels of trifluoroacetic acid (i.e. a metabolite generated from trifluoroacetyl chloride) tended to be higher in morbidly obese patients compared to lean individuals (Bentley, Vaughan, Gandolfi, & Cork, 1982). Another study performed in morbidly obese individuals reported higher halothane biotransformation to the ionic fluoride metabolite (Young, Stoelting, Peterson, & Madura, 1975). Unfortunately, no experimental investigations have been performed in in vivo or in vitro models of NAFLD in order to confirm that higher hepatic CYP2E1 activity is responsible for increased halothane (or isoflurane) hepatotoxicity in obesity.

4.5 Irinotecan

The topoisomerase 1 inhibitor irinotecan, also known as CPT11, is primarily used for the treatment of advanced colorectal cancer. This antineoplastic drug is also used before resection of hepatic colorectal metastases. Actually, irinotecan is a prodrug that is converted to the active molecule 7-ethyl-10-hydroxycamptothecin, also referred to as SN-38. The most frequent hepatic lesions induced by irinotecan are macrovacuolar steatosis and steatohepatitis (Massart et al., 2013; Ramachandran & Kakar, 2009).

According to different experimental investigations, irinotecan-induced liver fat accumulation could be induced by mitochondrial dysfunction, impairment of autophagy and increased DNL (Mahli et al., 2018; Sawano et al., 2015). In the last study, irinotecan treatment in rat (200 mg/kg) rapidly enhanced the mRNA expression of different genes involved in fatty acid and cholesterol synthesis (Sawano et al., 2015). Whereas enhanced fatty acid levels could explain the occurrence of steatosis via triglyceride formation, increased liver cholesterol is deemed to participate to the pathogenesis of steatohepatitis by several mechanisms including mitochondrial dysfunction, ER stress, ROS overproduction and inflammation (Ioannou, 2016; Tirosh, 2018).

Two independent clinical studies reported that irinotecan administration before liver resection could induce steatohepatitis (sometimes severe) in treated patients, with a greater risk in overweight or obese individuals (Fernandez et al., 2005; Vauthey et al., 2006). Recent investigations in mice also showed that a 6-day treatment with irinotecan (50 mg/kg) was able to aggravate fatty liver when the animals were fed a diet enriched in saturated fatty acids and sucrose (saccharose) (Mallick et al., 2018). Moreover, this effect was associated with hepatic inflammation. In contrast, irinotecan did not induce steatosis when mice were fed diets with lower content in saturated fatty acids and sucrose (Mallick et al., 2018). Notably, determination of irinotecan and SN-38 plasma concentrations in mice fed the different diets indicated that liver injury was not associated with higher SN-38 levels (Mallick et al., 2018). Unfortunately, the mechanism(s) whereby irinotecan was able to worsen fatty liver was not determined in this study.

4.6 Methotrexate

Methotrexate is a folate antagonist used in the treatment of some malignancies and different inflammatory and autoimmune diseases such as psoriasis, psoriatic arthritis and rheumatoid arthritis. Notably, methotrexate-induced liver toxicity is commonly associated with its long-term use for the treatment of inflammatory diseases (Massart et al., 2017; Rabinowich & Shibolet, 2015). Indeed, although acute hepatitis (with marked increase in plasma transaminases and hepatocellular necrosis) has been reported in a few patients treated with high doses of intravenous methotrexate, this drug mostly induces chronic forms of liver lesions such as steatosis, steatohepatitis, fibrosis and even cirrhosis (Massart et al., 2017; Rabinowich & Shibolet, 2015; Ramachandran & Kakar, 2009). Besides obesity and related diseases (see below), other factors seem to increase the risk of methotrexate-induced hepatotoxicity including cumulative dose and duration of methotrexate therapy, lack of folate supplementation, psoriasis, alcohol abuse and genetic factors (Massart et al., 2017; Schmajuk et al., 2014; Shetty, Cho, Alazawi, & Syn, 2017).

Although the exact mechanism whereby methotrexate can induce steatosis, steatohepatitis and fibrosis is still poorly understood, one attractive hypothesis is mitochondrial dysfunction (Massart et al., 2017). Indeed, methotrexate-induced impairment of mitochondrial function, in particular at the level of MRC and mitochondrial FAO, has been shown in different experiments models (Massart et al., 2013; Yamamoto, Lopes, Campello, & Klüppel, 1989; Zhang et al., 2018). Increased intracellular levels of homocysteine, ROS overproduction and oxidative stress might also be involved in steatohepatitis and fibrosis (Aithal, 2007; Fayez, Zakaria, & Moustafa, 2018; Massart et al., 2017). Actually, experimental investigations showed that methotrexate can promote oxidative stress through mechanisms that seem to involve both mitochondrial and extra-mitochondrial pathways (Aithal, 2007; Prestigiacomo, Weston, Messner, Lampart, & Suter-Dick, 2017; Sramek, Neradil, & Veselska, 2017; Tabassum, Parvez, Pasha, Banerjee, & Raisuddin, 2010). Lastly, methotrexate might favor fibrosis by activating the complement system in liver including C3, C5 and C8a, as recently discussed (Massart et al., 2017).

Different studies reported that obesity, NAFLD and T2D could increase the risk of methotrexate-induced hepatotoxicity as assessed by increased plasma transaminases, or the presence of hepatic histologic alterations indicating chronic liver injury such as steatohepatitis, fibrosis or cirrhosis (Berends et al., 2006; Kent, Luthra, & Michet, 2004; Rosenberg et al., 2007;

Schmajuk et al., 2014; Shetty et al., 2017). In addition, some data suggested that methotrexate might aggravate pre-existing NAFLD. Indeed, in a study carried out in a small group ($n=21$) of obese and/or diabetic patients for whom serial liver biopsies were performed, fibrosis was aggravated in three-quarter of the treated patients, whereas steatosis and necroinflammation were worsened in the remaining individuals (Langman, Hall, & Todd, 2001). However, the aforementioned investigations are retrospective and sometimes did not include comparable control groups and baseline liver biopsies, as already pointed out by different authors (Aithal, 2007; Shetty et al., 2017). Hence, prospective studies are required in order to better characterize the exact profile of methotrexate-induced liver injury in patients with obesity and related diseases. Nonetheless, experimental investigations in a rat model of steatohepatitis induced by a methionine choline-deficient (MCD) diet showed that a single injection of methotrexate was able to induce liver fibrosis in the MCD rats whereas no fibrosis was observed in rats fed with a control diet (Hardwick et al., 2014; Kyriakides et al., 2014). Although these data are interesting, it should be underlined that the MCD model of NASH does not reflect the metabolic context of obesity, as previously mentioned.

4.7 Rosiglitazone and troglitazone

The thiazolidinedione derivatives troglitazone and rosiglitazone are PPARγ agonists that have been developed for the treatment of T2D, in particular due to their beneficial effects on insulin sensitivity. However, troglitazone, the first derivative of this pharmacological class, has been withdrawn from the market in 2000 because of the occurrence of several cases of severe (and sometimes fatal) ALI (Ikeda, 2011; Kohlroser, Mathai, Reichheld, Banner, & Bonkovsky, 2000). Although rosiglitazone is safer than troglitazone, several cases of hepatotoxicity, sometimes severe, were reported in treated patients (Al-Salman, Arjomand, Kemp, & Mittal, 2000; Biour et al., 2004).

Several studies suggested that mitochondrial dysfunction, in particular at the level of MRC, could play a major role in troglitazone-induced hepatotoxicity (Hu et al., 2015; Massart et al., 2017). Interestingly, rosiglitazone also induces mitochondrial dysfunction but to a lesser extent compared to troglitazone (Hu et al., 2015; Nadanaciva, Dykens, Bernal, Capaldi, & Will, 2007). Pioglitazone, another thiazolidinedione derivative, presents a hepatotoxicity profile and an ability to impair mitochondrial dysfunction that seems about similar to rosiglitazone (Biour et al., 2004; Hu et al., 2015).

Rosiglitazone and pioglitazone have been tested in the treatment of NASH (Massart et al., 2017; Soccio, Chen, & Lazar, 2014). However, although pioglitazone showed beneficial effects on NASH progression, rosiglitazone was found to be without benefit (Massart et al., 2017; Musso, Cassader, Paschetta, & Gambino, 2017). In addition, worsening of steatosis, necroinflammation and perisinusoidal fibrosis was observed in some patients (Neuschwander-Tetri, Brunt, Wehmeier, Oliver, & Bacon, 2003; Ratziu et al., 2010). Interestingly, increased hepatic expression of different pro-inflammatory genes (i.e. TLR4, IL-8 and CCL2) was reported in patients treated with rosiglitazone (Lemoine, Serfaty, Cervera, Capeau, & Ratziu, 2014).

Several investigations performed in different murine models of obesity and T2D consistently reported that rosiglitazone was able to worsen liver triglyceride accumulation and hepatic steatosis (Gao, Ma, Alsaggar, & Liu, 2016; Garcia-Ruiz et al., 2007; Massart et al., 2017; Watkins, Reifsnyder, Pan, German, & Leiter, 2002). Interestingly, two of these studies reported that aggravation of steatosis was associated with increased circulating ALT levels, thus suggesting that necroinflammation could also be exacerbated by rosiglitazone (Garcia-Ruiz et al., 2007; Watkins et al., 2002). The exact mechanism(s) whereby rosiglitazone is able to aggravate liver steatosis in obese and diabetic mice is unknown. However, some data suggest an exacerbation of hepatic DNL (Watkins et al., 2002), possibly favored by the high expression of PPARγ already present in the obese liver (Gao et al., 2016; Garcia-Ruiz et al., 2007). Further impairment of MRC complex I activity and exacerbation of oxidative stress might have been involved in the possible worsening of hepatic necroinflammation in rosiglitazone-treated obese mice (Garcia-Ruiz et al., 2007).

By using a cellular model of NAFL induced by lipid overload, we recently showed that troglitazone was significantly more cytotoxic in steatotic cells compared with nonsteatotic cells, as assessed by measuring cellular ATP levels (Le Guillou et al., 2018). Indeed, in human differentiated HepaRG cells treated for 2 weeks with troglitazone, the IC_{50} values were 70 and 59 μM in nonsteatotic and steatotic HepaRG cells, respectively (Le Guillou et al., 2018). Moreover, another recent study showed that troglitazone-induced mitochondrial toxicity was increased in a rat model of obesity, T2D and NAFLD (Segawa, Sekine, Sato, & Ito, 2018). Taken together, these experimental data suggest that troglitazone-induced severe hepatotoxicity in obese patients with T2D might have been favored by pre-existing NAFL in these individuals (Le Guillou et al., 2018).

4.8 Tamoxifen

Tamoxifen is a selective estrogen receptor modulator used for the treatment of breast cancer. Tamoxifen can induce different types of chronic liver lesion including steatosis, steatohepatitis, fibrosis, cirrhosis and hepatocellular carcinoma (Biour et al., 2004; Massart et al., 2017; Yang et al., 2016). Tamoxifen-induced steatosis could be favored by different factors including CYP2D6 polymorphisms reducing tamoxifen biotransformation (Wickramage, Tennekoon, Ariyaratne, Hewage, & Sundralingam, 2017) and a body mass index >22 kg/m^2 (Chang, Pan, & Lee, 2018). Whereas steatosis can be detected in at least one-third of the treated patients (Hong et al., 2017; Ogawa, Murata, Nishioka, Inomata, & Yoshida, 1998), tamoxifen-induced steatohepatitis and cirrhosis seem to be uncommon (Massart et al., 2017). Similarly, tamoxifen-induced acute hepatitis seems to be rare (Biour et al., 2004).

The exact mechanism whereby tamoxifen could induce steatosis and steatohepatitis is currently unknown, but several investigations pointed to mitochondrial dysfunction. Indeed, tamoxifen is able to inhibit mitochondrial FAO, at least in part by impairing carnitine palmitoyl-transferase 1 (CPT1) activity (Grünig, Duthaler, & Krähenbühl, 2018; Larosche et al., 2007). In addition, tamoxifen-induced inhibition of several MRC complexes could also participate to the impairment of mitochondrial FAO (Larosche et al., 2007; Massart et al., 2017; Ribeiro, Santos, & Custódio, 2014). Impairment of MRC activity might explain why tamoxifen is able to induce oxidative stress in liver, including at the mitochondrial level (Larosche et al., 2007; Massart et al., 2017; Parvez, Tabassum, Banerjee, & Raisuddin, 2008). Besides mitochondrial dysfunction, tamoxifen-induced steatosis might also be due to increased DNL (Cole, Jacobs, & Vance, 2010; Zhao et al., 2014) and reduced VLDL secretion (Birzniece, Barrett, & Ho, 2017; Grünig et al., 2018).

Several studies reported that obesity increased the risk of tamoxifen hepatotoxicity as assessed by increased plasma transaminases, or the presence of hepatic histologic alterations (Bruno et al., 2005; Elefsiniotis et al., 2004; Saphner, Triest-Robertson, Li, & Holzman, 2009). Two of these studies showed that obesity more specifically enhanced the risk of tamoxifen-induced steatohepatitis (Bruno et al., 2005; Saphner et al., 2009). Interestingly, in a study reporting three cases of tamoxifen-induced steatohepatitis, all patients were overweight, or obese (Pinto et al., 1995). It is noteworthy that the study from Saphner et al. (2009) suggested that tamoxifen did not worsen pre-existing NASH in a small subgroup of patients. Further investigations in larger series of obese patients would be needed in order to confirm or not these results. This could be clinically relevant because a previous study reported a case of NASH aggravation in a female patient treated with raloxifene (Takamura et al., 2007), a selective estrogen receptor modulator used to treat osteoporosis. Notably, in contrast to pre-existing NASH, a recent study showed that tamoxifen was able to worsen pre-existing NAFL in a significant number of treated patients (Pan, Chang, & Lee, 2016).

4.9 Other drugs

In a 6-year prospective study carried out in 74 patients with NAFLD and 174 patients with HCV-related chronic hepatitis, Tarantino et al. reported that NAFLD was an independent risk of DILI with an odds ratio of almost four (Tarantino et al., 2007). In this study, ALI was observed in obese patients treated with fosinopril and losartan (antihypertensive agents), piperacillin/tazobactam and telithromycin (antibiotics), omeprazole (proton pump inhibitor) and ticlopidine (inhibitor of platelet aggregation) (Tarantino et al., 2007). Another study reported a case of acute liver failure induced by the anticancer agent sorafenib in a patient with advanced hepatocellular carcinoma related to NASH, but without underlying cirrhosis (Brandi et al., 2015). ALI has also been reported with Kombiglyze (metformin and saxagliptin) in a young patient with T2D and NAFLD (Thalha, Mahadeva, Boon Tan, & Mun, 2018). Although these reports are interesting, prospective studies on larger population are needed in order to determine whether NAFLD is a bona fide independent risk of hepatotoxicity induced by these drugs.

In addition to benzbromarone and rosiglitazone and other above-mentioned drugs, some others have been shown to worsen NAFLD in different experimental models. These drugs, which have recently been discussed in detail (Massart et al., 2017), include tetracycline (Ito et al., 2006), pentoxifylline (Massart et al., 2012) and phenobarbital (Zannikos, Bandyopadhyay, Robertson, & Blouin, 1993). Other investigations in obese mice also showed that the weight-loss supplement *Garcinia cambogia* exacerbates hepatic inflammation and collagen accumulation (Kim et al., 2013). Finally, the antiretroviral nucleoside reverse transcriptase inhibitors stavudine and didanosine are suspected to worsen NAFLD in treated patients (Larrain & Rinella, 2012; Lemoine, Serfaty, & Capeau, 2012; Massart et al., 2017).

In contrast to all the aforementioned investigations, some studies suggest that different drugs might be safe in the context of obesity and NAFLD. This is for instance the case for statins (Bays, Cohen, Chalasani, & Harrison, 2014; Chalasani, Aljadhey, Kesterson, Murray, & Hall, 2004) and amiodarone (Mattar, Juliar, Gradus-Pizlo, & Kwo, 2009), although further clinical studies are warranted to confirm the safety of these drugs in obese patients. Nonetheless, these clinical data are in keeping with our recent investigations performed in HepaRG cells overloaded or not with mixture of fatty acids for 2 weeks. Indeed, in this NAFL model, we found that atorvastatin, lovastatin and amiodarone-induced cytotoxicity were similar in nonsteatotic and steatotic cells (Le Guillou et al., 2018). In the same study, we also found that carbamazepine, imipramine, perhexiline and terbinafine-induced cytotoxicity were comparable between nonsteatotic and steatotic HepaRG cells (Le Guillou et al., 2018). In addition, whereas troglitazone-induced cytotoxicity was higher in steatotic HepaRG cells, as previously mentioned, ritonavir was more cytotoxic in nonsteatotic cells (Le Guillou et al., 2018). Finally, a recent study performed in mice fed a MCD diet suggested that the antimalarial amodiaquine might be safe in NAFLD (Mak, Cho, & Uetrecht, 2018). Hence, although further studies are warranted to confirm the innocuousness of these drugs in obese patients, these investigations suggest that NAFLD might not increase the risk of liver injury for all hepatotoxic drugs.

5. Conclusion

DILI in the context of obesity and NAFLD is a growing concern for practitioners because of the high prevalence of these metabolic diseases but also because obese patients are consuming on average more drugs than non-obese individuals (Fromenty, 2013; Pais, Rusu, & Ratziu, 2014). The current pharmacopeia includes >350 potential hepatotoxic drugs (Björnsson & Hoofnagle, 2016; Massart et al., 2017), without mentioning the numerous herbals and dietary supplements that can also induce liver injury (Seeff, Bonkovsky, Navarro, & Wang, 2015; Stickel & Shouval, 2015). However, except for some drugs discussed in this review, other still unidentified molecules might pose a risk in obese patients. Hence, there is an urgent need to determine what are the drugs (or other compounds) that can pose a specific risk in obese patients and also to decipher the involved mechanisms.

Actually, two different but complementary strategies can be implemented to collect further information regarding DILI in obesity and NAFLD:

(1) Prospective clinical studies might be designed but it should be kept in mind that DILI is a rare event. Indeed, it is estimated that this adverse effect occurs at the most in about 1 per 10,000 individuals taking the drug (Chalasani et al., 2008; Sgro et al., 2002). Hence, it will be hard to draw valid

conclusion for some drugs because the very low number of DILI cases will preclude to statistically ascertain that obesity and/or NAFLD actually increases the risk of hepatotoxicity. In contrast, aggravation of NAFL by some drugs might be more frequent, as illustrated with tamoxifen, and thus such adverse effect might be easier to detect in prospective clinical studies.

(2) Experimental in vivo and in vitro investigations can allow to screen a great number of compounds and to perform mechanistic investigations. For instance, it will be interesting to determine whether mitochondrial dysfunction is a central mechanism involved in drug-induced aggravation of NAFLD. As already mentioned, drug-induced mitochondrial dysfunction might explain not only why hepatic fat can further accumulate but also why necroinflammation and fibrosis can be worsened in some patients. Mitochondrial dysfunction might also explain why some xenobiotics could favor the progression of simple fatty liver to steatohepatitis, as illustrated by our recent investigations on ethanol/benzo[*a*]pyrene co-exposure (Bucher, Le Guillou, et al., 2018; Bucher, Tête, et al., 2018). Importantly, numerous drugs have been shown to disturb mitochondrial function in liver via different mechanisms (Begriche et al., 2011; Massart et al., 2013; Porceddu et al., 2012; Schon & Fromenty, 2016).

Additional mechanisms of NAFLD aggravation can also be sought such as induction of CYP2E1 induction, ER stress, JNK activation, impairment of autophagy and the accumulation of certain lipid intermediates (e.g. free fatty acids, cholesterol) since these events could play a significant role in NAFLD progression (Masarone et al., 2018; Massart et al., 2017; Neuschwander-Tetri, 2010). Ongoing investigations in our laboratory also suggest that VLDL secretion is worth to be studied, in keeping with previous investigations reporting that impairment of triglyceride secretion is frequently observed with different drugs inducing steatosis (Bellringer, Rahman, & Coleman, 1988; Grünig et al., 2018; Labbe et al., 1991; Lettéron et al., 1997; Lettéron, Sutton, Mansouri, Fromenty, & Pessayre, 2003). Interestingly, ER stress can impair VLDL formation and export (Fu, Watkins, & Hotamisligil, 2012; Zhang, Xu, Yu, Chen, & Li, 2014) and numerous drugs are able to induce ER stress (Chen, Melchior, & Guo, 2014; Foufelle & Fromenty, 2016). Hence, it would be interesting to determine whether ER stress and impairment of VLDL secretion are common mechanisms leading to NAFLD worsening.

Acknowledgments

J.A. was a recipient of a fellowship from the Agence Nationale de la Recherche (ANR-16-CE18-0010 MITOXDRUGS). We are grateful to INSERM (Institut National de la Recherche et de la Santé Médicale) for its constant financial support.

Conflict of interest

The authors declare that they have no conflict of interest in relation to this work.

References

Abdelmegeed, M. A., Choi, Y., Godlewski, G., Ha, S. K., Banerjee, A., Jang, S., et al. (2017). Cytochrome P450-2E1 promotes fast food-mediated hepatic fibrosis. *Scientific Reports*, *7*, 39764.

Aithal, G. P. (2007). Dangerous liaisons: Drug, host and the environment. *Journal of Hepatology*, *46*, 995–998.

Aithal, G. P., Watkins, P. B., Andrade, R. J., Larrey, D., Molokhia, M., Takikawa, H., et al. (2011). Case definition and phenotype standardization in drug-induced liver injury. *Clinical Pharmacology & Therapeutics*, *89*, 806–815.

Al-Salman, J., Arjomand, H., Kemp, D. G., & Mittal, M. (2000). Hepatocellular injury in a patient receiving rosiglitazone. A case report. *Annals of Internal Medicine*, *132*, 121–124.

Amatruda, J. M., Danahy, S. A., & Chang, C. L. (1983). The effects of glucocorticoids on insulin-stimulated lipogenesis in primary cultures of rat hepatocytes. *Biochemical Journal*, *212*, 135–141.

Aninat, C., Piton, A., Glaise, D., Le Charpentier, T., Langouët, S., Morel, F., et al. (2006). Expression of cytochromes P450, conjugating enzymes and nuclear receptors in human hepatoma HepaRG cells. *Drug Metabolism and Disposition*, *34*, 75–83.

Anthérieu, S., Chesné, C., Li, R., Guguen-Guillouzo, C., & Guillouzo, A. (2012). Optimization of the HepaRG cell model for drug metabolism and toxicity studies. *Toxicology In Vitro*, *26*, 1278–1285.

Aubert, J., Begriche, K., Delannoy, M., Morel, I., Pajaud, J., Ribault, C., et al. (2012). Differences in early acetaminophen hepatotoxicity between obese ob/ob and db/db mice. *Journal of Pharmacology and Experimental Therapeutics*, *342*, 676–687.

Aubert, J., Begriche, K., Knockaert, L., Robin, M. A., & Fromenty, B. (2011). Increased expression of cytochrome P450 2E1 in nonalcoholic fatty liver disease: Mechanisms and pathophysiological role. *Clinics and Research in Hepatology and Gastroenterology*, *35*, 630–637.

Bays, H., Cohen, D. E., Chalasani, N., & Harrison, S. A. (2014). An assessment by the statin liver safety task force: 2014 update. *Journal of Clinical Lipidology*, *8*, S47–S57.

Begriche, K., Massart, J., Robin, M. A., Bonnet, F., & Fromenty, B. (2013). Mitochondrial adaptations and dysfunctions in nonalcoholic fatty liver disease. *Hepatology*, *58*, 1497–1507.

Begriche, K., Massart, J., Robin, M. A., Borgne-Sanchez, A., & Fromenty, B. (2011). Drug-induced toxicity on mitochondria and lipid metabolism: Mechanistic diversity and deleterious consequences for the liver. *Journal of Hepatology*, *54*, 773–794.

Bellringer, M. E., Rahman, K., & Coleman, R. (1988). Sodium valproate inhibits the movement of secretory vesicles in rat hepatocytes. *Biochemical Journal*, *249*, 513–519.

Bentley, J. B., Vaughan, R. W., Gandolfi, A. J., & Cork, R. C. (1982). Halothane biotransformation in obese and nonobese patients. *Anesthesiology*, *57*, 94–97.

Berends, M. A., Snoek, J., de Jong, E. M., van de Kerkhof, P. C., van Oijen, M. G., van Krieken, J. H., et al. (2006). Liver injury in long-term methotrexate treatment in psoriasis is relatively infrequent. *Alimentary Pharmacology & Therapeutics*, *24*, 805–811.

Bessone, F., Dirchwolf, M., Rodil, M. A., Razori, M. V., & Roma, M. G. (2018). Review article: Drug-induced liver injury in the context of nonalcoholic fatty liver disease—A physiopathological and clinical integrated view. *Alimentary Pharmacology & Therapeutics*, *48*, 892–913.

Biour, M., Ben Salem, C., Chazouillères, O., Grangé, J. D., Serfati, L., & Poupon, R. (2004). Drug-induced liver injury; fourteenth updated edition of the bibliographic database of liver injuries and related drugs. *Gastroentérologie Clinique et Biologique*, *28*, 720–759.

Birzniece, V., Barrett, P. H., & Ho, K. K. (2017). Tamoxifen reduces hepatic VLDL production and GH secretion in women: A possible mechanism for steatosis development. *European Journal of Endocrinology, 177*, 137–143.

Björnsson, E. S., & Hoofnagle, J. H. (2016). Categorization of drugs implicated in causing liver injury: Critical assessment based on published case reports. *Hepatology, 63*, 590–603.

Brandi, G., De Lorenzo, S., Di Girolamo, S., Bellentani, S., Saccoccio, G., & Biasco, G. (2015). Fulminant hepatitis in a patient with hepatocellular carcinoma related to non-alcoholic steatohepatitis treated with sorafenib. *Tumori, 101*, e46–e48.

Brill, M. J., Diepstraten, J., van Rongen, A., van Kralingen, S., van den Anker, J. N., & Knibbe, C. A. (2012). Impact of obesity on drug metabolism and elimination in adults and children. *Clinical Pharmacokinetics, 51*, 277–304.

Bruno, S., Maisonneuve, P., Castellana, P., Rotmensz, N., Rossi, S., Maggioni, M., et al. (2005). Incidence and risk factors for non-alcoholic steatohepatitis: Prospective study of 5408 women enrolled in Italian tamoxifen chemoprevention trial. *British Medical Journal, 330*, 932.

Brunt, E. M., White, H., Marsh, J. W., Holtmann, B., & Peters, M. G. (1991). Fulminant hepatic failure after repeated exposure to isoflurane anesthesia: A case report. *Hepatology, 13*, 1017–1021.

Bucher, S., Le Guillou, D., Allard, J., Pinon, G., Begriche, K., Tête, A., et al. (2018). Possible involvement of mitochondrial dysfunction and oxidative stress in a cellular model of NAFLD progression induced by benzo[a]pyrene/ethanol co-exposure. *Oxidative Medicine and Cellular Longevity, 2018*, 4396403.

Bucher, S., Tête, A., Podechard, N., Liamin, M., Le Guillou, D., Chevanne, M., et al. (2018). Co-exposure to benzo[a]pyrene and ethanol induces a pathological progression of liver steatosis in vitro and in vivo. *Scientific Reports, 8*, 5963.

Cao, Q., Zhu, X., Zhai, X., Ji, L., Cheng, F., Zhu, Y., et al. (2018). Leptin suppresses microRNA-122 promoter activity by phosphorylation of foxO1 in hepatic stellate cell contributing to leptin promotion of mouse liver fibrosis. *Toxicology and Applied Pharmacology, 339*, 143–150.

Chalasani, N., Aljadhey, H., Kesterson, J., Murray, M. D., & Hall, S. D. (2004). Patients with elevated liver enzymes are not at higher risk for statin hepatotoxicity. *Gastroenterology, 126*, 1287–1292.

Chalasani, N., Fontana, R. J., Bonkovsky, H. L., Watkins, P. B., Davern, T., Serrano, J., et al. (2008). Causes, clinical features, and outcomes from a prospective study of drug-induced liver injury in the United States. *Gastroenterology, 135*, 1924–1934.

Chang, H. T., Pan, H. J., & Lee, C. H. (2018). Prevention of tamoxifen-related nonalcoholic fatty liver disease in breast cancer patients. *Clinical Breast Cancer, 18*, e677–e685.

Chen, S., Melchior, W. B., & Guo, L. (2014). Endoplasmic reticulum stress in drug- and environmental toxicant-induced liver toxicity. *Journal of Environmental Science and Health. Part C, Environmental Carcinogenesis & Ecotoxicology Reviews, 32*, 83–104.

Chen, Y. Y., Zhang, C. L., Zhao, X. L., Xie, K. Q., & Zeng, T. (2014). Inhibition of cytochrome P4502E1 by chlormethiazole attenuated acute ethanol-induced fatty liver. *Chemico-Biological Interactions, 222*, 18–26.

Chomchai, S., & Chomchai, C. (2018). Being overweight or obese as a risk factor for acute liver injury secondary to acute acetaminophen overdose. *Pharmacoepidemiology and Drug Safety, 27*, 19–24.

Chowdhary, V., Teng, K. Y., Thakral, S., Zhang, B., Lin, C. H., & Wani, N. (2017). miRNA-122 protects mice and human hepatocytes from acetaminophen toxicity by regulating cytochrome P450 family 1 subfamily A member 2 and family 2 subfamily E member 1 expression. *American Journal of Pathology, 187*, 2758–2774.

Cobbina, E., & Akhlaghi, F. (2017). Non-alcoholic fatty liver disease (NAFLD)—Pathogenesis, classification, and effect on drug metabolizing enzymes and transporters. *Drug Metabolism Reviews, 49*, 197–211.

Cole, L. K., Jacobs, R. L., & Vance, D. E. (2010). Tamoxifen induces triacylglycerol accumulation in the mouse liver by activation of fatty acid synthesis. *Hepatology*, *52*, 1258–1265.

Denk, H., Abuja, P. M., & Zatloukal, K. (2019). Animal models of NAFLD from the pathologist's point of view. *Biochimica et Biophysica Acta—Molecular Basis of Disease*. https://doi.org/10.1016/j.bbadis.2018.04.024. in press.

D'souza, A. M., Beaudry, J. L., Szigiato, A. A., Trumble, S. J., Snook, L. A., Bonen, A., et al. (2012). Consumption of a high-fat diet rapidly exacerbates the development of fatty liver disease that occurs with chronically elevated glucocorticoids. *American Journal of Physiology—Gastrointestinal and Liver Physiology*, *302*, G850–G863.

Duval, C., Teixeira-Clerc, F., Leblanc, A. F., Touch, S., Emond, C., Guerre-Millo, M., et al. (2017). Chronic exposure to low doses of dioxin promotes liver fibrosis development in the C57BL/6J diet-induced obesity mouse model. *Environmental Health Perspectives*, *125*, 428–436.

Elefsiniotis, I. S., Pantazis, K. D., Ilias, A., Pallis, L., Mariolis, A., Glynou, I., et al. (2004). Tamoxifen induced hepatotoxicity in breast cancer patients with pre-existing liver steatosis: The role of glucose intolerance. *European Journal of Gastroenterology & Hepatology*, *16*, 593–598.

Emery, M. G., Fisher, J. M., Chien, J. Y., Kharasch, E. D., Dellinger, E. P., Kowdley, K. V., et al. (2003). CYP2E1 activity before and after weight loss in morbidly obese subjects with nonalcoholic fatty liver disease. *Hepatology*, *38*, 428–435.

Fayez, A. M., Zakaria, S., & Moustafa, D. (2018). Alpha lipoic acid exerts antioxidant effect via Nrf2/HO-1 pathway activation and suppresses hepatic stellate cells activation induced by methotrexate in rats. *Biomedicine & Pharmacotherapy*, *105*, 428–433.

Felser, A., Lindinger, P. W., Schnell, D., Kratschmar, D. V., Odermatt, A., Mies, S., et al. (2014). Hepatocellular toxicity of benzbromarone: Effects on mitochondrial function and structure. *Toxicology*, *324*, 136–146.

Feng, R., Wang, Y., Liu, C., Yan, C., Zhang, H., Su, H., et al. (2018). Acetaminophen-induced liver injury is attenuated in transgenic fat-1 mice endogenously synthesizing long-chain n-3 fatty acids. *Biochemical Pharmacology*, *154*, 75–88.

Fernandez, F. G., Ritter, J., Goodwin, J. W., Linehan, D. C., Hawkins, W. G., & Strasberg, S. M. (2005). Effect of steatohepatitis associated with irinotecan or oxaliplatin pretreatment on resectability of hepatic colorectal metastases. *Journal of the American College of Surgeons*, *200*, 845–853.

Foufelle, F., & Fromenty, B. (2016). Role of endoplasmic reticulum stress in drug-induced toxicity. *Pharmacology Research & Perspectives*, *4*, e00211.

Fromenty, B. (2013). Drug-induced liver injury in obesity. *Journal of Hepatology*, *58*, 824–826.

Fu, S., Watkins, S. M., & Hotamisligil, G. S. (2012). The role of endoplasmic reticulum in hepatic lipid homeostasis and stress signaling. *Cell Metabolism*, *15*, 623–634.

Gade, C., Dalhoff, K., Petersen, T. S., Riis, T., Schmeltz, C., Chabanova, E., et al. (2018). Higher chlorzoxazone clearance in obese children compared with nonobese peers. *British Journal of Clinical Pharmacology*, *84*, 1738–1747.

Gao, M., Ma, Y., Alsaggar, M., & Liu, D. (2016). Dual outcomes of rosiglitazone treatment on fatty liver. *The AAPS Journal*, *18*, 1023–1031.

Garcia-Ruiz, I., Rodríguez-Juan, C., Díaz-Sanjuán, T., Martínez, M. A., Muñoz-Yagüe, T., & Solís-Herruzo, J. A. (2007). Effects of rosiglitazone on the liver histology and mitochondrial function in ob/ob mice. *Hepatology*, *46*, 414–423.

Grünig, D., Duthaler, U., & Krähenbühl, S. (2018). Effect of toxicants on fatty acid metabolism in HepG2 cells. *Frontiers in Pharmacology*, *9*, 257.

Gutkowski, K., Chwist, A., & Hartleb, M. (2011). Liver injury induced by high-dose methylprednisolone therapy: A case report and brief review of the literature. *Hepatitis Monthly*, *11*, 656–661.

Haczeyni, F., Yeh, M. M., Ioannou, G. N., Leclercq, I. A., Goldin, R., Dan, Y. Y., et al. (2018). Mouse models of non-alcoholic steatohepatitis: A reflection on recent literature. *Journal of Gastroenterology and Hepatology*, *33*, 1312–1320.

Hardwick, R. N., Clarke, J. D., Lake, A. D., Canet, M. J., Anumol, T., Street, S. M., et al. (2014). Increased susceptibility to methotrexate-induced toxicity in nonalcoholic steatohepatitis. *Toxicological Sciences*, *142*, 45–55.

Hardy, T., Oakley, F., Anstee, Q. M., & Day, C. P. (2016). Nonalcoholic fatty liver disease: Pathogenesis and disease spectrum. *Annual Review of Pathology: Mechanisms of Disease*, *11*, 451–496.

Hartman, J. H., Miller, G. P., & Meyer, J. N. (2017). Toxicological implications of mitochondrial localization of CYP2E1. *Toxicology Research*, *6*, 273–289.

Hong, N., Yoon, H. G., Seo, D. H., Park, S., Kim, S. I., Sohn, J. H., et al. (2017). Different patterns in the risk of newly developed fatty liver and lipid changes with tamoxifen versus aromatase inhibitors in postmenopausal women with early breast cancer: A propensity score-matched cohort study. *European Journal of Cancer*, *82*, 103–114.

Hu, D., Wu, C. Q., Li, Z. J., Liu, Y., Fan, X., Wang, Q. J., et al. (2015). Characterizing the mechanism of thiazolidinedione-induced hepatotoxicity: An in vitro model in mitochondria. *Toxicology and Applied Pharmacology*, *284*, 134–141.

Ijiri, Y., Kato, R., Sadamatsu, M., Takano, M., Yasuda, Y., Tanaka, F., et al. (2018). Contributions of caspase-8 and -9 to liver injury from CYP2E1-produced metabolites of halogenated hydrocarbons. *Xenobiotica*, *48*, 60–72.

Ikeda, T. (2011). Drug-induced idiosyncratic hepatotoxicity: Prevention strategy developed after the troglitazone case. *Drug Metabolism and Pharmacokinetics*, *26*, 60–70.

Ioannou, G. N. (2016). The role of cholesterol in the pathogenesis of NASH. *Trends in Endocrinology and Metabolism*, *27*, 84–95.

Ito, M., Suzuki, J., Sasaki, M., Watanabe, K., Tsujioka, S., Takahashi, Y., et al. (2006). Development of nonalcoholic steatohepatitis model through combination of high-fat diet and tetracycline with morbid obesity in mice. *Hepatology Research*, *34*, 92–98.

Jamwal, R., de la Monte, S. M., Ogasawara, K., Adusumalli, S., Barlock, B. B., & Akhlaghi, F. (2018). Nonalcoholic fatty liver disease and diabetes are associated with decreased CYP3A4 protein expression and activity in human liver. *Molecular Pharmaceutics*, *15*, 2621–2632.

Jha, P., Knopf, A., Koefeler, H., Mueller, M., Lackner, C., Hoefler, G., et al. (2014). Role of adipose tissue in methionine-choline-deficient model of non-alcoholic steatohepatitis (NASH). *Biochimica et Biophysica Acta—Molecular Basis of Disease*, *1842*, 959–970.

Kanuri, G., & Bergheim, I. (2013). In vitro and in vivo models of non-alcoholic fatty liver disease (NAFLD). *International Journal of Molecular Sciences*, *14*, 11963–11980.

Kaufmann, P., Török, M., Hänni, A., Roberts, P., Gasser, R., & Krähenbühl, S. (2005). Mechanisms of benzarone and benzbromarone-induced hepatic toxicity. *Hepatology*, *41*, 925–935.

Kent, P. D., Luthra, H. S., & Michet, C. (2004). Risk factors for methotrexate-induced abnormal laboratory monitoring results in patients with rheumatoid arthritis. *The Journal of Rheumatology*, *31*, 1727–1731.

Kharasch, E. D., Hankins, D. C., & Cox, K. (1999). Clinical isoflurane metabolism by cytochrome P450 2E1. *Anesthesiology*, *90*, 766–771.

Kim, T. H., Choi, D., Kim, J. Y., Lee, J. H., & Koo, S. H. (2017). Fast food diet-induced non-alcoholic fatty liver disease exerts early protective effect against acetaminophen intoxication in mice. *BMC Gastroenterology*, *17*, 124.

Kim, Y. J., Choi, M. S., Park, Y. B., Kim, S. R., Lee, M. K., & Jung, U. J. (2013). Garcinia Cambogia attenuates diet-induced adiposity but exacerbates hepatic collagen accumulation and inflammation. *World Journal of Gastroenterology*, *19*, 4689–4701.

Kim, H., Oh, E., Im, H., Mun, J., Yang, M., Khim, J. Y., et al. (2006). Oxidative damages in the DNA, lipids, and proteins of rats exposed to isofluranes and alcohols. *Toxicology, 220*, 169–178.

Knockaert, L., Fromenty, B., & Robin, M. A. (2011). Mechanisms of mitochondrial targeting of cytochrome P450 2E1, physiopathological role in liver injury and obesity. *FEBS Journal, 278*, 4252–4260.

Kohlroser, J., Mathai, J., Reichheld, J., Banner, B. F., & Bonkovsky, H. L. (2000). Hepatotoxicity due to troglitazone: Report of two cases and review of adverse events reported to the United States Food and Drug Administration. *American Journal of Gastroenterology, 95*, 272–276.

Kyriakides, M., Hardwick, R. N., Jin, Z., Goedken, M. J., Holmes, E., Cherrington, N. J., et al. (2014). Systems level metabolic phenotype of methotrexate administration in the context of non-alcoholic steatohepatitis in the rat. *Toxicological Sciences, 142*, 105–116.

Labbe, G., Fromenty, B., Freneaux, E., Morzelle, V., Letteron, P., Berson, A., et al. (1991). Effects of various tetracycline derivatives on in vitro and in vivo beta-oxidation of fatty acids, egress of triglycerides from the liver, accumulation of hepatic triglycerides, and mortality in mice. *Biochemical Pharmacology, 41*, 638–641.

Labbe, G., Pessayre, D., & Fromenty, B. (2008). Drug-induced liver injury through mitochondrial dysfunction: Mechanisms and detection during preclinical safety studies. *Fundamental & Clinical Pharmacology, 22*, 335–353.

Lammert, C., Imler, T., Teal, E., & Chalasani, N. (2019). Patients with chronic liver disease suggestive of nonalcoholic fatty liver disease may be at higher risk for drug-induced liver injury. *Clinical Gastroenterology and Hepatology*. https://doi.org/10.1016/j.cgh.2018.12.013. in press.

Langman, G., Hall, P. M., & Todd, G. (2001). Role of non-alcoholic steatohepatitis in methotrexate-induced liver injury. *Journal of Gastroenterology and Hepatology, 16*, 1395–1401.

Larosche, I., Lettéron, P., Fromenty, B., Vadrot, N., Abbey-Toby, A., Feldmann, G., et al. (2007). Tamoxifen inhibits topoisomerases, depletes mitochondrial DNA, and triggers steatosis in mouse liver. *Journal of Pharmacology and Experimental Therapeutics, 321*, 526–535.

Larrain, S., & Rinella, M. E. (2012). A myriad of pathways to NASH. *Clinics in Liver Disease, 16*, 525–548.

Le Guillou, D., Bucher, S., Begriche, K., Hoët, D., Lombès, A., Labbe, G., et al. (2018). Drug-induced alterations of mitochondrial DNA homeostasis in steatotic and nonsteatotic HepaRG cells. *Journal of Pharmacology and Experimental Therapeutics, 365*, 711–726.

Lee, M. H., Graham, G. G., Williams, K. M., & Day, R. O. (2008). A benefit-risk assessment of benzbromarone in the treatment of gout. Was its withdrawal from the market in the best interest of patients? *Drug Safety, 31*, 643–665.

Lee, J., Homma, T., Kurahashi, T., Kang, E. S., & Fujii, J. (2015). Oxidative stress triggers lipid droplet accumulation in primary cultured hepatocytes by activating fatty acid synthesis. *Biochemical and Biophysical Research Communications, 464*, 229–235.

Lemoine, M., Serfaty, L., & Capeau, J. (2012). From nonalcoholic fatty liver to nonalcoholic steatohepatitis and cirrhosis in HIV-infected patients: Diagnosis and management. *Current Opinion in Infectious Diseases, 25*, 10–16.

Lemoine, M., Serfaty, L., Cervera, P., Capeau, J., & Ratziu, V. (2014). Hepatic molecular effects of rosiglitazone in human non-alcoholic steatohepatitis suggest long-term pro-inflammatory damage. *Hepatology Research, 44*, 1241–1247.

Lettéron, P., Brahimi-Bourouina, N., Robin, M. A., Moreau, A., Feldmann, G., & Pessayre, D. (1997). Glucocorticoids inhibit mitochondrial matrix acyl-CoA dehydrogenases and fatty acid beta-oxidation. *American Journal of Physiology—Gastrointestinal and Liver Physiology, 272*, G1141–G1150.

Lettéron, P., Sutton, A., Mansouri, A., Fromenty, B., & Pessayre, D. (2003). Inhibition of microsomal triglyceride transfer protein: Another mechanism for drug-induced steatosis in mice. *Hepatology, 38*, 133–140.

Li, H., Toth, E., & Cherrington, N. J. (2018). Asking the right questions with animal models: Methionine- and choline-deficient model in predicting adverse drug reactions in human NASH. *Toxicological Sciences, 161*, 23–33.

Lu, Y., Zhuge, J., Wang, X., Bai, J., & Cederbaum, A. I. (2008). Cytochrome P450 2E1 contributes to ethanol-induced fatty liver in mice. *Hepatology, 47*, 1483–1494.

Lucas, D., Farez, C., Bardou, L. G., Vaisse, J., Attali, J. R., & Valensi, P. (1998). Cytochrome P450 2E1 activity in diabetic and obese patients as assessed by chlorzoxazone hydroxylation. *Fundamental & Clinical Pharmacology, 12*, 553–558.

Luo, Y., Rana, P., & Will, Y. (2012). Palmitate increases the susceptibility of cells to drug-induced toxicity: An in vitro method to identify drugs with potential contraindications in patients with metabolic disease. *Toxicological Sciences, 129*, 346–362.

Maes, M., Vinken, M., & Jaeschke, H. (2016). Experimental models of hepatotoxicity related to acute liver failure. *Toxicology and Applied Pharmacology, 290*, 86–97.

Mahli, A., Saugspier, M., Koch, A., Sommer, J., Dietrich, P., Lee, S., et al. (2018). ERK activation and autophagy impairment are central mediators of irinotecan-induced steatohepatitis. *Gut, 67*, 746–756.

Mak, A., Cho, T., & Uetrecht, J. (2018). Use of an animal model to test whether non-alcoholic fatty liver disease increases the risk of idiosyncratic drug-induced liver injury. *Journal of Immunotoxicology, 15*, 90–95.

Mallick, P., Shah, P., Ittmann, M. M., Trivedi, M., Hu, M., Gao, S., et al. (2018). Impact of diet on irinotecan toxicity in mice. *Chemico-Biological Interactions, 291*, 87–94.

Masarone, M., Rosato, V., Dallio, M., Gravina, A. G., Aglitti, A., Loguercio, C., et al. (2018). Role of oxidative stress in pathophysiology of nonalcoholic fatty liver disease. *Oxidative Medicine and Cellular Longevity, 2018*, 9547613.

Massart, J., Begriche, K., Buron, N., Porceddu, M., Borgne-Sanchez, A., & Fromenty, B. (2013). Drug-induced inhibition of mitochondrial fatty acid oxidation and steatosis. *Current Pathobiology Reports, 1*, 147–157.

Massart, J., Begriche, K., Moreau, C., & Fromenty, B. (2017). Role of nonalcoholic fatty liver disease as risk factor for drug-induced hepatotoxicity. *Journal of Clinical and Translational Research, 3*(Suppl. 1), 212–232.

Massart, J., Robin, M. A., Noury, F., Fautrel, A., Lettéron, P., Bado, A., et al. (2012). Pentoxifylline aggravates fatty liver in obese and diabetic ob/ob mice by increasing intestinal glucose absorption and activating hepatic lipogenesis. *British Journal of Pharmacology, 165*, 1361–1374.

Mattar, W., Juliar, B., Gradus-Pizlo, I., & Kwo, P. Y. (2009). Amiodarone hepatotoxicity in the context of the metabolic syndrome and right-sided heart failure. *Journal of Gastrointestinal and Liver Diseases, 18*, 419–423.

Merrell, M. D., & Cherrington, N. J. (2011). Drug metabolism alterations in nonalcoholic fatty liver disease. *Drug Metabolism Reviews, 43*, 317–334.

Michaut, A., Le Guillou, D., Moreau, C., Bucher, S., McGill, M. R., Martinais, S., et al. (2016). A cellular model to study drug-induced liver injury in nonalcoholic fatty liver disease: Application to acetaminophen. *Toxicology and Applied Pharmacology, 292*, 40–55.

Michaut, A., Moreau, C., Robin, M. A., & Fromenty, B. (2014). Acetaminophen-induced liver injury in obesity and nonalcoholic fatty liver disease. *Liver International, 34*, e171–e179.

Mota, M., Banini, B. A., Cazanave, S. C., & Sanyal, A. J. (2016). Molecular mechanisms of lipotoxicity and glucotoxicity in nonalcoholic fatty liver disease. *Metabolism, 65*, 1049–1061.

Moult, P. J., & Sherlock, S. (1975). Halothane-related hepatitis. A clinical study of twenty-six cases. *Quarterly Journal of Medicine, 44*, 99–114.

Musso, G., Cassader, M., Paschetta, E., & Gambino, R. (2017). Thiazolidinediones and advanced liver fibrosis in nonalcoholic steatohepatitis: A meta-analysis. *JAMA Internal Medicine*, *177*, 633–640.

Myers, R. P., & Shaheen, A. A. (2009). Hepatitis C, alcohol abuse, and unintentional overdoses are risk factors for acetaminophen-related hepatotoxicity. *Hepatology*, *49*, 1399–1400.

Nadanaciva, S., Dykens, J. A., Bernal, A., Capaldi, R. A., & Will, Y. (2007). Mitochondrial impairment by PPAR agonists and statins identified via immunocaptured OXPHOS complex activities and respiration. *Toxicology and Applied Pharmacology*, *223*, 277–287.

Neuschwander-Tetri, B. A. (2010). Hepatic lipotoxicity and the pathogenesis of nonalcoholic steatohepatitis: The central role of nontriglyceride fatty acid metabolites. *Hepatology*, *52*, 774–788.

Neuschwander-Tetri, B. A., Brunt, E. M., Wehmeier, K. R., Oliver, D., & Bacon, B. R. (2003). Improved nonalcoholic steatohepatitis after 48 weeks of treatment with the PPAR-γ ligand rosiglitazone. *Hepatology*, *38*, 1008–1017.

Nguyen, G. C., Sam, J., & Thuluvath, P. J. (2008). Hepatitis C is a predictor of acute liver injury among hospitalizations for acetaminophen overdose in the United States: A nationwide analysis. *Hepatology*, *48*, 1336–1341.

Niedfeldt, M. W. (2018). Anabolic steroid effect on the liver. *Current Sports Medicine Reports*, *17*, 97–102.

Ogawa, Y., Murata, Y., Nishioka, A., Inomata, T., & Yoshida, S. (1998). Tamoxifen-induced fatty liver in patients with breast cancer. *Lancet*, *351*, 725.

Pais, R., Rusu, E., & Ratziu, V. (2014). The impact of obesity and metabolic syndrome on chronic hepatitis B and drug-induced liver disease. *Clinics in Liver Disease*, *18*, 165–178.

Pan, H. J., Chang, H. T., & Lee, C. H. (2016). Association between tamoxifen treatment and the development of different stages of nonalcoholic fatty liver disease among breast cancer patients. *Journal of the Formosan Medical Association*, *115*, 411–417.

Parvez, S., Tabassum, H., Banerjee, B. D., & Raisuddin, S. (2008). Taurine prevents tamoxifen-induced mitochondrial oxidative damage in mice. *Basic & Clinical Pharmacology & Toxicology*, *102*, 382–387.

Peyta, L., Jarnouen, K., Pinault, M., Guimaraes, C., Pais de Barros, J. P., Chevalier, S., et al. (2016). Reduced cardiolipin content decreases respiratory chain capacities and increases ATP synthesis yield in the human HepaRG cells. *Biochimica et Biophysica Acta—Bioenergetics*, *1857*, 443–453.

Pinto, H. C., Baptista, A., Camilo, M. E., de Costa, E. B., Valente, A., & de Moura, M. C. (1995). Tamoxifen-associated steatohepatitis-report of three cases. *Journal of Hepatology*, *23*, 95–97.

Poggioli, R., Ueta, C. B., Drigo, R. A., Castillo, M., Fonseca, T. L., & Bianco, A. C. (2013). Dexamethasone reduces energy expenditure and increases susceptibility to diet-induced obesity in mice. *Obesity*, *21*, E415–E420.

Porceddu, M., Buron, N., Roussel, C., Labbe, G., Fromenty, B., & Borgne-Sanchez, A. (2012). Prediction of liver injury induced by chemicals in human with a multiparametric assay on isolated mouse liver mitochondria. *Toxicological Sciences*, *129*, 332–345.

Prestigiacomo, V., Weston, A., Messner, S., Lampart, F., & Suter-Dick, L. (2017). Pro-fibrotic compounds induce stellate cell activation, ECM-remodelling and Nrf2 activation in a human 3D-multicellular model of liver fibrosis. *PLoS One*, *12*, e0179995.

Rabinowich, L., & Shibolet, O. (2015). Drug induced steatohepatitis: An uncommon culprit of a common disease. *BioMed Research International*, *2015*, 168905.

Radosevich, J. J., Patanwala, A. E., & Erstad, B. L. (2016). Hepatotoxicity in obese versus nonobese patients with acetaminophen poisoning who are treated with intravenous N-acetylcysteine. *American Journal of Therapeutics*, *23*, e714–e719.

Rafacho, A., Ortsäter, H., Nadal, A., & Quesada, I. (2014). Glucocorticoid treatment and endocrine pancreas function: Implications for glucose homeostasis, insulin resistance and diabetes. *Journal of Endocrinology, 223*, R49–R62.

Ramachandran, A., & Jaeschke, H. (2017). Mechanisms of acetaminophen hepatotoxicity and their translation to the human pathophysiology. *Journal of Clinical and Translational Research, 3*(Suppl. 1), 157–169.

Ramachandran, R., & Kakar, S. (2009). Histological patterns in drug-induced liver disease. *Journal of Clinical Pathology, 62*, 481–492.

Ratziu, V., Charlotte, F., Bernhardt, C., Giral, P., Halbron, M., Lenaour, G., et al. (2010). Long-term efficacy of rosiglitazone in nonalcoholic steatohepatitis: Results of the fatty liver improvement by rosiglitazone therapy (FLIRT 2) extension trial. *Hepatology, 51*, 445–453.

Ribeiro, M. P., Santos, A. E., & Custódio, J. B. (2014). Mitochondria: The gateway for tamoxifen-induced liver injury. *Toxicology, 323*, 10–18.

Rosenberg, P., Urwitz, H., Johannesson, A., Ros, A. M., Lindholm, J., Kinnman, N., et al. (2007). Psoriasis patients with diabetes type 2 are at high risk of developing liver fibrosis during methotrexate treatment. *Journal of Hepatology, 46*, 1111–1118.

Rutherford, A., Davern, T., Hay, J. E., Murray, N. G., Hassanein, T., Lee, W. M., et al. (2006). Influence of high body mass index on outcome in acute liver failure. *Clinical Gastroenterology and Hepatology, 4*, 1544–1549.

Sadler, N. C., Webb-Robertson, B. M., Clauss, T. R., Pounds, J. G., Corley, R., & Wright, A. T. (2018). High-fat diets alter the modulatory effects of xenobiotics on cytochrome P450 activities. *Chemical Research in Toxicology, 31*, 308–318.

Santhekadur, P. K., Kumar, D. P., & Sanyal, A. J. (2018). Preclinical models of non-alcoholic fatty liver disease. *Journal of Hepatology, 68*, 230–237.

Santos, J. D., Mendonça, A. A., Sousa, R. C., Silva, T. G., Bigonha, S. M., Santos, E. C., et al. (2018). Food-drug interaction: Anabolic steroids aggravate hepatic lipotoxicity and nonalcoholic fatty liver disease induced by trans fatty acids. *Food and Chemical Toxicology, 116*, 360–368.

Saphner, T., Triest-Robertson, S., Li, H., & Holzman, P. (2009). The association of nonalcoholic steatohepatitis and tamoxifen in patients with breast cancer. *Cancer, 115*, 3189–3195.

Satapati, S., Kucejova, B., Duarte, J. A., Fletcher, J. A., Reynolds, L., Sunny, N. E., et al. (2015). Mitochondrial metabolism mediates oxidative stress and inflammation in fatty liver. *Journal of Clinical Investigation, 125*, 4447–4462.

Sawano, T., Shimizu, T., Yamada, T., Nanashima, N., Miura, T., Morohashi, S., et al. (2015). Fatty acid synthase-positive hepatocytes and subsequent steatosis in rat livers by irinotecan. *Oncology Reports, 33*, 2151–2160.

Schmajuk, G., Miao, Y., Yazdany, J., Boscardin, W. J., Daikh, D. I., & Steinman, M. A. (2014). Identification of risk factors for elevated transaminases in methotrexate users through an electronic health record. *Arthritis Care & Research, 66*, 1159–1166.

Schon, E., & Fromenty, B. (2016). Alterations of mitochondrial DNA in liver diseases. In D. Han & N. Kaplowitz (Eds.), *Mitochondria in liver disease* (pp. 283–313). Boca Raton: CRC Press.

Seeff, L. B., Bonkovsky, H. L., Navarro, V. J., & Wang, G. (2015). Herbal products and the liver: A review of adverse effects and mechanisms. *Gastroenterology, 148*, 517–532.

Segawa, M., Sekine, S., Sato, T., & Ito, K. (2018). Increased susceptibility to troglitazone-induced mitochondrial permeability transition in type 2 diabetes mellitus model rat. *Journal of Toxicological Sciences, 43*, 339–351.

Sekiya, M., Hiraishi, A., Touyama, M., & Sakamoto, K. (2008). Oxidative stress induced lipid accumulation via SREBP1c activation in HepG2 cells. *Biochemical and Biophysical Research Communications, 375*, 602–607.

Seth, R. K., Das, S., Dattaroy, D., Chandrashekaran, V., Alhasson, F., Michelotti, G., et al. (2017). TRPV4 activation of endothelial nitric oxide synthase resists nonalcoholic fatty liver disease by blocking CYP2E1-mediated redox toxicity. *Free Radical Biology and Medicine, 102*, 260–273.

Sgro, C., Clinard, F., Ouazir, K., Chanay, H., Allard, C., & Guilleminet, C. (2002). Incidence of drug-induced hepatic injuries: A French population-based study. *Hepatology, 36*, 451–455.

Shetty, A., Cho, W., Alazawi, W., & Syn, W. K. (2017). Methotrexate hepatotoxicity and the impact of nonalcoholic fatty liver disease. *American Journal of the Medical Sciences, 354*, 172–181.

Soccio, R. E., Chen, E. R., & Lazar, M. A. (2014). Thiazolidinediones and the promise of insulin sensitization in type 2 diabetes. *Cell Metabolism, 20*, 573–591.

Sramek, M., Neradil, J., & Veselska, R. (2017). Much more than you expected: The non-DHFR-mediated effects of methotrexate. *Biochimica et Biophysica Acta—General Subjects, 1861*, 499–503.

Stickel, F., & Shouval, D. (2015). Hepatotoxicity of herbal and dietary supplements: An update. *Archives of Toxicology, 89*, 851–865.

Sun, P., Zhu, J. J., Wang, T., Huang, Q., Zhou, Y. R., Yu, B. W., et al. (2018). Benzbromarone aggravates hepatic steatosis in obese individuals. *Biochimica et Biophysica Acta—Molecular Basis of Disease, 1864*, 2067–2077.

Tabassum, H., Parvez, S., Pasha, S. T., Banerjee, B. D., & Raisuddin, S. (2010). Protective effect of lipoic acid against methotrexate-induced oxidative stress in liver mitochondria. *Food and Chemical Toxicology, 48*, 1973–1979.

Takahashi, Y., Soejima, Y., & Fukusato, T. (2012). Animal models of nonalcoholic fatty liver disease/nonalcoholic steatohepatitis. *World Journal of Gastroenterology, 18*, 2300–2308.

Takamura, T., Shimizu, A., Komura, T., Ando, H., Zen, Y., Minato, H., et al. (2007). Selective estrogen receptor modulator raloxifene-associated aggravation of nonalcoholic steatohepatitis. *Internal Medicine, 46*, 579–581.

Tarantino, G., Conca, P., Basile, V., Gentile, A., Capone, D., Polichetti, G., et al. (2007). A prospective study of acute drug-induced liver injury in patients suffering from non-alcoholic fatty liver disease. *Hepatology Research, 37*, 410–415.

Teratani, T., Tomita, K., Suzuki, T., Furuhashi, H., Irie, R., Hida, S., et al. (2017). Free cholesterol accumulation in liver sinusoidal endothelial cells exacerbates acetaminophen hepatotoxicity via TLR9 signaling. *Journal of Hepatology, 67*, 780–790.

Thalha, A. M., Mahadeva, S., Boon Tan, A. T., & Mun, K. S. (2018). Kombiglyze (metformin and saxagliptin)-induced hepatotoxicity in a patient with non-alcoholic fatty liver disease. *JGH Open, 2*, 242–245.

Tirosh, O. (2018). Hypoxic signaling and cholesterol lipotoxicity in fatty liver disease progression. *Oxidative Medicine and Cellular Longevity, 2018*, 2548154.

Trak-Smayra, V., Paradis, V., Massart, J., Nasser, S., Jebara, V., & Fromenty, B. (2011). Pathology of the liver in obese and diabetic ob/ob and db/db mice fed a standard or high-calorie diet. *International Journal of Experimental Pathology, 92*, 413–421.

van Rongen, A., Välitalo, P. A., Peeters, M. Y., Boerma, D., Huisman, F. W., van Ramshorst, B., et al. (2016). Morbidly obese patients exhibit increased CYP2E1-mediated oxidation of acetaminophen. *Clinical Pharmacokinetics, 55*, 833–847.

Vauthey, J. N., Pawlik, T. M., Ribero, D., Wu, T. T., Zorzi, D., Hoff, P. M., et al. (2006). Chemotherapy regimen predicts steatohepatitis and an increase in 90-day mortality after surgery for hepatic colorectal metastases. *Journal of Clinical Oncology, 24*, 2065–2072.

Wahlang, B., Song, M., Beier, J. I., Cameron Falkner, K., Al-Eryani, L., Clair, H. B., et al. (2014). Evaluation of Aroclor 1260 exposure in a mouse model of diet-induced obesity and non-alcoholic fatty liver disease. *Toxicology and Applied Pharmacology, 279*, 380–390.

Wang, Z., Hall, S. D., Maya, J. F., Li, L., Asghar, A., & Gorski, J. C. (2003). Diabetes mellitus increases the in vivo activity of cytochrome P450 2E1 in humans. *British Journal of Clinical Pharmacology, 55*, 77–85.

Wang, Y., Lin, Z., Liu, Z., Harris, S., Kelly, R., Zhang, J., et al. (2013). A unifying ontology to integrate histological and clinical observations for drug-induced liver injury. *The American Journal of Pathology, 182*, 1180–1187.

Wang, H., Peng, Y., Zhang, T., Lan, Q., Zhao, H., Wang, W., et al. (2017). Metabolic epoxidation is a critical step for the development of benzbromarone-induced hepatotoxicity. *Drug Metabolism and Disposition, 45*, 1354–1363.

Watkins, S. M., Reifsnyder, P. R., Pan, H. J., German, J. B., & Leiter, E. H. (2002). Lipid metabolome-wide effects of the PPARγ agonist rosiglitazone. *Journal of Lipid Research, 43*, 1809–1817.

Wickramage, I., Tennekoon, K. H., Ariyaratne, M. A., Hewage, A. S., & Sundralingam, T. (2017). CYP2D6 polymorphisms may predict occurrence of adverse effects to tamoxifen: A preliminary retrospective study. *Breast Cancer (Dove Medical Press), 9*, 111–120.

Woods, C. P., Hazlehurst, J. M., & Tomlinson, J. W. (2015). Glucocorticoids and non-alcoholic fatty liver disease. *The Journal of Steroid Biochemistry and Molecular Biology, 154*, 94–103.

Woolsey, S. J., Mansell, S. E., Kim, R. B., Tirona, R. G., & Beaton, M. D. (2015). CYP3A activity and expression in nonalcoholic fatty liver disease. *Drug Metabolism and Disposition, 43*, 1484–1490.

Yamamoto, N., Lopes, L. C., Campello, A. P., & Klüppel, M. L. (1989). Methotrexate: Studies on cellular metabolism. II—Effects on mitochondrial oxidative metabolism and ion transport. *Cell Biochemistry and Function, 7*, 129–134.

Yang, Y. J., Kim, K. M., An, J. H., Lee, D. B., Shim, J. H., Lim, Y. S., et al. (2016). Clinical significance of fatty liver disease induced by tamoxifen and toremifene in breast cancer patients. *Breast, 28*, 67–72.

Young, S. R., Stoelting, R. K., Peterson, C., & Madura, J. A. (1975). Anesthetic biotransformation and renal function in obese patients during and after methoxyflurane or halothane anesthesia. *Anesthesiology, 42*, 451–457.

Zannikos, P. N., Bandyopadhyay, A. M., Robertson, L. W., & Blouin, R. A. (1993). Effect of nutritional obesity on the induction of CYP2B enzymes following phenobarbital treatment. *Drug Metabolism and Disposition, 21*, 782–787.

Zeng, T., Zhang, C. L., Song, F. Y., Zhao, X. L., & Xie, K. Q. (2014). CMZ reversed chronic ethanol-induced disturbance of PPAR-α possibly by suppressing oxidative stress and PGC-1α acetylation, and activating the MAPK and GSK3β pathway. *PLoS One, 9*, e98658.

Zhang, K., Kim, H., Fu, Z., Qiu, Y., Yang, Z., Wang, J., et al. (2018). Deficiency of the mitochondrial NAD kinase causes stress-induced hepatic steatosis in mice. *Gastroenterology, 154*, 224–237.

Zhang, X. Q., Xu, C. F., Yu, C. H., Chen, W. X., & Li, Y. M. (2014). Role of endoplasmic reticulum stress in the pathogenesis of nonalcoholic fatty liver disease. *World Journal of Gastroenterology, 20*, 1768–1776.

Zhao, F., Xie, P., Jiang, J., Zhang, L., An, W., & Zhan, Y. (2014). The effect and mechanism of tamoxifen-induced hepatocyte steatosis in vitro. *International Journal of Molecular Sciences, 15*, 4019–4030.

Zhou, P. Z., Zhu, Y. M., Zou, G. H., Sun, Y. X., Xiu, X. L., Huang, X., et al. (2016). Relationship between glucocorticoids and insulin resistance in healthy individuals. *Medical Science Monitor, 22*, 1887–1894.

CHAPTER FOUR

Role and mechanisms of autophagy in alcohol-induced liver injury

Xiaojuan Chao, Wen-Xing Ding[1]
Department of Pharmacology, Toxicology and Therapeutics, University of Kansas Medical Center, Kansas City, KS, United States
[1]Corresponding author: e-mail address: wxding@kumc.edu

Contents

Abstract

Alcoholic liver disease (ALD) is one of the major causes of chronic liver disease worldwide. Currently, no successful treatments are available for ALD. The pathogenesis of ALD is characterized as simple steatosis, fibrosis, cirrhosis, alcoholic hepatitis (AH), and eventually hepatocellular carcinoma (HCC). Autophagy is a highly conserved intracellular catabolic process, which aims at recycling cellular components and removing damaged organelles in response to starvation and stresses. Therefore, autophagy is considered as an important cellular adaptive and survival mechanism under various pathophysiological conditions. Recent studies from our lab and others suggest that chronic alcohol consumption may impair autophagy and contribute to the pathogenesis of ALD. In this

Advances in Pharmacology, Volume 85
ISSN 1054-3589
https://doi.org/10.1016/bs.apha.2019.01.008
© 2019 Elsevier Inc.
All rights reserved.

chapter, we summarize recent progress on the role and mechanisms of autophagy in the development of ALD. Understanding the roles of autophagy in ALD may offer novel therapeutic avenues against ALD by targeting these pathways.

Abbreviations

3-MA	3-methyladenine
ADH	alcohol dehydrogenase
AH	alcoholic hepatitis
ALD	alcoholic liver disease
ALDH1/2	aldehyde dehydrogenase 1/2
ALT	alanine aminotransferase
AMPK	AMP-activated protein kinase
AST	aspartate aminotransferase
Atg	autophagy-related gene
CYP2E1	cytochrome P450 2E1
EM	electron microscope
ER	endoplasmic reticulum
FAEE	fatty acid ethyl ester
HCC	hepatocellular carcinoma
HO-1	heme oxygenase-1
KO	knockout
Lamp1	lysosome-associated membrane protein 1
LC3/MAP1-LC3	microtubule-associated protein 1A/1B light chain 3
LIR	LC3 interacting region
MAPK14/p38	mitogen-activated protein kinase 14
MDB	Mallory-Denk bodies
Mfn1	mitofusin 1
mTORC1	mechanistic target of rapamycin complex 1
MTS	mitochondrial targeting sequence
NAD^+	nicotinamide adenine dinucleotide
ROS	reactive oxygen species
NAFLD	non-alcoholic fatty liver disease
NIAAA	National Institute on alcohol abuse and alcoholism
PA	phosphatidic acid
PAS	phagophore assembly site
PE	phosphatidylethanolamine
PINK1	phosphatase and tensin homolog (PTEN)-induced kinase 1
PLD	phospholipase D
PI3K	phosphoinositide 3-kinase
PtdIns3P	phosphatidylinositol-3-phosphate
RB1CC1/FIP200	RB1-inducible coiled-coil 1
SNARE	soluble NSF [*N*-ethyl-maleimide-sensitive fusion protein] attachment protein receptor
TFEB	transcription factor EB
TIM	translocase of mitochondrial inner membrane

TOM	translocase of mitochondrial outer membrane
Ubl	ubiquitin-like
ULK1/2	Unc-51 like autophagy activating kinase 1/2
VDAC	voltage-dependent anion channel

1. Introduction

Alcoholic liver disease (ALD) is a major health problem and a significant source of chronic liver injury worldwide. In 2012, about 3.3 million deaths, or 5.9% of all global deaths, were attributed to alcohol consumption (WHO). The latest surveillance report published by the National Institute on Alcohol Abuse and Alcoholism (NIAAA) showed that liver cirrhosis was the 12th leading cause of death in the United States, with a total of 42,443 deaths in 2015, 49.5% of which were estimated to be attributed to ALD (Yoon, 2018). ALD comprises a spectrum of disorders and pathologic changes in individuals with acute and chronic alcohol consumption, ranging from alcoholic steatosis to liver fibrosis, cirrhosis, alcoholic hepatitis (AH) and liver cancer (Gao & Bataller, 2011; Nagy, Ding, Cresci, Saikia, & Shah, 2016; Williams, Manley, & Ding, 2014).

Macroautophagy (hereafter referred to as autophagy) is an evolutionarily conserved and programmed intracellular degradation pathway in response to starvation and stresses. It is involved in the trafficking of long-lived proteins and cellular organelles via the formation of autophagosomes, which then fuse with lysosomes for degradation to maintain cellular homeostasis. Autophagy is generally considered as a pro-survival mechanism in response to various stress conditions and plays a critical role in normal liver physiology and liver diseases (Czaja et al., 2013; Ding, 2010; Yin, Ding, & Gao, 2008).

Accumulating evidence has shown that altered autophagy is implicated in the pathogenesis and protection of alcohol-induced tissue injury (Czaja et al., 2013; Ding, Li, & Yin, 2011; Ding, Manley, & Ni, 2011; Dolganiuc, Thomes, Ding, Lemasters, & Donohue, 2012; Li, Wang, Ni, Huang, & Ding, 2014). In this chapter, we summarize recent findings about the roles and the underlying molecular mechanisms of autophagy in the development of ALD.

2. Alcohol metabolism

Metabolism of alcohol has been extensively studied (Cederbaum, 2012; Zakhari, 2006; Zelner, Matlow, Natekar, & Koren, 2013). Briefly, it is metabolized mainly in the liver and through both major oxidative and minor non-oxidative pathways. The most common oxidative pathway of alcohol metabolism in the liver is catalyzed by alcohol dehydrogenase (ADH), which converts alcohol into highly reactive metabolite, acetaldehyde (Crabb, Matsumoto, Chang, & You, 2004). Alcohol can also be oxidized into acetaldehyde by cytochrome P450 family 2, subfamily E, polypeptide 1 (Cyp2E1) and catalase (Crabb et al., 2004; Lu & Cederbaum, 2008). The highly reactive acetaldehyde forms adducts with other macromolecules, such as proteins, leading to alteration of protein functions, loss of activity and subsequent liver injury (Setshedi, Wands, & Monte, 2010). Acetaldehyde is further metabolized by mitochondrial aldehyde dehydrogenase 2 (ALDH2) into more harmless acetate and acetyl-CoA for use in metabolic pathways (Crabb et al., 2004). The metabolism of alcohol through this pathway increases the conversion of nicotinamide adenine dinucleotide (NAD^+) into its reduced form, NADH, resulting in an increased $NADH/NAD^+$ ratio, alteration of cellular redox status and decreased NAD^+-dependent enzyme activities (Bailey & Cunningham, 2002). In addition, metabolism of alcohol by Cyp2E1 results in production of reactive oxygen species (ROS), which also leads to liver injury (Cederbaum, Lu, & Wu, 2009).

In addition to the oxidative metabolism, a minimal portion of alcohol can also be metabolized via two non-oxidative pathways. Alcohol can directly interact with fatty acid and generates fatty acid ethyl ester (FAEE) through FAEE synthase (Zelner et al., 2013). FAEE was thought to have minor effects and mainly considered as a diagnostic marker, but increasing evidences showed that FAEE exacerbates alcohol-induced injury in various tissues including liver (Wu et al., 2006), pancreas (Werner et al., 2002; Wu, Bhopale, Ansari, & Kaphalia, 2008), and heart (Beckemeier & Bora, 1998; Wu et al., 2008, 2006). FAEE induces mitochondria damage by binding to mitochondria membrane and uncoupling oxidative phosphorylation (Lange & Sobel, 1983). Alcohol also reacts with phospholipase D (PLD), which normally breaks down phospholipids to generate phosphatidic acid (PA). The reaction of ethanol with PLD leads to the formation of phosphatidyl ethanol, which is poorly metabolized and its impact on cellular functions remain to be established (Zakhari, 2006).

3. Autophagy

Autophagy is an evolutionarily conserved degradation pathway for cytosolic macromolecules and damaged/excess organelles. It is first described by de Duve and Wattiaux in the 1960s (De Duve & Wattiaux, 1966). However, until 1990s, the molecular characterization of autophagy began by Ohsumi's laboratory using yeast genetic screens that led to the discovery of a group of essential autophagy-related genes (Atg) in yeast (Thumm et al., 1994; Tsukada & Ohsumi, 1993). So far, more than 30 different Atg have been identified in yeast, and most of them are found to be highly conserved in mammals. The process of autophagy starts from the formation of a transient double-membrane structure, the phagophore, which is the active sequestering compartment. Following the expansion and closure, the phagophore becomes a complete autophagosome. Autophagosomes then subsequently fuse with lysosomes to form autolysosomes where the enwrapped contents are degraded by lysosomal enzymes (Klionsky & Emr, 2000; Nakatogawa, Suzuki, Kamada, & Ohsumi, 2009; Parzych & Klionsky, 2014). Several multimolecular complexes have been found to contribute to autophagosome formation including: (1) ULK1 protein-kinase complex, (2) Becline-VPS34 class III PI3K complex, (3) Atg5-Atg12-Atg16 and Atg8/LC3 conjugation systems, and (4) Atg9-Atg2-Atg18 complex.

The ULK1 (Unc-51 like autophagy activating kinase 1 or 2, mammalian homologs of Atg1, hereafter we only refer to as ULK1) kinase complex is the most upstream component of the core autophagy machinery. In mammalian cells, this complex is composed of ULK1, Atg13, RB1CC1/FIP200 (RB1-inducible coiled-coil 1, a putative yeast Atg17 homolog) and C12orf44/Atg101 (Mizushima, 2010). The initiation of autophagy requires the formation of the ULK1 kinase complex at the phagophore assembly site (PAS) to allow the recruitment and activation of other Atg proteins. ULK1 interacts with Atg13, which directly binds to FIP200 and mediates the interaction between FIP200 and ULK1. The activity of ULK1 kinase complex can be regulated by both mechanistic target of rapamycin complex 1 (mTORC1) and the AMP-activated protein kinase (AMPK). When nutrients are sufficient, mTORC1 is activated and negatively regulates autophagy by directly phosphorylating ULK1 (S757) and inhibiting its activity (Egan, Kim, Shaw, & Guan, 2011, Egan et al., 2011; Kim, Kundu, Viollet, & Guan, 2011). In contrast, when cells suffer from energy deficiency, AMPK is activated and phosphorylates ULK1 at different sites (S317, S467, S555, T574, S637 and S777), which activates ULK1 to promote autophagy resulting in the catabolic degradation of cellular components to generate ATP (Egan, Kim, et al., 2011, Egan, Shackelford, et al., 2011; Kim et al., 2011; Loffler et al., 2011).

Once activated, ULK1 further phosphorylates Beclin1 (mammalian homologs of Atg6) on S14 (Russell et al., 2013). Beclin1 is a component of the autophagy-promoting class III phosphoinositide 3 (PI3)-kinase complexes, which also contains Atg14L, p150 (the yeast ortholog is Vps15) and the class-III PI3 kinase VPS34 (Kihara, Noda, Ishihara, & Ohsumi, 2001). This complex is responsible for the production of phosphatidylinositol-3-phosphate (PtdIns3P) directly from phosphatidylinositol (Burman & Ktistakis, 2010). PtdIns3P serves as a landmark on the membrane to recruit other factors, such as Atg18, involved in the process of autophagosome formation (Obara, Sekito, Niimi, & Ohsumi, 2008). After the activation of Beclin1-VPS34 class III PI3K complex, phagophore expands and elongates by membrane addition, which is accomplished by the Atg5-Atg12-Atg16 and Atg8/LC3 conjugation systems.

These two essential ubiquitin-like (Ubl) conjugation systems involve the Ubl proteins Atg12 and microtubule-associated protein 1A/1B light chain 3 (MAP1-LC3 or LC3, a homolog of Atg8) (Ohsumi, 2001). In the ubiquitin system, Atg12 is the first Ubl and its carboxy-terminal glycine is first activated by an E1-like enzyme, Atg7. Subsequently, Atg12 is transferred to an E2-like conjugating enzyme, Atg10, and conjugates with Atg5. This conjugation requires no known E3 enzyme, and further binds to Atg16L1 (the ortholog of yeast Atg16) to form the Atg12-Atg5-Atg16L1 complex. The Atg12-Atg5-Atg16L1 complex localizes to the isolation membrane throughout its elongation process and serves as an E3 ligase to promote LC3 conjugation with phosphatidylethanolamine (PE). Nascent LC3 is first processed by a protease, Atg4, to expose its C-terminus glycine, which is called LC3-I form that resides in the cytosol. LC3-I is then further activated by E1-like enzyme, Atg7, then transferred to an E2-like conjugating enzyme, Atg3. Finally, LC3 conjugates with PE to form a membrane associated LC3-II form, with the Atg12-Atg5-Atg16L1 complex participating as an E3-like ligase.

In addition to Ubl conjugation system, a Atg9-Atg2-Atg18 complex containing the core protein Atg9, Atg2 and WIPI1/2 (mammalian homologs of Atg18) acts as a cycling system. It contributes to the elongation of the phagophore (Polson et al., 2010). Atg9 is thought to participate in membrane delivery from donor sources, such as the trans-Golgi network or late endosomes, to the expanding phagophore. The movement of Atg9 is dependent on the activity of the ULK1, class III PI3K VPS34, and mitogen-activated protein kinase (MAPK/p38) (Papinski et al., 2014; Webber & Tooze, 2010). Eventually, the expanding membrane closes around its cargo to form a complete autophagosome. The latter moves along microtubules in a dynein motor-dependent manner and cluster closed to the microtubule-organizing center near the nucleus, where it fuses with a lysosome to form an autolysosome. The mechanism that controls the timing of fusion is not known at present. UVRAG, which is part of the PtdIns3K complex, can activate the GTPase Rab7, which promotes fusion with lysosomes (Jager et al., 2004; Liang et al., 2008). Other components of the SNARE (soluble NSF [*N*-ethyl-maleimide-sensitive fusion protein] attachment protein receptor) family proteins, such as VAMP7, VAMP8, VAMP9 and STX17/syntaxin 17, are also implicated in autophagosome fusion with lysosomes (Fader, Sanchez, Mestre, & Colombo, 2009; Furuta, Fujita, Noda, Yoshimori, & Amano, 2010; Itakura, Kishi-Itakura, & Mizushima, 2012). In addition, LAMP-2A, a lysosomal membrane protein, is also required for the fusion of autophagosomes with lysosomes. Lack of LAMP-2A prevents the localization of STX17 and SNAP-29 on the autophagosomes resulting in defective fusion of autophagosomes with lysosomes (Hubert et al., 2016). After the sequestered cargo is delivered inside the lysosome, it is broken down by resident hydrolases of the lysosome and the resulting macromolecules are released back into the cytosol as new energy sources for cell survival. In addition to providing new building blocks and energy sources, autophagy also helps to remove damaged organelles such as mitochondria as another important mechanism for cell survival (Williams & Ding, 2018).

4. Autophagy in ALD mouse models

While many species have been used to study ALD including baboons, pigs and rats, mice have been used predominantly in current ALD research. This is due to the availability of numerous transgenic and knockout mice that can easily help scientists determine the role of a particular molecule or signaling pathway in the pathogenesis of ALD. In addition, mice have more than 85% genetic similarity to humans, and their physiology and genetics have been extensively studied. Moreover, mice can reproduce quickly and are relatively inexpensive compared to baboons and pigs. Several mouse models have been used to study alcoholic liver injury that include acute oral gavage, ad libitum oral alcohol in drinking water, intragastric infusion (Tsukamoto-French model) (Tsukamoto, Reidelberger, French, & Largman, 1984), chronic Lieber-DeCarli diet ethanol feeding and the most recent NIAAA chronic-binge ethanol model, which was developed by Bin Gao's group (hereafter referred to as Gao-binge model).

4.1 Acute alcohol exposure

Alcohol binge drinking can result in mitochondrial damage, inhibition of insulin signaling, steatosis, apoptotic and necrotic cell death, all of which can be regulated by autophagy. Acute alcohol treatment significantly increased both mRNA and protein levels of various essential Atg in mouse livers (Ni, Du, You, & Ding, 2013). Induction of the expression of Atg in hepatocytes by acute alcohol is mediated by the transcription factor FoxO3 and hypoxia-inducing factor-1 beta (Ni et al., 2014, 2013). Using GFP-LC3 transgenic mice, we demonstrated that acute ethanol treatment induced a significant elevation of GFP-LC3 positive autophagosomes and autophagic flux in mouse livers. Similarly, an enrichment of PE-conjugated LC3 was particularly found in the LAMP1-positive heavy membrane fraction, where lysosomes are located, indicating that autophagosomes have been fused with the lysosomes to form the degradative autolysosomes (Ding et al., 2010; Ding, Li, & Yin, 2011; Ding, Manley, & Ni, 2011). Electron microscope (EM) analysis also indicated an accumulation of autophagosomes in acute alcohol treated mouse livers. This induction of autophagy is suppressed after siRNA-mediated knockdown of Atg7 (Ding et al., 2010). In accordance with our findings, several recent studies also found that acute alcohol exposure induces autophagy in mouse livers (Lin et al., 2013; Thomes et al., 2012).

4.2 Chronic alcohol exposure

In a chronic alcohol mouse model, male SV129 mice were fed with Lieber-DeCarli liquid dextrose diet containing gradually increased alcohol for 4 weeks. Fatty liver, elevation of Cyp2E1 and oxidative stress were induced by alcohol feeding in these mice (Lu & Cederbaum, 2015). Inhibition of autophagy by administration of 3-methyladenine (3-MA) enhanced alcohol-induced hepatotoxicity, steatosis and oxidant stress. In contrast, activation of autophagy by rapamycin blunted the elevated steatosis produced by alcohol feeding (Lu & Cederbaum, 2015). In similar studies from another research group, GFP-LC3 transgenic mice were fed control and ethanol-containing liquid diets for 4–6 weeks. Alcohol feeding increased hepatomegaly, steatosis and elevated liver proteins, suggesting slower catabolism in alcohol fed-GFP-LC3 mice (Lin et al., 2013; Thomes et al., 2012). Hepatocytes from mice chronically consuming alcohol exhibited a fourfold rise in GFP-LC3 puncta, which represents autophagosomes, compared with hepatocytes from pair-fed control mice. Cyp2E1 activity and content are elevated in alcohol-fed mice, suggesting enhanced ethanol metabolism may contribute to the augmented autophagosome contents. It should be noted that hepatic proteasome activity was also suppressed in livers of alcohol-fed mice, which may also contribute to a portion of the net protein gain in the liver (Thomes et al., 2012). There is evidence that chronic ethanol consumption also inhibits the degradative phase (i.e. autophagosome degradation by lysosomes) of autophagy, which could account, in part, for the rise in autophagosomes (Thomes, Trambly, Fox, Tuma, & Donohue, 2015).

Isolated primary hepatocytes from rats after 6 weeks of Lieber-Decarli ethanol feeding showed decreased lipid droplet (LD) breakdown in response to starvation. Mechanistically, it is found that chronic ethanol exposure inhibited lysosome mobility and decreased Rab7 activity. Moreover, chronic ethanol also decreased Src kinase activity and Dyn2 (a GTPase involved in scission of cell membrane and formation of microtubule bundle) activities resulting decreased lysosome-mediated LD turnover (Li & Ding, 2017; Rasineni et al., 2017; Schroeder et al., 2015; Schulze, Drizyte, Casey, & McNiven, 2017, Schulze et al., 2017).

4.3 Gao-binge model

Most recently, a novel mouse model (Gao-binge model or NIAAA model) that combines chronic alcohol feeding with acute alcohol exposure was developed by Bin Gao's group (Bertola, Mathews, Ki, Wang, & Gao, 2013, Bertola, Park, & Gao, 2013). In this model, mice are fed a control Lieber-DeCarli liquid diet for 5-days before switching them to a 10-days ethanol Lieber-DeCarli diet (1–5%) followed by one oral gavage of ethanol (31.5% v/v, 5 g/kg) in the morning of day 11 for 9 h. Control animals are fed a calorie-matched diet and receive a maltose dextran gavage (45%) on day 11 (Bertola, Mathews, et al., 2013; Bertola, Park, & Gao, 2013). In this model, mice showed markedly elevated alanine aminotransferase (ALT), aspartate aminotransferase (AST) and steatosis along with significant inflammation in mouse livers compared with either the chronic 10-days feeding or the acute binge alone (Bertola, Mathews, et al., 2013; Bertola, Park, & Gao, 2013).

Using GFP-LC3 transgenic mice, we recently characterized autophagic flux in the mouse livers after Gao-binge treatment (Chao, Ni, & Ding, 2018). We found that the number of GFP-LC3 puncta increased in hepatocytes of ethanol feeding plus binge mice. In the presence of leupeptin, a lysosomal inhibitor that blocks autolysosomal degradation, the number of

GFP-LC3 puncta and levels of GFP-LC3-II further increased compared with either leupeptin alone or ethanol group alone, suggesting that Gao-binge alcohol increases autophagic flux in mouse livers. Increased autophagic flux often leads to the degradation of p62, a substrate protein of autophagy. However, to our surprise, the levels of hepatic p62 were not altered in Gao-binge alcohol-treated mice, suggesting that Gao-binge alcohol-induced autophagy is not sufficient to degrade p62. Subsequently, we found that Gao-binge alcohol decreased hepatic TFEB, a master transcription factor that regulates lysosomal biogenesis, resulting in the decreased lysosome numbers in hepatocytes. Decreased hepatic TFEB is likely mediated by the activation of mTOR and pharmacological inhibition of mTOR partially rescued TFEB signaling and protected against Gao-binge alcohol-induced steatosis and liver injury. Overexpression of TFEB enhanced not only hepatic lysosomal biogenesis but also mitochondrial biogenesis as overexpression of TFEB also markedly upregulated PGC-1α expression. As a result, activation of TFEB protected against Gao-binge alcohol-induced steatosis and liver injury. More importantly, we also found that nuclear TFEB levels decreased in human ALD liver samples compared with healthy human liver donors (Chao et al., 2018). These findings suggest that targeting TFEB may be a promising strategy for treating ALD.

5. Potential therapeutic approaches to treat ALD by modulating autophagy

Alcohol consumption can alter autophagy and modulating autophagy may help to improve the pathogenesis of ALD (Ding et al., 2010; Lin et al., 2013; Thomes et al., 2012; Wu, Wang, Zhou, Yang, & Cederbaum, 2012). Suppression of autophagy with pharmacologic agent chloroquine or siRNA against Atg7 significantly increases hepatocyte apoptosis and liver injury (Ding et al., 2010; Lin et al., 2013). In contrast, pharmacological activation of autophagy protects against alcohol-induced steatosis and liver injury (Chao, Ni, & Ding, 2018; Ding et al., 2010). How autophagy protects against alcohol-induced liver injury is not fully understood, but it could involve selective degradation of damaged mitochondrial and/or lipids (Ding, Li, & Yin, 2011, Ding, Manley, & Ni, 2011; Williams, Ni, Ding, & Ding, 2015; Williams & Ding, 2015).

Autophagy can be either selective or nonselective. Traditionally autophagy is viewed as a non-selective process under nutrient and/or energy deprivation condition. While nonselective autophagic bulk degradation of cellular components provides nutrients and energy to support anabolic metabolism in response to starvation, selective autophagy targets specific substrates and organelles such as intracellular aggregated proteins, mitochondria (mitophagy), endoplasmic reticulum (ER-phagy), pathogens, peroxisomes (pexophagy), ribosomes (ribophagy) and lipid droplets (lipophagy), in either nutrient rich or poor conditions (Green & Levine, 2014; Reggiori, Komatsu, Finley, & Simonsen, 2012). The selective functions of autophagy indicate that it is important for maintaining cellular homeostasis by removing superfluous or injured organelles.

5.1 Mitophagy

The selectively removal of damaged mitochondria is a specific form of autophagy termed as mitophagy. Mitophagy is mediated by autophagy receptor proteins, which typically can bind both damaged mitochondria (usually are ubiquitinated) and LC3-decorated phagophores (Behrends & Fulda, 2012; Ding & Yin, 2012; Ni, Williams, & Ding, 2015; Williams & Ding, 2018).

Several signaling pathways are responsible for the progression of mitophagy, among which, so far, the phosphatase and tensin homolog (PTEN)-induced kinase 1 (PINK1)/Parkin pathway is the best characterized. PINK1, containing a mitochondrial targeting sequence (MTS), is a 64-kDa mitochondrial serine/threonine kinase and is recruited to mitochondria immediately after synthesis. In healthy mitochondria, PINK1 is imported through the outer and inner mitochondrial membranes via the translocase of the outer mitochondrial membrane (TOM) complex and translocase of the inner mitochondrial membrane (TIM) complex respectively. It is then first processed by the matrix processing peptidase (Greene et al., 2012) and then cleaved between amino acids A103 and F104 by the inner mitochondrial membrane protease PARL (Deas et al., 2011; Jin et al., 2010; Meissner, Lorenz, Weihofen, Selkoe, & Lemberg, 2011). The new truncated form of PINK1 is released into the cytosol for N-terminal recognition and degraded by the proteasome (Yamano & Youle, 2013). The cleaved PINK1 fragments in the cytosol may also inhibit Parkin translocation to mitochondria (Fedorowicz et al., 2014). When mitochondria are damaged, in particular with depolarized mitochondrial membrane potential, PINK1 is no longer imported into the inner membrane or cleaved by PARL, resulting in its accumulation on the outer mitochondrial membrane (Matsuda et al., 2010; Narendra et al., 2010;

Vives-Bauza et al., 2010). The accumulated PINK1 on the outer mitochondrial membrane then phosphorylates Ser65 within Parkin's UBL domain that leads to the recruitment and tethering of Parkin to mitochondria. Besides of Parkin phosphorylation, PINK1 also phosphorylates Ser65 on ubiquitin and promotes the Parkin E3 ligase activity resulting in greater Parkin-induced ubiquitination of outer mitochondrial membrane protein, including the mitochondrial fusion proteins mitofusin 1 (Mfn1) and Mfn2, the mitochondrial trafficking protein Miro1, TOM20, and the voltage-dependent anion channel (VDAC) (Koyano et al., 2014). Degradation of Mfn1/Mfn2 causes imbalance of mitochondrial dynamic, resulting in mitochondrial fragmentation (Chan et al., 2011; Gegg et al., 2010; Geisler et al., 2010; Thomas et al., 2011). Ubiquitination and degradation of Miro1 lead to mitochondrial arrest, which can separate damaged mitochondria from healthy mitochondria. Both of mitochondrial fragmentation and mitochondrial arrest may further facilitate mitophagy since smaller mitochondria are likely more readily to be engulfed by autophagosomes (Ni et al., 2015; Wang et al., 2011).

Mitochondrial damage is well defined in alcoholic liver disease (Serviddio, Bellanti, Sastre, Vendemiale, & Altomare, 2010; Williams & Ding, 2015). As we discussed above, during the major oxidative metabolism of alcohol, excess NADH is generated and oxidized indirectly by mitochondrial electron transport system. The excessive amount of NADH and thus the reducing capacity in the mitochondrial electron transport system is thought to cause an increased leakage of mitochondrial ROS, causing alcohol-induced oxidative stress in livers. This has been shown to alter oxidative phosphorylation, mitochondrial proteome and mitochondrial dynamics. Mitochondrial fragmentation was observed in ethanol-treated hepatocytes (Ding, Li, & Yin, 2011; Ding, Manley, & Ni, 2011). Ethanol treatment also increased the sensitivity of mitochondrial permeability transition (King et al., 2014) and mitochondrial DNA depletion in livers of ethanol-treated mouse (Mansouri et al., 1999; Mansouri, Demeilliers, Amsellem, Pessayre, & Fromenty, 2001). Chronic ethanol consumption enhances oxidative damage to mtDNA along with increased strand breakage, and other alterations in the structural integrity of mitochondrial DNA (Cahill, Stabley, Wang, & Hoek, 1999), which has been thought to cause ethanol-related liver pathology. Mitophagy may be important to eliminate dysfunctional and potentially deleterious mitochondria (Williams & Ding, 2015). Alcohol-induced autophagy can selectively target to the damaged mitochondria as observed in both acute (Ding et al., 2010; Ding, Li, &

Yin, 2011; Ding, Manley, & Ni, 2011) and chronic (Eid, Ito, Maemura, & Otsuki, 2013) as well as Gao-binge alcohol (Williams et al., 2015). Alcohol-induced GFP-LC3 positive autophagosomes specifically envelop mitochondria have been documented (Ding et al., 2010; Ding, Li, & Yin, 2011; Ding, Manley, & Ni, 2011). What is the mechanism of this selectivity has yet to be determined. It is possible that the PINK1-Parkin signaling pathway may be involved. Immunoelectron microscopic studies indicated that expression of PINK1 was increased in mitochondria from ethanol-treated rats (Eid et al., 2013). To investigate the role of Parkin in alcohol-induced liver injury and steatosis, we recently used WT and Parkin KO mice that were treated with acute and Gao-binge alcohol model (Williams et al., 2015). We demonstrated that the translocation of Parkin to mitochondria and mitophagy increased after Gao-binge alcohol treatment in mouse livers, but not in acute alcohol treated mouse livers (Williams et al., 2015). Alcohol caused greater mitochondrial damage and oxidative stress in Parkin KO mouse livers compared with WT mouse livers. Furthermore, Parkin KO mice had decreased mitophagy, β-oxidation, mitochondrial respiration, and cytochrome c oxidase activity after acute alcohol treatment compared with WT mice. Interestingly, liver mitochondria seemed to be able to adapt to alcohol treatment, but mitochondria in Parkin KO mouse liver had less capacity to adapt to Gao-binge treatment compared with mitochondria in WT mouse liver. These data suggest that Parkin-mediated mitophagy may be protective against alcohol-induced liver injury by removing alcohol-induced damaged mitochondria. In addition to decreasing mitophagy, after alcohol treatment, Parkin KO mice had severely swollen and damaged mitochondria that lacked cristae, which were not seen in WT mice, suggesting that Parkin may have other roles in maintaining healthy mitochondria population (Williams et al., 2015). Other group also found that alcohol-mediated oxidative stress can also cause the translocation of the inducible form of heme oxygenase-1 (HO-1) to mitochondria, which in turn increases the recruitment of LC3 to the mitochondria (Bansal, Biswas, & Avadhani, 2014). The recognition of the damaged mitochondria could be mediated by multiple mechanisms after alcohol exposure and elucidation of these mechanisms is one of the important future works.

5.2 Removal of lipid droplet by autophagy

Excessive accumulation of hepatic triglycerides and fatty acids is one of the main features of alcoholic fatty liver diseases. Free fatty acids can be detrimental to hepatocytes. The esterified lipids are sequestered in LD and would be considered harmless, although de-esterification can occur, which would increase levels of cellular free fatty acids. Autophagosomes can transport the content of LD to the lysosome, in which lipids are degraded by the lysosomal acid lipase. This process, known as lipophagy (Singh et al., 2009), is still far from a complete understanding. Nevertheless, lipophagy occurs in alcohol-treated mouse livers although it could be impaired or insufficient (Ding, Li, & Yin, 2011; Ding, Manley, & Ni, 2011; Rasineni et al., 2017). Alcohol-induced GFP-LC3 positive autophagosomes specifically envelop LD have been observed in vivo and in vitro (Ding et al., 2010; Lin et al., 2013). While activating autophagy by rapamycin reduced hepatic TG level, inhibiting autophagy by chloroquine elevated hepatic TG level in both acute and chronic ALD models (Ding et al., 2010; Lin et al., 2013). Notably, similar observations can be made in a HFD-induced non-alcoholic fatty liver disease (NAFLD) model (Lin et al., 2013), suggesting that a common mechanism of lipophagy may be involved in the removal of lipids. In addition to the canonical lipophagy that may involve the autophagosomes, more recent evidence suggests that β-adrenergic (β-AR)/cAMP pathway-mediated LD lipolysis via cytosolic adipose triglyceride lipase (ATGL) and hormone-sensitive lipase (HSL) may be important for LD turnover (Schott et al., 2017). ATGL-mediated lipolysis may breakdown large LD into small LD that are favorable for the engulfment of autophagosomes that deliver the LD to lysosomes. Alternatively, small LD can be enveloped directly by lysosomes via microlipophagy or nanolipophagy (Schulze, Drizyte, et al., 2017; Schulze, Rasineni, et al., 2017). Indeed, we recently found that LD can directly penetrate into single membrane vesicles in hepatocytes during fasting (Li et al., 2018). Our unpublished data also show that the majority of isolated lysosomes from Gao-binge-treated mouse livers contain LD, suggesting a role of microlipophagy in regulating LD homeostasis. Interestingly, chronic ethanol exposure impaired (β-AR)/cAMP-mediated LD lipolysis and in turn blocked the mobilization of LD to lysosomes (Schott et al., 2017). Impaired LD lipolysis together with the impaired TFEB-mediated lysosomal biogenesis thus could be major contributors for the hepatic LD accumulation in the development of ALD.

5.3 Removal of protein aggregates by autophagy

It is well documented that chronic alcohol consumption can inhibit proteasome activity and induce endoplasmic reticulum (ER) stress resulting in the accumulation of aggregated proteins, which are called Mallory-Denk bodies (MDB) in the liver (Baraona, Leo, Borowsky, & Lieber, 1975; Donohue et al., 2007; Ji, 2008; Kaplowitz & Ji, 2006; Riley et al., 2002; Zatloukal et al., 2007). Early studies showed the rate of hepatic protein degradation in ethanol-fed animals declined significantly (Donohue, Zetterman, & Tuma, 1989), which might be due to declines in both proteasome and autophagy function, contributing to the development of hepatomegaly and the formation of MDB. These cytosolic inclusion bodies are characteristic hall markers of ALD, which are also often seen in autophagy deficiency. MDB is enriched with cytokeratin 8 and 18, and in association with other proteins including ubiquitin and p62 (Lahiri et al., 2016). p62 is able to polymerize via an N-terminal PB1 domain, and interacts with ubiquitinated proteins via the C-terminal UBA domain. p62 also binds directly to LC3 via its LC3 interacting region (LIR). p62 is an autophagy substrate protein and usually degraded by autophagy. p62 also acts as an autophagy receptor for selective autophagy such as selective autophagy for protein aggregates via its interaction with ubiquitinated proteins and LC3. The presence of MDB suggests that autophagy activity may be impaired in chronic alcohol consumption. Indeed, pharmacological activation autophagy by rapamycin, an mTORC1 inhibitor, increased the clearance of MDB in a keratin 8-overexpressing transgenic mouse model of MDB pathology (Harada, Hanada, Toivola, Ghori, & Omary, 2008). In another classical protein aggregates-induced liver injury model, the α1-antitrypsin deficiency, carbamazepine (CBZ) induced autophagy and decreased the hepatic load of α1-antitrypsin mutant proteins as well as hepatic fibrosis (Hidvegi et al., 2010). In contrast to rapamycin, CBZ induces autophagy in the liver independent of mTOR, suggesting that various autophagy pathways could be targeted to remove aggregated proteins and/or to treat liver diseases including ALD.

6. Conclusion

In summary, increasing evidence has indicated that alcohol may increase the formation of autophagosomes but may also impair either the lysosome functions or lysosomal biogenesis resulting in insufficient autophagy in hepatocytes. Pharmacological targeting lysosomal biogenesis or autophagy may protect against alcohol-induced liver injury by removing damaged mitochondria, protein aggregates and LD. Since ALD is a chronic liver disease, it remains to be studied whether activation of lysosomal

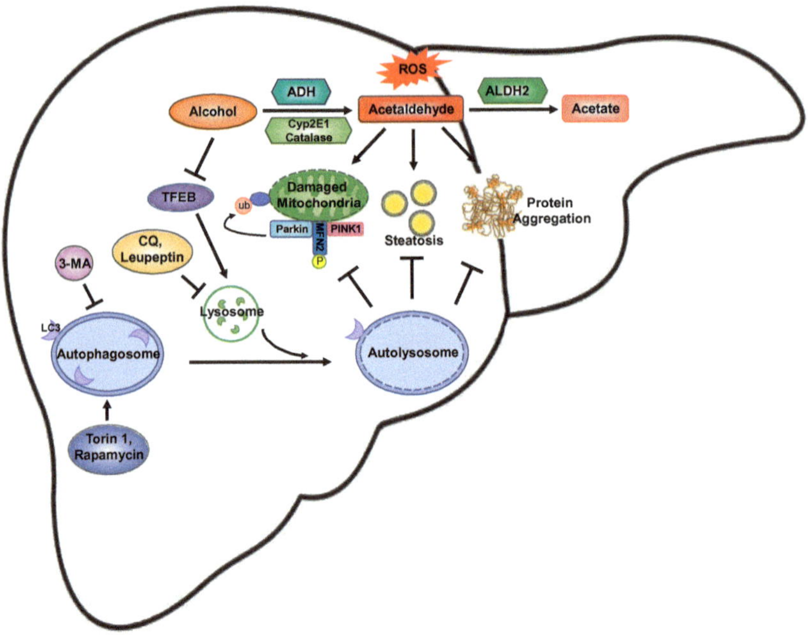

Fig. 1 A proposed model for the molecular events and mechanisms underlying the protection of autophagy against alcoholic liver disease. Alcohol is mainly metabolized in the liver through a major oxidative pathway. In this pathway, alcohol is catalyzed by alcohol dehydrogenase (ADH), which converts alcohol into highly reactive metabolite, acetaldehyde. A small portion of alcohol can also be oxidized into acetaldehyde by cytochrome P450 family 2, subfamily E, polypeptide 1 (Cyp2E1) and catalase. Acetaldehyde is further metabolized by mitochondrial aldehyde dehydrogenase 2 (ALDH2) into more harmless acetate. Alcohol consumption leads to mitochondria damage due to increased reactive oxygen species, lipid accumulation and formation of protein aggregates. Autophagy can be induced as an adapted protective mechanism to remove damaged mitochondria, accumulated lipid droplets and protein aggregates. The removal of damaged mitochondria is through selective mitophagy, which is mediated by the PINK1/Parkin pathway that promotes mitochondrial ubiquitination. However, chronic alcohol drinking inhibits the activity of transcription factor EB, which is a master regulator of lysosomal biogenesis and autophagy, leading to insufficient autophagy. Pharmacological induction of autophagy (Torin 1 or rapamycin) or inhibition of autophagy (Leupeptin, CQ or 3-MA) protects or exacerbates alcohol-induced liver injury and steatosis, respectively.

degradation and autophagy can reverse the chronic alcoholic pathogenesis such as fibrosis and inflammation by promoting liver repair and regeneration. The possible molecular events associated with autophagy that could be altered by alcohol consumption and the possible targets that can be manipulated to prevent and treat ALD are summarized in Fig. 1.

Acknowledgments

This work was partially supported by NIH grants: R01 AA020518, R01 DK102142, U01 AA024733 and P20GM103549 & P30GM118247 (W.X.D.), and CSC (No. 201708040024) (X.C.).

Conflict of interest

The authors declare no conflict of interest.

References

Bailey, S. M., & Cunningham, C. C. (2002). Contribution of mitochondria to oxidative stress associated with alcoholic liver disease. *Free Radical Biology & Medicine*, *32*, 11–16.

Bansal, S., Biswas, G., & Avadhani, N. G. (2014). Mitochondria-targeted heme oxygenase-1 induces oxidative stress and mitochondrial dysfunction in macrophages, kidney fibroblasts and in chronic alcohol hepatotoxicity. *Redox Biology*, *2*, 273–283.

Baraona, E., Leo, M. A., Borowsky, S. A., & Lieber, C. S. (1975). Alcoholic hepatomegaly: Accumulation of protein in the liver. *Science*, *190*, 794–795.

Beckemeier, M. E., & Bora, P. S. (1998). Fatty acid ethyl esters: Potentially toxic products of myocardial ethanol metabolism. *Journal of Molecular and Cellular Cardiology*, *30*, 2487–2494.

Behrends, C., & Fulda, S. (2012). Receptor proteins in selective autophagy. *International Journal of Cell Biology*, *2012*, 673290.

Bertola, A., Mathews, S., Ki, S. H., Wang, H., & Gao, B. (2013). Mouse model of chronic and binge ethanol feeding (the NIAAA model). *Nature Protocols*, *8*, 627–637.

Bertola, A., Park, O., & Gao, B. (2013). Chronic plus binge ethanol feeding synergistically induces neutrophil infiltration and liver injury in mice: A critical role for E-selectin. *Hepatology*, *58*, 1814–1823.

Burman, C., & Ktistakis, N. T. (2010). Regulation of autophagy by phosphatidylinositol 3-phosphate. *FEBS Letters*, *584*, 1302–1312.

Cahill, A., Stabley, G. J., Wang, X., & Hoek, J. B. (1999). Chronic ethanol consumption causes alterations in the structural integrity of mitochondrial DNA in aged rats. *Hepatology*, *30*, 881–888.

Cederbaum, A. I. (2012). Alcohol metabolism. *Clinics in Liver Disease*, *16*, 667–685.

Cederbaum, A. I., Lu, Y., & Wu, D. (2009). Role of oxidative stress in alcohol-induced liver injury. *Archives of Toxicology*, *83*, 519–548.

Chan, N. C., Salazar, A. M., Pham, A. H., Sweredoski, M. J., Kolawa, N. J., Graham, R. L., et al. (2011). Broad activation of the ubiquitin-proteasome system by Parkin is critical for mitophagy. *Human Molecular Genetics*, *20*, 1726–1737.

Chao, X., Ni, H. M., & Ding, W. X. (2018). Insufficient autophagy: A novel autophagic flux scenario uncovered by impaired liver TFEB-mediated lysosomal biogenesis from chronic alcohol-drinking mice. *Autophagy*, *14*, 1646–1648.

Chao, X., Wang, S., Zhao, K., Li, Y., Williams, J. A., Li, T., et al. (2018). Impaired TFEB-mediated lysosome biogenesis and autophagy promote chronic ethanol-induced liver injury and steatosis in mice. *Gastroenterology*, *155*, 865–879.e12.

Crabb, D. W., Matsumoto, M., Chang, D., & You, M. (2004). Overview of the role of alcohol dehydrogenase and aldehyde dehydrogenase and their variants in the genesis of alcohol-related pathology. *The Proceedings of the Nutrition Society*, *63*, 49–63.

Czaja, M. J., Ding, W. X., Donohue, T. M., Jr., Friedman, S. L., Kim, J. S., Komatsu, M., et al. (2013). Functions of autophagy in normal and diseased liver. *Autophagy*, *9*, 1131–1158.

De Duve, C., & Wattiaux, R. (1966). Functions of lysosomes. *Annual Review of Physiology*, *28*, 435–492.
Deas, E., Plun-Favreau, H., Gandhi, S., Desmond, H., Kjaer, S., Loh, S. H., et al. (2011). PINK1 cleavage at position A103 by the mitochondrial protease PARL. *Human Molecular Genetics*, *20*, 867–879.
Ding, W. X. (2010). Role of autophagy in liver physiology and pathophysiology. *World Journal of Biological Chemistry*, *1*, 3–12.
Ding, W. X., Li, M., Chen, X., Ni, H. M., Lin, C. W., Gao, W., et al. (2010). Autophagy reduces acute ethanol-induced hepatotoxicity and steatosis in mice. *Gastroenterology*, *139*, 1740–1752.
Ding, W. X., Li, M., & Yin, X. M. (2011). Selective taste of ethanol-induced autophagy for mitochondria and lipid droplets. *Autophagy*, *7*, 248–249.
Ding, W. X., Manley, S., & Ni, H. M. (2011). The emerging role of autophagy in alcoholic liver disease. *Experimental Biology and Medicine (Maywood, N.J.)*, *236*, 546–556.
Ding, W. X., & Yin, X. M. (2012). Mitophagy: Mechanisms, pathophysiological roles, and analysis. *Biological Chemistry*, *393*, 547–564.
Dolganiuc, A., Thomes, P. G., Ding, W. X., Lemasters, J. J., & Donohue, T. M., Jr. (2012). Autophagy in alcohol-induced liver diseases. *Alcoholism, Clinical and Experimental Research*, *36*, 1301–1308.
Donohue, T. M., Jr., Cederbaum, A. I., French, S. W., Barve, S., Gao, B., & Osna, N. A. (2007). Role of the proteasome in ethanol-induced liver pathology. *Alcoholism, Clinical and Experimental Research*, *31*, 1446–1459.
Donohue, T. M., Jr., Zetterman, R. K., & Tuma, D. J. (1989). Effect of chronic ethanol administration on protein catabolism in rat liver. *Alcoholism, Clinical and Experimental Research*, *13*, 49–57.
Egan, D., Kim, J., Shaw, R. J., & Guan, K. L. (2011). The autophagy initiating kinase ULK1 is regulated via opposing phosphorylation by AMPK and mTOR. *Autophagy*, *7*, 643–644.
Egan, D. F., Shackelford, D. B., Mihaylova, M. M., Gelino, S., Kohnz, R. A., Mair, W., et al. (2011). Phosphorylation of ULK1 (hATG1) by AMP-activated protein kinase connects energy sensing to mitophagy. *Science*, *331*, 456–461.
Eid, N., Ito, Y., Maemura, K., & Otsuki, Y. (2013). Elevated autophagic sequestration of mitochondria and lipid droplets in steatotic hepatocytes of chronic ethanol-treated rats: An immunohistochemical and electron microscopic study. *Journal of Molecular Histology*, *44*, 311–326.
Fader, C. M., Sanchez, D. G., Mestre, M. B., & Colombo, M. I. (2009). TI-VAMP/VAMP7 and VAMP3/cellubrevin: Two v-SNARE proteins involved in specific steps of the autophagy/multivesicular body pathways. *Biochimica et Biophysica Acta*, *1793*, 1901–1916.
Fedorowicz, M. A., de Vries-Schneider, R. L., Rub, C., Becker, D., Huang, Y., Zhou, C., et al. (2014). Cytosolic cleaved PINK1 represses Parkin translocation to mitochondria and mitophagy. *EMBO Reports*, *15*, 86–93.
Furuta, N., Fujita, N., Noda, T., Yoshimori, T., & Amano, A. (2010). Combinational soluble N-ethylmaleimide-sensitive factor attachment protein receptor proteins VAMP8 and Vti1b mediate fusion of antimicrobial and canonical autophagosomes with lysosomes. *Molecular Biology of the Cell*, *21*, 1001–1010.
Gao, B., & Bataller, R. (2011). Alcoholic liver disease: Pathogenesis and new therapeutic targets. *Gastroenterology*, *141*, 1572–1585.
Gegg, M. E., Cooper, J. M., Chau, K. Y., Rojo, M., Schapira, A. H., & Taanman, J. W. (2010). Mitofusin 1 and mitofusin 2 are ubiquitinated in a PINK1/parkin-dependent manner upon induction of mitophagy. *Human Molecular Genetics*, *19*, 4861–4870.

Geisler, S., Holmstrom, K. M., Skujat, D., Fiesel, F. C., Rothfuss, O. C., Kahle, P. J., et al. (2010). PINK1/Parkin-mediated mitophagy is dependent on VDAC1 and p62/SQSTM1. *Nature Cell Biology*, *12*, 119–131.

Green, D. R., & Levine, B. (2014). To be or not to be? How selective autophagy and cell death govern cell fate. *Cell*, *157*, 65–75.

Greene, A. W., Grenier, K., Aguileta, M. A., Muise, S., Farazifard, R., Haque, M. E., et al. (2012). Mitochondrial processing peptidase regulates PINK1 processing, import and Parkin recruitment. *EMBO Reports*, *13*, 378–385.

Harada, M., Hanada, S., Toivola, D. M., Ghori, N., & Omary, M. B. (2008). Autophagy activation by rapamycin eliminates mouse Mallory-Denk bodies and blocks their proteasome inhibitor-mediated formation. *Hepatology*, *47*, 2026–2035.

Hidvegi, T., Ewing, M., Hale, P., Dippold, C., Beckett, C., Kemp, C., et al. (2010). An autophagy-enhancing drug promotes degradation of mutant alpha1-antitrypsin Z and reduces hepatic fibrosis. *Science*, *329*, 229–232.

Hubert, V., Peschel, A., Langer, B., Groger, M., Rees, A., & Kain, R. (2016). LAMP-2 is required for incorporating syntaxin-17 into autophagosomes and for their fusion with lysosomes. *Biology Open*, *5*, 1516–1529.

Itakura, E., Kishi-Itakura, C., & Mizushima, N. (2012). The hairpin-type tail-anchored SNARE syntaxin 17 targets to autophagosomes for fusion with endosomes/lysosomes. *Cell*, *151*, 1256–1269.

Jager, S., Bucci, C., Tanida, I., Ueno, T., Kominami, E., Saftig, P., et al. (2004). Role for Rab7 in maturation of late autophagic vacuoles. *Journal of Cell Science*, *117*, 4837–4848.

Ji, C. (2008). Dissection of endoplasmic reticulum stress signaling in alcoholic and non-alcoholic liver injury. *Journal of Gastroenterology and Hepatology*, *23*(Suppl. 1), S16–S24.

Jin, S. M., Lazarou, M., Wang, C., Kane, L. A., Narendra, D. P., & Youle, R. J. (2010). Mitochondrial membrane potential regulates PINK1 import and proteolytic destabilization by PARL. *The Journal of Cell Biology*, *191*, 933–942.

Kaplowitz, N., & Ji, C. (2006). Unfolding new mechanisms of alcoholic liver disease in the endoplasmic reticulum. *Journal of Gastroenterology and Hepatology*, *21*(Suppl. 3), S7–S9.

Kihara, A., Noda, T., Ishihara, N., & Ohsumi, Y. (2001). Two distinct Vps34 phosphatidylinositol 3-kinase complexes function in autophagy and carboxypeptidase Y sorting in *Saccharomyces cerevisiae*. *The Journal of Cell Biology*, *152*, 519–530.

Kim, J., Kundu, M., Viollet, B., & Guan, K. L. (2011). AMPK and mTOR regulate autophagy through direct phosphorylation of Ulk1. *Nature Cell Biology*, *13*, 132–141.

King, A. L., Swain, T. M., Mao, Z., Udoh, U. S., Oliva, C. R., Betancourt, A. M., et al. (2014). Involvement of the mitochondrial permeability transition pore in chronic ethanol-mediated liver injury in mice. *American Journal of Physiology. Gastrointestinal and Liver Physiology*, *306*, G265–G277.

Klionsky, D. J., & Emr, S. D. (2000). Autophagy as a regulated pathway of cellular degradation. *Science*, *290*, 1717–1721.

Koyano, F., Okatsu, K., Kosako, H., Tamura, Y., Go, E., Kimura, M., et al. (2014). Ubiquitin is phosphorylated by PINK1 to activate parkin. *Nature*, *510*, 162–166.

Lahiri, P., Schmidt, V., Smole, C., Kufferath, I., Denk, H., Strnad, P., et al. (2016). p62/Sequestosome-1 is indispensable for maturation and stabilization of Mallory-Denk bodies. *PLoS One*, *11*, e0161083.

Lange, L. G., & Sobel, B. E. (1983). Mitochondrial dysfunction induced by fatty acid ethyl esters, myocardial metabolites of ethanol. *The Journal of Clinical Investigation*, *72*, 724–731.

Li, Y., Chao, X., Yang, L., Lu, Q., Li, T., Ding, W. X., et al. (2018). Impaired fasting-induced adaptive lipid droplet biogenesis in liver-specific Atg5-deficient mouse liver is mediated by persistent nuclear factor-like 2 activation. *The American Journal of Pathology*, *188*, 1833–1846.

Li, Y., & Ding, W. X. (2017). Impaired Rab7 and dynamin2 block fat turnover by autophagy in alcoholic fatty livers. *Hepatology Communications*, *1*, 473–476.

Li, Y., Wang, S., Ni, H. M., Huang, H., & Ding, W. X. (2014). Autophagy in alcohol-induced multiorgan injury: Mechanisms and potential therapeutic targets. *BioMed Research International*, *2014*, 498491.

Liang, C., Lee, J. S., Inn, K. S., Gack, M. U., Li, Q., Roberts, E. A., et al. (2008). Beclin1-binding UVRAG targets the class C Vps complex to coordinate autophagosome maturation and endocytic trafficking. *Nature Cell Biology*, *10*, 776–787.

Lin, C. W., Zhang, H., Li, M., Xiong, X., Chen, X., Chen, X., et al. (2013). Pharmacological promotion of autophagy alleviates steatosis and injury in alcoholic and non-alcoholic fatty liver conditions in mice. *Journal of Hepatology*, *58*, 993–999.

Loffler, A. S., Alers, S., Dieterle, A. M., Keppeler, H., Franz-Wachtel, M., Kundu, M., et al. (2011). Ulk1-mediated phosphorylation of AMPK constitutes a negative regulatory feedback loop. *Autophagy*, *7*, 696–706.

Lu, Y., & Cederbaum, A. I. (2008). CYP2E1 and oxidative liver injury by alcohol. *Free Radical Biology & Medicine*, *44*, 723–738.

Lu, Y., & Cederbaum, A. I. (2015). Autophagy protects against CYP2E1/chronic ethanol-induced hepatotoxicity. *Biomolecules*, *5*, 2659–2674.

Mansouri, A., Demeilliers, C., Amsellem, S., Pessayre, D., & Fromenty, B. (2001). Acute ethanol administration oxidatively damages and depletes mitochondrial dna in mouse liver, brain, heart, and skeletal muscles: Protective effects of antioxidants. *The Journal of Pharmacology and Experimental Therapeutics*, *298*, 737–743.

Mansouri, A., Gaou, I., De Kerguenec, C., Amsellem, S., Haouzi, D., Berson, A., et al. (1999). An alcoholic binge causes massive degradation of hepatic mitochondrial DNA in mice. *Gastroenterology*, *117*, 181–190.

Matsuda, N., Sato, S., Shiba, K., Okatsu, K., Saisho, K., Gautier, C. A., et al. (2010). PINK1 stabilized by mitochondrial depolarization recruits Parkin to damaged mitochondria and activates latent Parkin for mitophagy. *The Journal of Cell Biology*, *189*, 211–221.

Meissner, C., Lorenz, H., Weihofen, A., Selkoe, D. J., & Lemberg, M. K. (2011). The mitochondrial intramembrane protease PARL cleaves human Pink1 to regulate Pink1 trafficking. *Journal of Neurochemistry*, *117*, 856–867.

Mizushima, N. (2010). The role of the Atg1/ULK1 complex in autophagy regulation. *Current Opinion in Cell Biology*, *22*, 132–139.

Nagy, L. E., Ding, W. X., Cresci, G., Saikia, P., & Shah, V. H. (2016). Linking pathogenic mechanisms of alcoholic liver disease with clinical phenotypes. *Gastroenterology*, *150*, 1756–1768.

Nakatogawa, H., Suzuki, K., Kamada, Y., & Ohsumi, Y. (2009). Dynamics and diversity in autophagy mechanisms: Lessons from yeast. *Nature Reviews. Molecular Cell Biology*, *10*, 458–467.

Narendra, D. P., Jin, S. M., Tanaka, A., Suen, D. F., Gautier, C. A., Shen, J., et al. (2010). PINK1 is selectively stabilized on impaired mitochondria to activate Parkin. *PLoS Biology*, *8*, e1000298.

Ni, H. M., Bhakta, A., Wang, S., Li, Z., Manley, S., Huang, H., et al. (2014). Role of hypoxia inducing factor-1beta in alcohol-induced autophagy, steatosis and liver injury in mice. *PLoS One*, *9*, e115849.

Ni, H. M., Du, K., You, M., & Ding, W. X. (2013). Critical role of FoxO3a in alcohol-induced autophagy and hepatotoxicity. *The American Journal of Pathology*, *183*, 1815–1825.

Ni, H. M., Williams, J. A., & Ding, W. X. (2015). Mitochondrial dynamics and mitochondrial quality control. *Redox Biology*, *4*, 6–13.

Obara, K., Sekito, T., Niimi, K., & Ohsumi, Y. (2008). The Atg18-Atg2 complex is recruited to autophagic membranes via phosphatidylinositol 3-phosphate and exerts an essential function. *The Journal of Biological Chemistry*, *283*, 23972–23980.

Ohsumi, Y. (2001). Molecular dissection of autophagy: Two ubiquitin-like systems. *Nature Reviews. Molecular Cell Biology*, *2*, 211–216.

Papinski, D., Schuschnig, M., Reiter, W., Wilhelm, L., Barnes, C. A., Maiolica, A., et al. (2014). Early steps in autophagy depend on direct phosphorylation of Atg9 by the Atg1 kinase. *Molecular Cell*, *53*, 471–483.

Parzych, K. R., & Klionsky, D. J. (2014). An overview of autophagy: Morphology, mechanism, and regulation. *Antioxidants & Redox Signaling*, *20*, 460–473.

Polson, H. E., de Lartigue, J., Rigden, D. J., Reedijk, M., Urbe, S., Clague, M. J., et al. (2010). Mammalian Atg18 (WIPI2) localizes to omegasome-anchored phagophores and positively regulates LC3 lipidation. *Autophagy*, *6*, 506–522.

Rasineni, K., Donohue, T. M., Jr., Thomes, P. G., Yang, L., Tuma, D. J., McNiven, M. A., et al. (2017). Ethanol-induced steatosis involves impairment of lipophagy, associated with reduced Dynamin2 activity. *Hepatology Communications*, *1*, 501–512.

Reggiori, F., Komatsu, M., Finley, K., & Simonsen, A. (2012). Selective types of autophagy. *International Journal of Cell Biology*, *2012*, 156272.

Riley, N. E., Li, J., Worrall, S., Rothnagel, J. A., Swagell, C., van Leeuwen, F. W., et al. (2002). The Mallory body as an aggresome: In vitro studies. *Experimental and Molecular Pathology*, *72*, 17–23.

Russell, R. C., Tian, Y., Yuan, H., Park, H. W., Chang, Y. Y., Kim, J., et al. (2013). ULK1 induces autophagy by phosphorylating Beclin-1 and activating VPS34 lipid kinase. *Nature Cell Biology*, *15*, 741–750.

Schott, M. B., Rasineni, K., Weller, S. G., Schulze, R. J., Sletten, A. C., Casey, C. A., et al. (2017). Beta-adrenergic induction of lipolysis in hepatocytes is inhibited by ethanol exposure. *The Journal of Biological Chemistry*, *292*, 11815–11828.

Schroeder, B., Schulze, R. J., Weller, S. G., Sletten, A. C., Casey, C. A., & McNiven, M. A. (2015). The small GTPase Rab7 as a central regulator of hepatocellular lipophagy. *Hepatology*, *61*, 1896–1907.

Schulze, R. J., Drizyte, K., Casey, C. A., & McNiven, M. A. (2017). Hepatic lipophagy: New insights into autophagic catabolism of lipid droplets in the liver. *Hepatology Communications*, *1*, 359–369.

Schulze, R. J., Rasineni, K., Weller, S. G., Schott, M. B., Schroeder, B., Casey, C. A., et al. (2017). Ethanol exposure inhibits hepatocyte lipophagy by inactivating the small guanosine triphosphatase Rab7. *Hepatology Communications*, *1*, 140–152.

Serviddio, G., Bellanti, F., Sastre, J., Vendemiale, G., & Altomare, E. (2010). Targeting mitochondria: A new promising approach for the treatment of liver diseases. *Current Medicinal Chemistry*, *17*, 2325–2337.

Setshedi, M., Wands, J. R., & Monte, S. M. (2010). Acetaldehyde adducts in alcoholic liver disease. *Oxidative Medicine and Cellular Longevity*, *3*, 178–185.

Singh, R., Kaushik, S., Wang, Y., Xiang, Y., Novak, I., Komatsu, M., et al. (2009). Autophagy regulates lipid metabolism. *Nature*, *458*, 1131–1135.

Thomas, K. J., McCoy, M. K., Blackinton, J., Beilina, A., van der Brug, M., Sandebring, A., et al. (2011). DJ-1 acts in parallel to the PINK1/parkin pathway to control mitochondrial function and autophagy. *Human Molecular Genetics*, *20*, 40–50.

Thomes, P. G., Trambly, C. S., Fox, H. S., Tuma, D. J., & Donohue, T. M., Jr. (2015). Acute and chronic ethanol administration differentially modulate hepatic autophagy and transcription factor EB. *Alcoholism, Clinical and Experimental Research*, *39*, 2354–2363.

Thomes, P. G., Trambly, C. S., Thiele, G. M., Duryee, M. J., Fox, H. S., Haorah, J., et al. (2012). Proteasome activity and autophagosome content in liver are reciprocally regulated by ethanol treatment. *Biochemical and Biophysical Research Communications*, *417*, 262–267.

Thumm, M., Egner, R., Koch, B., Schlumpberger, M., Straub, M., Veenhuis, M., et al. (1994). Isolation of autophagocytosis mutants of *Saccharomyces cerevisiae*. *FEBS Letters*, *349*, 275–280.

Tsukada, M., & Ohsumi, Y. (1993). Isolation and characterization of autophagy-defective mutants of *Saccharomyces cerevisiae*. *FEBS Letters, 333*, 169–174.
Tsukamoto, H., Reidelberger, R. D., French, S. W., & Largman, C. (1984). Long-term cannulation model for blood sampling and intragastric infusion in the rat. *The American Journal of Physiology, 247*, R595–R599.
Vives-Bauza, C., Zhou, C., Huang, Y., Cui, M., de Vries, R. L., Kim, J., et al. (2010). PINK1-dependent recruitment of Parkin to mitochondria in mitophagy. *Proceedings of the National Academy of Sciences of the United States of America, 107*, 378–383.
Wang, X., Winter, D., Ashrafi, G., Schlehe, J., Wong, Y. L., Selkoe, D., et al. (2011). PINK1 and Parkin target Miro for phosphorylation and degradation to arrest mitochondrial motility. *Cell, 147*, 893–906.
Webber, J. L., & Tooze, S. A. (2010). Coordinated regulation of autophagy by p38alpha MAPK through mAtg9 and p38IP. *The EMBO Journal, 29*, 27–40.
Werner, J., Saghir, M., Warshaw, A. L., Lewandrowski, K. B., Laposata, M., Iozzo, R. V., et al. (2002). Alcoholic pancreatitis in rats: Injury from nonoxidative metabolites of ethanol. *American Journal of Physiology. Gastrointestinal and Liver Physiology, 283*, G65–G73.
Williams, J. A., & Ding, W. X. (2015). A mechanistic review of mitophagy and its role in protection against alcoholic liver disease. *Biomolecules, 5*, 2619–2642.
Williams, J. A., & Ding, W. X. (2018). Mechanisms, pathophysiological roles and methods for analyzing mitophagy—Recent insights. *Biological Chemistry, 399*, 147–178.
Williams, J. A., Manley, S., & Ding, W. X. (2014). New advances in molecular mechanisms and emerging therapeutic targets in alcoholic liver diseases. *World Journal of Gastroenterology, 20*, 12908–12933.
Williams, J. A., Ni, H. M., Ding, Y., & Ding, W. X. (2015). Parkin regulates mitophagy and mitochondrial function to protect against alcohol-induced liver injury and steatosis in mice. *American Journal of Physiology. Gastrointestinal and Liver Physiology, 309*, G324–G340.
Wu, H., Bhopale, K. K., Ansari, G. A., & Kaphalia, B. S. (2008). Ethanol-induced cytotoxicity in rat pancreatic acinar AR42J cells: Role of fatty acid ethyl esters. *Alcohol and Alcoholism, 43*, 1–8.
Wu, H., Cai, P., Clemens, D. L., Jerrells, T. R., Ansari, G. A., & Kaphalia, B. S. (2006). Metabolic basis of ethanol-induced cytotoxicity in recombinant HepG2 cells: Role of nonoxidative metabolism. *Toxicology and Applied Pharmacology, 216*, 238–247.
Wu, D., Wang, X., Zhou, R., Yang, L., & Cederbaum, A. I. (2012). Alcohol steatosis and cytotoxicity: The role of cytochrome P4502E1 and autophagy. *Free Radical Biology & Medicine, 53*, 1346–1357.
Yamano, K., & Youle, R. J. (2013). PINK1 is degraded through the N-end rule pathway. *Autophagy, 9*, 1758–1769.
Yin, X. M., Ding, W. X., & Gao, W. (2008). Autophagy in the liver. *Hepatology, 47*, 1773–1785.
Yoon, Y.-H. C. C. (2018). *Liver cirrhosis mortality in the United States: National, state, and regional trends, 2000–2015*. Surveillance Report #111. Available at: https://pubs.niaaa.nih.gov/publications/surveillance111/Cirr115.htm.
Zakhari, S. (2006). Overview: How is alcohol metabolized by the body? *Alcohol Research & Health, 29*, 245–254.
Zatloukal, K., French, S. W., Stumptner, C., Strnad, P., Harada, M., Toivola, D. M., et al. (2007). From Mallory to Mallory-Denk bodies: What, how and why? *Experimental Cell Research, 313*, 2033–2049.
Zelner, I., Matlow, J. N., Natekar, A., & Koren, G. (2013). Synthesis of fatty acid ethyl esters in mammalian tissues after ethanol exposure: A systematic review of the literature. *Drug Metabolism Reviews, 45*, 277–299.

Further reading

Kim, J., & Guan, K. L. (2011). Regulation of the autophagy initiating kinase ULK1 by nutrients: Roles of mTORC1 and AMPK. *Cell Cycle*, *10*, 1337–1338.
WHO. Management of substance abuse, Available at: http://www.who.int/substance_abuse/facts/alcohol/en/.

CHAPTER FIVE

Mechanisms of idiosyncratic drug-induced liver injury

Jack Uetrecht[1]
Faculties of Pharmacy and Medicine, University of Toronto, Toronto, ON, Canada
[1]Corresponding author: e-mail address: jack.uetrecht@utoronto.ca

Contents

Abstract

Idiosyncratic drug-induced liver injury (IDILI) is a significant problem. Little is known with certainty about the mechanisms of IDILI. However, there is growing evidence that most IDILI is immune mediated and caused by reactive metabolites. The two major and complementary hypotheses that link reactive metabolite formation with the induction of an immune response that can lead to IDILI are the hapten and danger hypotheses. Specifically, a reactive metabolite can bind to proteins and make them foreign; however, without activation of antigen presenting cells (APCs), the immune response will be immune tolerance. Not all reactive metabolites are associated with the same risk of causing IDILI. If the reactive metabolite can also cause some cell damage, this can lead to the release of danger-associated molecular pattern molecules (DAMPs) that activate APCs. Other hypotheses for the mechanism of IDILI include mitochondrial injury,

Advances in Pharmacology, Volume 85
ISSN 1054-3589
https://doi.org/10.1016/bs.apha.2018.12.001
© 2019 Elsevier Inc.
All rights reserved.

inhibition of the bile salt export pump, and endoplasmic reticulum stress. These mechanisms may be complementary to the danger hypothesis in that they may cause the release of DAMPs. None of these hypotheses has been adequately tested. Previous animal models have had characteristics very different from IDILI in humans and are unlikely to involve the same mechanism. However, impairment of immune tolerance has led to a model with characteristics very similar to IDILI in humans. This will make it possible to rigorously test hypotheses. A better mechanistic understanding of IDILI should lead to better methods to screen drug candidates for IDILI risk and treat IDILI when it occurs.

Abbreviations

ADRs adverse drug reactions
ALP alkaline phosphatase
ALT alanine transaminase
APC antigen presenting cell
AST aspartate transaminase
ATF activating transcription factor
BiP binding immunoglobulin protein
BSEP bile salt export pump
CD cluster of differentiation
CREBH to cAMP response element-binding protein H
CTLA-4 cytotoxic T lymphocyte-associated protein 4
CYP cytochrome P450 gene
DAMP danger-associated molecular pattern molecule
DRESS drug reaction with eosinophilia and systemic symptoms
eIF2α eukaryotic translation initiation factor2α
EP endoplasmic reticulum
GRP78 glucose regulatory protein 78
HLA human leukocyte antigen
IDILI idiosyncratic drug-induced liver injury
IDRs idiosyncratic drug reactions
IKK IκB kinase
IL interleukin
INR international ratio
IRE1 inositol-requiring enzyme 1
MHC major histocompatibility complex
MRP multidrug resistance protein
NASH nonalcoholic steatohepatitis
NF-κB nuclear factor light-chain-enhancer of activated B cells
NK natural killer
P450 cytochromes P450
PD-1 programmed cell death protein-1
PERK protein kinase RNA-like ER kinase
PKR protein kinase RNA-activated
ROS reactive oxygen species

TCR	T cell receptor
THP-1	a human monocyte cell line
TNF-α	tumor necrosis factor-alpha
Tregs	T regulatory cells
UPR	unfolded protein response

1. Introduction

1.1 Significance

Adverse drug reactions (ADRs) are a major cause of patient morbidity and mortality (Pirmohamed et al., 2004). Although most ADRs can be predicted based on the pharmacology of the drug (often referred to as type A reactions), many are unrelated to the therapeutic effect of the drug and do not occur in most patients treated with the drug at any dose; these are referred to as type B or idiosyncratic drug reactions (IDRs). Although less common than type A reactions, the unpredictable nature of IDRs make them more difficult to avoid. They are especially problematic for drug development because they significantly increase the risk of drug development. For example, if a drug is associated with a 1/10,000 incidence of a life-threatening IDR its use would be unacceptable except for very serious conditions such as cancer or HIV infections. Yet clinical trials usually involve <10,000 patients and so serious IDRs are often not detected until a drug has been on the market for some time and a very large number of patients have been treated. This can result in the withdrawal of the drug after a very large amount of resources have been spent on its development. In addition, even if a drug is ultimately successful, there are often "signals" during drug development such as evidence of liver injury in animals that suggest a drug may cause serious IDRs, and this can significantly delay development. The major IDR leading to drug candidate failure is idiosyncratic drug-induced liver injury (IDILI), which is the focus of this review.

1.2 Clinical characteristics of IDILI

There are three major types of IDILI: hepatocellular liver injury, cholestatic liver injury, and autoimmune hepatitis. There can be overlap between the types, and the same drug can cause a different pattern in different patients. It is very important to be familiar with the clinical characteristics of IDILI because they provide mechanistic clues, and any mechanistic hypothesis should be consistent with these characteristics. Although idiosyncratic drug reactions can be limited to the liver, IDILI can be part of a systemic adverse reaction such as drug reaction with eosinophilia and systemic symptoms (DRESS) or toxic epidermal necrolysis (Roujeau, 2005).

1.2.1 Hepatocellular IDILI

The most common type of IDILI leading to liver failure is hepatocellular IDILI (Hayashi et al., 2017). Like most other IDRs, hepatocellular IDILI is characterized by a delay between starting a drug and the onset of liver injury. This delay is typically 1–3 months, but it can be longer. The onset of liver injury can even be delayed for as much as a month after stopping a drug (Keisu & Andersson, 2010), and in serious cases the injury can progress after the drug has been discontinued. With a few drugs, especially telithromycin (Clay et al., 2006) and the fluoroquinolones, the delay can be very short, i.e., a matter of days, and with other drugs such as troglitazone, a longer delay of several months to a year is not uncommon (Watkins & Whitcomb, 1998). Mild injury that often resolves despite continued treatment with the drug is more common than serious liver injury, and if a drug does not cause mild injury in ~1% or more of patients it is unlikely to be associated with a significant incidence of serious liver injury (Temple's corollary) (Watkins et al., 2011). However, some drugs such as the statins commonly cause mild injury but rarely cause liver failure; there is not a good correlation between the incidence of mild injury and serious liver injury.

The liver injury can be asymptomatic or it can be associated with constitutional symptoms such as nausea, fatigue, and right upper quadrant abdominal pain. In some cases IDILI can also be accompanied by a fever and rash. This is uncommon with most drugs, although hepatocellular liver injury can be part of a more generalized immune-mediated IDR such as DRESS as mentioned above.

The liver injury is associated with an increase in alanine transaminase (ALT) and aspartate transaminase (AST), and the ALT is generally higher than the AST. The transaminases are often referred to as liver function tests, but they are not a measure of liver function; rather they represent a measure of liver injury. There is not even a good correlation between the height of the ALT and the degree of liver injury because liver injury with a relatively modest increase in ALT spread over a long period of time can lead to liver failure, while a very high ALT representing acute injury that resolves rapidly will not lead to a decrease in liver function. The function of the liver includes clearance of bilirubin and ammonia and synthesis of clotting factors. Therefore, elevated conjugated bilirubin and ammonia as well as an increased prothrombin time (commonly expressed as a international ratio, INR) are an indication of decreased liver function. In the case of hepatocellular IDILI, if there is an increase in bilirubin along with an increase in ALT, and there is no other potential cause for the increase in bilirubin, it is associated with a ~10% mortality. This is referred to as Hy's law or rule, because it was first noted by Hyman Zimmerman (Senior, 2006). Originally the increase in bilirubin used for this assessment by Hyman Zimmerman was jaundice, which is about 3 times the upper limit of normal, but now the increase in bilirubin used to define Hy's law is 2 times the upper limit of normal.

The liver histology in hepatocellular IDILI is characterized by piecemeal hepatocyte necrosis with a mononuclear leukocyte infiltrate consisting mostly of T cells and macrophages (Foureau et al., 2015). The histology is similar to viral hepatitis, but the number of natural killer (NK) cells is generally less than with viral hepatitis. Eosinophils are present in up to 50% of cases, and the presence of eosinophils was associated with a better outcome (Kleiner et al., 2014).

1.2.2 Cholestatic IDILI

Clinically, cholestatic IDILI is differentiated from hepatocellular IDILI by the ratio of ALT to alkaline phosphatase (ALP). Both the ALT and ALP are expressed as the ratio compared to the upper limit of normal; therefore, the ALT/ALP used for the determination is a ratio of ratios. In hepatocellular IDILI this ratio is >5, and with cholestatic IDILI the ratio is <2 (Kleiner et al., 2014). If the ALT/ALP ratio is between 2 and 5 it is considered mixed hepatocellular/cholestatic injury. Cholestatic IDILI is associated with a significantly lower risk of death (Zimmerman, 1999), although this has been questioned (Bjornsson & Olsson, 2005). Cholestatic injury is more common in older patients, and resolution is usually slow and can take a month or more.

1.2.3 Autoimmune IDILI

Drugs can also cause IDILI that resembles idiopathic autoimmune hepatitis (Bjornsson et al., 2010; Czaja, 2011; deLemos et al., 2014). As with idiopathic autoimmune hepatitis, the incidence is higher in females. The delay in onset is usually significantly longer that with other types of IDILI: often more than a year. Although many drugs may cause autoimmune IDILI, the two most common causes are minocycline and nitrofurantoin. More recently, therapeutic antibodies such as anti-tumor necrosis factor-alpha (TNF-α) (Favalli, Varenna, & Sinigaglia, 2005) and anti-CD25 antibodies

(Giovannoni et al., 2014) have also been associated with autoimmune IDLIL. Although there are no absolute criteria, a major diagnostic feature of autoimmune IDILI is the presence of autoantibodies such as anti-nuclear antibodies and anti-smooth muscle antibodies as well as hypergammaglobulinemia. The histology of autoimmune IDILI is similar to that of idiopathic autoimmune hepatitis, which is characterized by interface hepatitis and an increase in plasma cells. As with idiopathic autoimmune hepatitis, response to corticosteroids is usually good, but one differentiating feature is that autoimmune IDILI is unlikely to recur when the steroid treatment is stopped.

2. Involvement of reactive metabolites in the mechanism of IDILI

There is a large amount of circumstantial evidence that the mechanism of most IDILI involves the intrinsic chemical reactivity of drugs such as β-lactams, or is caused by reactive metabolites of drugs. Examples of reactive metabolites that are associated with IDILI are provided in the review by Leung, Kalgutkar, and Obach (2012). However, given the difficulty in performing mechanistic studies, it is difficult to adequately test this hypothesis. In addition, many drugs form more than one reactive metabolite, and it is difficult to be confident which of the several reactive metabolites is responsible for a specific IDILI. For example, carbamazepine can form epoxide, arene oxide, iminoquinone and quinone reactive metabolites (Pearce, Uetrecht, & Leeder, 2005; Pearce, Vakkalagadda, & Leeder, 2002; Yip et al., 2017). It is likely that the site and reactivity of a reactive metabolite determines what type of IDR a drug will cause. Two different reactive metabolites formed by the same drug can be responsible for two different types of IDRs. For example, nevirapine forms a reactive sulfate conjugate in the skin that is responsible for nevirapine-induced skin rash, and a quinone methide is formed in the liver that is likely responsible for nevirapine-induced IDILI (Chen, Mannargudi, Xu, & Uetrecht, 2008). Presumably one reason that the liver is a common target of IDRs is that it is the site of most drug metabolism and reactive metabolite formation. In addition, many drugs are concentrated by the liver. There is some correlation between the amount of covalent binding to human hepatocytes when corrected for daily dose (Nakayama et al., 2009), but the correlation is far from perfect (Obach, Kalgutkar, Soglia, & Zhao, 2008). In part this is because not all covalent binding has the same potential to cause IDRs, and which proteins are modified is also an important determinant as discussed in Section 4.3. Attempts have been made to correlate the targets of covalent binding with toxicity; however, these studies tested drugs associated with direct cytotoxicity rather than IDILI (Hanzlik, Koen, & Fang, 2013).

3. Immune system involvement in IDILI

There is little question that some types of IDRs such as skin rashes, autoimmune IDRs, and β-lactam-induced anaphylaxis are immune mediated. Hyman Zimmerman classed IDILI into two categories: immune idiosyncrasy and metabolic idiosyncrasy based on whether they had characteristics of an allergic reaction (Zimmerman, 1999). However, even the drugs that he classed as metabolic idiosyncrasy appear to be immune mediated. For example, the prototypic IDILI classed as metabolic idiosyncrasy is isoniazid-induced IDILI. However, it is associated with anti-drug antibodies and antibodies against the cytochromes P450 (P450) that metabolize the drug (Metushi, Sanders, Lee, & Uetrecht, 2014). Isoniazid DILI is also associated with a positive lymphocyte transformation test (Warrington, Tse, Gorski, Schwenk, & Sehon, 1978). Furthermore, patients who are treated with isoniazid resulting in a small increase in ALT also have an increase in peripheral lymphocytes that produce interleukin-17 (IL-17), and other T cells that produce IL-10 (Metushi et al., 2014). One of the reasons that isoniazid was not believed to be immune mediated is that patients can often be rechallenged without recurrence of injury. However, this is the pattern with mild injury, which usually resolves even when the drug is continued. With more severe injury, rechallenge can result in an immediate recurrence (Maddrey & Boitnott, 1973). An immune mechanism is also the most likely explanation for the idiosyncratic nature of IDILI; we are familiar with the fact that only a minority of individuals have a severe immune response to things such as peanuts. The observation that virtually all IDILI is associated with a delay between starting the drug and the onset of the liver injury is also consistent with an immune mechanism, although there are other potential mechanisms for a delay in onset. In addition, the fact that the onset can occur or progress well after the drug has been discontinued is also consistent with an immune response, which either has an autoimmune component or involves an immune response to a drug-modified protein that persists longer than the drug itself. Furthermore, the liver histology of IDILI is typical of an immune response (Kleiner et al., 2014). As mentioned above, it is similar to that of viral hepatitis, which is dominated by a mononuclear leukocyte infiltrate; however, the number of NK cells is usually less in IDILI than in viral hepatitis. This suggests that most IDILI is mediated by cytotoxic T cells. Eosinophils are also present in about a third of IDILI cases, either in the peripheral blood or liver histology (Kleiner et al., 2014). As mentioned above, there is a plausible link between the involvement of reactive metabolites and an immune mechanism of DILI, and antidrug antibodies and autoantibodies have been detected in halothane (Vergani et al., 1980) and isoniazid IDILI (Metushi et al., 2014).

A relatively recent finding is that many IDRs, including IDILI, are associated with specific HLA genotypes (Daly, 2013; Osanlou, Pirmohamed, & Daly, 2018). This provides very strong evidence for an immune mechanism. However, for most drugs, an association has not been studied because there have not been sufficient patient samples available for study, and in still other cases such as isoniazid, if there is an HLA association, it is quite weak. This is not surprising; if isoniazid IDILI represents an immune response against drug-modified proteins as suggested above, a major reactive metabolite of isoniazid reacts with amino groups and probably modifies most proteins (Metushi, Nakagawa, & Uetrecht, 2012). There should be some HLA in most patients that would recognize one of the many, probably thousands, of isoniazid-modified peptides that would be formed during processing of these proteins by antigen presenting cells. The more potential antigenic structures that are formed by a reactive metabolite, the less likely that the immune response will be limited to one or two HLA genotypes. Another point is that even when IDILI is associated with a specific HLA genotype, with the exception of abacavir-induced hypersensitivity, if a patient with the required HLA genotype takes a drug that can cause IDILI, it is still unlikely that they will develop IDILI. For example, it appears that 80% of patients who develop flucloxacillin IDILI carry the HLA-B*5701 genotype; however, if a patient with this genotype takes flucloxacillin, there is <1 in 500 chance that they will develop IDILI (Daly et al., 2009). Therefore, other risk factors must be important for the development of IDILI. Overall, the combined evidence is overwhelming that many cases of IDILI are immune mediated. Furthermore, the fact that the characteristics of most IDILI are very similar suggests that most IDILI is immune mediated; however, it is possible that some cases are not immune mediated.

If IDILI is immune mediated, and in many cases the immune response is initiated by a reactive metabolite formed in the liver, the question becomes how does a reactive metabolite induce an immune response that in some cases leads to IDILI. To borrow from the example of penicillin-induced hypersensitivity, it is known that penicillin is chemically reactive and covalently binds to proteins. Patients who develop penicillin-induced hypersensitivity have IgE antibodies that recognize penicillin-modified proteins, and these antibodies mediate the hypersensitivity reaction (Parker & Thiel, 1963). In contrast, it appears that IDILI is usually mediated by T cells (Kim & Naisbitt, 2016). It is more difficult to study cell-mediated immune responses, but the principle is the same. The observation that modification of proteins by small molecules can lead to an immune response is known as the hapten hypothesis, where the small molecule that binds to proteins represents the hapten (Landsteiner & Jacobs, 1935). Classic studies led to the idea that haptens make the proteins "foreign," and it is the role of the immune system to recognize and destroy things that were foreign. However, this hypothesis is incomplete because it was also recognized that foreign proteins rarely induce a strong immune response without something such as an adjuvant that activates antigen presenting cells (APCs). Janeway referred to adjuvants as the "immunologist's dirty little secret" because of this requirement (Janeway, 1989). This led to a second hypothesis to complement the hapten hypothesis, i.e., the danger hypothesis (Matzinger, 1994). This hypothesis posits that unless the "foreign" protein is associated with some damage to the organism, the immune system will ignore it. The damage leads to the release of danger-associated molecular pattern molecules (DAMPs) that activate APCs, and without this activation of APCs the immune response is tolerance. The recognition of antigen by T cells is referred to as signal 1 and the activation of APCs is referred to as signal 2. Both signals are required for an immune response. Applying these hypotheses to IDILI leads to a picture of IDILI in which drugs that form reactive metabolites in the liver can act as haptens and bind to hepatic proteins to make them foreign. However, this does not lead to a strong immune response unless the reactive metabolite also causes some damage to the hepatocyte leading to the release of DAMPs that activate APCs, i.e., signal 2. This could explain why not all reactive metabolite formation is associated with the same risk of IDILI. These concepts are presented in Fig. 1.

The location of a haptenated protein has a major effect on how it is presented to the immune system and what type of immune response results. A very reactive metabolite that binds to intracellular proteins close to where it is formed will be presented on the surface of a hepatocyte in the context of major histocompatibility complex I (MHC-I) and be recognized by a CD8 T cell leading to a cell-mediated immune response. For example, the quinone methide of nevirapine is so reactive that much of its covalent binding is to the P450 that formed it (Sharma, Li, Novalen, Hayes, & Uetrecht, 2012).

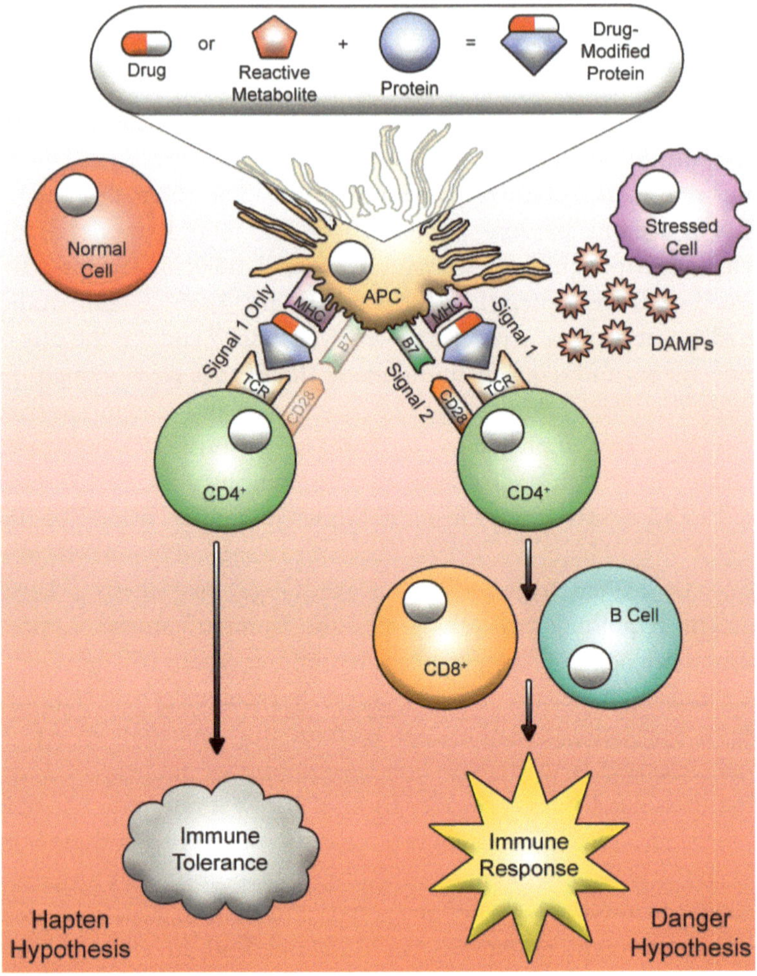

Fig. 1 The two major hypotheses that link the formation of a reactive metabolite and the induction of an immune response that can lead to IDILI are the hapten and danger hypotheses. The hapten hypothesis involves the modification of proteins to make them foreign. This produces signal 1. However, without signal 2 the result is immune tolerance. The danger hypothesis involves cell damage with the release of DAMPs. This activates APCs and produces signal 2, which when combined with signal 1 can lead to an immune response resulting in IDILI. *Reprinted with permission from Cho, T., & Uetrecht, J. (2017). How reactive metabolites induce an immune response that sometimes leads to an idiosyncratic drug reaction.* Chemical Research in Toxicology, 30, *295–314. Copyright 2017 American Chemical Society.*

In contrast, a less reactive drug or metabolite that can circulate and bind to extracellular proteins such as β-lactams or acyl glucuronides will be presented to the immune system by major histocompatibility complex-II (MHC-II) and be recognized by CD4 T cells. This is more likely to cause an antibody-mediated immune response, e.g., penicillin-induced IgE-mediated hypersensitivity reactions. Covalent binding to a high abundance protein may not cause much of an immune response, and if the binding to a protein can be removed from a protein during antigen processing, e.g., a disulfide bond, it may not result in any immune response.

However, the immune response is complex, and even if the immune response is predominantly mediated by cytotoxic T cells, antibodies are also usually formed. Furthermore, some drugs that cause IDILI such as ximelagatran do not appear to form reactive metabolites and appear to directly, but non-covalently, interact with MHC-II (Kindmark et al., 2008). Other potential mechanisms that do not involve a reactive metabolite include the mechanisms involved in the p-i hypothesis and the altered peptide presentation hypothesis (Cho & Uetrecht, 2017).

4. Other proposed mechanisms of IDILI

It is possible that not all IDILI are immune mediated. Several other mechanisms have been proposed as discussed below. However, these hypotheses are not mutually exclusive. Specifically, a mechanism such as bile salt export pump inhibition or the unfolded protein response could cause the release of DAMPs, which in turn, supply signal 2 and result in an immune response.

4.1 Mitochondrial injury

It has been proposed that IDILI is caused by mitochondrial injury (Boelsterli & Lim, 2007). Mitochondria play a very important role in cell death; therefore, it is plausible that mitochondrial injury could lead to hepatocyte injury. The liver injury caused by acetaminophen, which causes more liver failure than any other drug, involves mitochondrial injury (Hinson, Roberts, & James, 2010). However, acetaminophen-induced liver injury is acute and not idiosyncratic. Fialuridine, a drug developed for the treatment of hepatitis B, caused liver failure by inhibition of mitochondrial DNA synthesis (McKenzie et al., 1995). However, the injury was not limited to the liver, and it was not really idiosyncratic. Other drugs, mostly nucleoside-type antiviral drugs such as stavudine and zidovudine can also cause liver injury by inhibition of mitochondrial DNA synthesis (Brinkman, ter Hofstede, Burger, Smeitink, & Koopmans, 1998). The mitochondrial injury is cumulative, and the risk is a function of dose and duration of therapy. It is usually characterized by steatosis and lactic acidosis, which is characteristic of decreased mitochondrial dysfunction. Linezolid inhibits mitochondrial protein synthesis and can cause liver injury; however, the liver is not the major target of linezolid toxicity; anemias and neurotoxicity are more common, and again the injury is not really idiosyncratic (Vazquez, Arnold, Swanson, Biswas, & Bassetti, 2016). Given the function of mitochondria, a major clue to the mechanism of agents that cause liver injury by damaging mitochondria is the presence of lactic acidosis and/or microvesicular steatosis, which is not typical of most IDILI. The one drug that causes IDILI with a mechanism that clearly does involve mitochondria is valproate IDILI. Valproate IDILI is usually associated with microvesicular steatosis and often lactic acidosis (Bryant & Dreifuss, 1996). The IDILI caused by valproate is also different from most other IDILI in that it is much more common in infants than in adults. Further evidence of mitochondrial involvement is that a genetic polymorphism in mitochondrial DNA polymerase is a major risk factor for valproate IDILI (Stewart et al., 2010). In addition, valproate is a branched chain carboxylic acid, which inhibits fatty acid metabolism, which explains at least part of its effects on mitochondrial function (Silva et al., 2008). Although there is ample evidence that the mechanism of valproate IDILI involves mitochondrial injury, it is possible that there is also an immune component to the mechanism.

It has been proposed that many other drugs cause IDILI by inhibition of the mitochondrial electron transport chain (Dykens & Will, 2007). However, inhibition of the mitochondrial electron transport chain causes lactic acidosis, which is not a common feature of IDILI. In contrast, metformin clearly does inhibit complex I of the mitochondrial electron transport chain and can cause lactic acidosis, but rarely if ever causes IDILI. It is possible that inhibition of the mitochondrial electron transport chain causes cell damage leading to a danger signal, which promotes an immune response. If that were the case, then inhibition of the mitochondrial electron transport chain could play a role in the mechanism of IDILI, but be insufficient on its own to cause IDILI. However, there is no evidence that metformin increases the IDILI risk of co-administered drugs, and given the common use of metformin and the fact that patients with type II diabetes commonly use other medication, it is likely that if metformin did increase the risk of IDILI caused by co-administered drugs, such an interaction would be detected. Phenformin also inhibits complex I of the mitochondrial electron transport chain. It was withdrawn from the market because it is cleared by CYP 2D6, which is polymorphic, and poor metabolizers were at increased risk of lactic acidosis. As with metformin, phenformin was not associated with a significant risk of IDILI.

It was reported that the combination of isoniazid and rotenone was toxic to hepatocytes in vitro at concentrations that were not toxic individually

(Lee, Fujimoto, et al., 2013). Rotenone is the classic inhibitor of mitochondrial complex I, and hydrazine, a metabolite of isoniazid inhibits complex II. Rotenone may be more toxic than metformin because its inhibition is essentially irreversible, and it leads to more of an increase in reactive oxygen species than metformin (Siddiqui et al., 2013). It was proposed that drugs that inhibit complex I would increase the risk of isoniazid IDILI. We tested this hypothesis in vivo. We found that the combination of isoniazid and rotenone was indeed lethal in mice after about 8 days; however, there was no evidence of significant liver injury. As mentioned before, it is possible that inhibition of complex I would help to induce an immune response. However, in our impaired immune tolerance model where isoniazid does cause mild liver injury, addition of rotenone at half the lethal dose did not increase isoniazid-induced liver injury (Cho & Uetrecht, 2018).

Together, these data provide convincing evidence that inhibition of the mitochondrial electron transport chain is not involved in the mechanism of IDILI. However, inhibition of the mitochondrial electron transport chain is the basis for one of the tests to screen drug candidates for their potential to cause IDILI commonly used by the pharmaceutical industry; specifically, the effects of drugs on oxygen uptake by isolated mitochondria (Aleo et al., 2014). But the evidence that this assay helps to predict IDILI risk is weak, and simple properties of a molecule appear to be more accurate at predicting risk (Chan & Benet, 2018). It is possible that other types of mitochondrial injury leading to the release of DAMPs could be involved in the mechanism of IDILI. It is interesting that acetaminophen causes mitochondrial damage but does not cause IDILI as discussed in Section 4.3. It is possible that mitochondrial injury leads to apoptosis/necrosis rather than an immune response. However, valproate-induced IDILI clearly does involve mitochondria, and it is possible that some other drugs can cause some type of mitochondrial liver injury that leads to IDILI. With the exception of valproate we simply do not have compelling evidence that mitochondrial injury is a common mechanism of IDILI (specifically idiosyncratic liver injury, i.e., not through inhibition of mitochondria DNA or mitochondrial protein synthesis), either through a direct mechanism or through induction of an immune response.

4.2 Bile salt export pump (BSEP) inhibition

Bile acids are toxic, and genetic defects that lead to the absence of BSEP activity result in liver failure (Jacquemin, 2012). The most common clinical picture of patients who lack BSEP activity is cholestatic liver injury with an elevated serum alkaline phosphatase, but unlike most cholestatic liver injury, the serum γ-glutamyl transferase is usually normal. Several drugs can inhibit BSEP activity, and it has been proposed that this is a relatively common mechanism of IDILI (Morgan et al., 2010). Most drugs that have been proposed to cause IDILI through this mechanism cause mostly hepatocellular IDILI rather than cholestatic IDILI in that there is little increase in alkaline phosphatase. However, the definition of cholestatic IDILI used by hepatologists may not be appropriate in this context. It may be possible for bile acids to cause an increase in ALT in the absence of a significant increase in alkaline phosphatase. Genetic defects that lead to less severe impaired BSEP activity do not lead to significant liver injury (Köck et al., 2014), at least in part because there are other compensatory mechanisms and bile salt transport proteins such as multidrug resistance protein (MRP) 3 and MRP4 (Rodrigues et al., 2014). It is difficult to test this hypothesis in an animal model because the composition of bile acids in rodents is less toxic than human bile acids. These observations make it questionable that BSEP inhibition alone is a common mechanism of IDILI, but it is possible that BSEP inhibition, especially if the drug also inhibits other bile acid transporters, does lead to mild liver injury that promotes an immune response leading to IDILI as discussed previously. In fact, one study found that glyburide, which inhibits BSEP but is not associated with a significant incidence of IDILI, increased serum bile acids and the incidence of liver injury when combined with bosentan (Fattinger et al., 2001). The potential effects of BSEP inhibition on the mechanism of IDILI are summarized in Fig. 2.

4.3 Endoplasmic reticulum stress/unfolded protein response (UPR)

The enzymes involved in the formation of drug reactive metabolites, principally P450s are present in the smooth endoplasmic reticulum (ER). Therefore, if a reactive metabolite is very reactive it may bind mostly to the proteins in the ER leading to a change in their conformation, and this could lead to an UPR. It is relatively common for drugs to cause mechanism-based P450 inhibition by covalent binding of a reactive metabolite to the enzyme (Feng & He, 2013). The reactivity of the drug reactive metabolite may determine the type of toxicity it causes. Acetaminophen is probably a good example. It is a mystery why acetaminophen covalently binds to hepatic proteins and causes acute liver injury, but it is not associated with IDILI. There is substantive evidence that the mechanism of acetaminophen toxicity involves mitochondrial damage, and this leads to hepatocyte cell death (Hinson et al., 2010). The regioisomer of acetaminophen, 3′-hydroxyacetanilide, covalently binds to hepatocytes to a similar degree as acetaminophen, but it does not

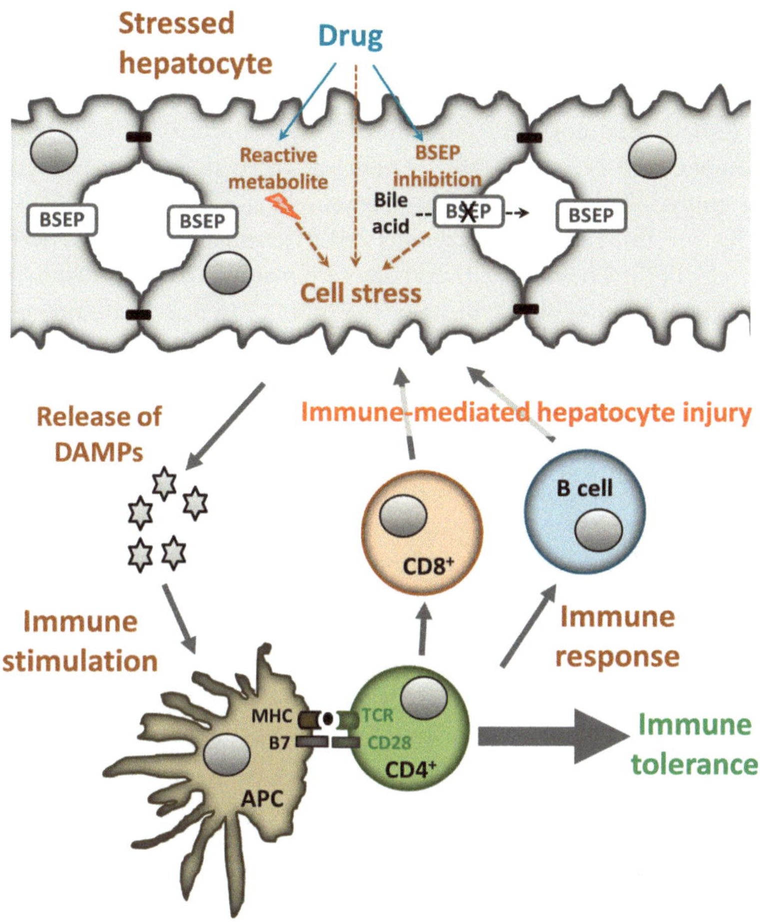

Fig. 2 BSEP inhibition can lead to hepatocyte damage and cell stress. This may cause IDILI, but it is more likely that it could cause the release of DAMPs, which promotes an immune response that is ultimately responsible for IDILI. However, in most patients the immune response in the liver results in immune tolerance. *Reprinted with permission from Kenna, J., & Uetrecht, J. (2018). Do in vitro assays predict drug candidate idiosyncratic drug-induced liver injury risk?* Drug Metabolism and Disposition, *46, 1658.*

cause acute hepatotoxicity. When the location of binding was compared, there is much more binding of acetaminophen in the mitochondrial fraction than the binding of 3′-hydroxyacetanilide (Tirmenstein & Nelson, 1989). This binding presumably is responsible for the acute toxicity of acetaminophen, and this acute mitochondrial-associated cell death may not provoke an adaptive immune response that can lead to IDILI. In contrast, although 3′-hydroxyacetanilide is said to be nontoxic, it is quite plausible that it would cause more UPR response, and it could cause IDILI if administered chronically.

This is another good illustration of the observation that not all covalent binding produces the same degree and type of toxicity.

The UPR is complex; for more comprehensive reviews, see Almanza et al. (2018), Bettigole and Glimcher (2015), Martins, Alves, Helguero, Domingues, and Neves (2016)). There are three major sensors involved in the unfolded protein response: protein kinase RNA-like ER kinase (PERK), inositol-requiring enzyme 1 (IRE1), and activating transcription factor 6 (ATF6). These three transducers are maintained in an inactive state by binding immunoglobulin protein (BiP) also known as glucose regulatory protein 78 (GRP78), which is a major protein chaperone in the ER. However, when there is an increase in unfolded proteins, these proteins compete with the transducers for binding to BiP. As binding of BiP to the transducers decreases, they are activated. Activation of PERK leads to its oligomerization and autophosphorylation. In turn, activated PERK phosphorylates eukaryotic translation initiation factor2α (eIF2α). This leads to a decrease in the synthesis of most proteins, but it causes an increase in antioxidant proteins and ER chaperones through activating transcription factor 4 (ATF4). Dissociation of BiP from IRE1 also leads to its oligomerization and autophosphorylation. Activation of IRE1 leads to activation of IκB kinase (IKK), which in turn leads to activation of nuclear factor light-chain-enhancer of activated B cells (NF-κB). Dissociation of BiP from ATF6 leads to its movement to the Golgi apparatus where it binds to cAMP response element-binding protein H (CREBH). This, in turn, leads to the upregulation of the synthesis of acute phase proteins. Another contribution to ER stress is the production of reactive oxygen species (ROS) and the release of DAMPs, which can lead to inflammasome activation through protein kinase RNA-activated (PKR). These events are summarized in Fig. 3.

It is unclear to what degree reactive metabolites can activate the UPR. In general, the absolute amount of protein modification is relatively low; however, some drugs generate sufficient reactive metabolite to cause mechanism-based inhibition of P450s. It seems likely that this could activate the UPR, but there is little direct evidence that this occurs. Likewise, although some reactive metabolites can redox cycle with the generation of ROS, there are many antioxidant mechanisms. It is interesting to note that although amodiaquine forms an iminoquinone reactive metabolite, which could redox cycle and reacts with glutathione, depletion of glutathione did not increase covalent binding, and it actually protected against amodiaquine-induced liver injury in mice (Liu et al., 2016). There must be several redundant antioxidant systems.

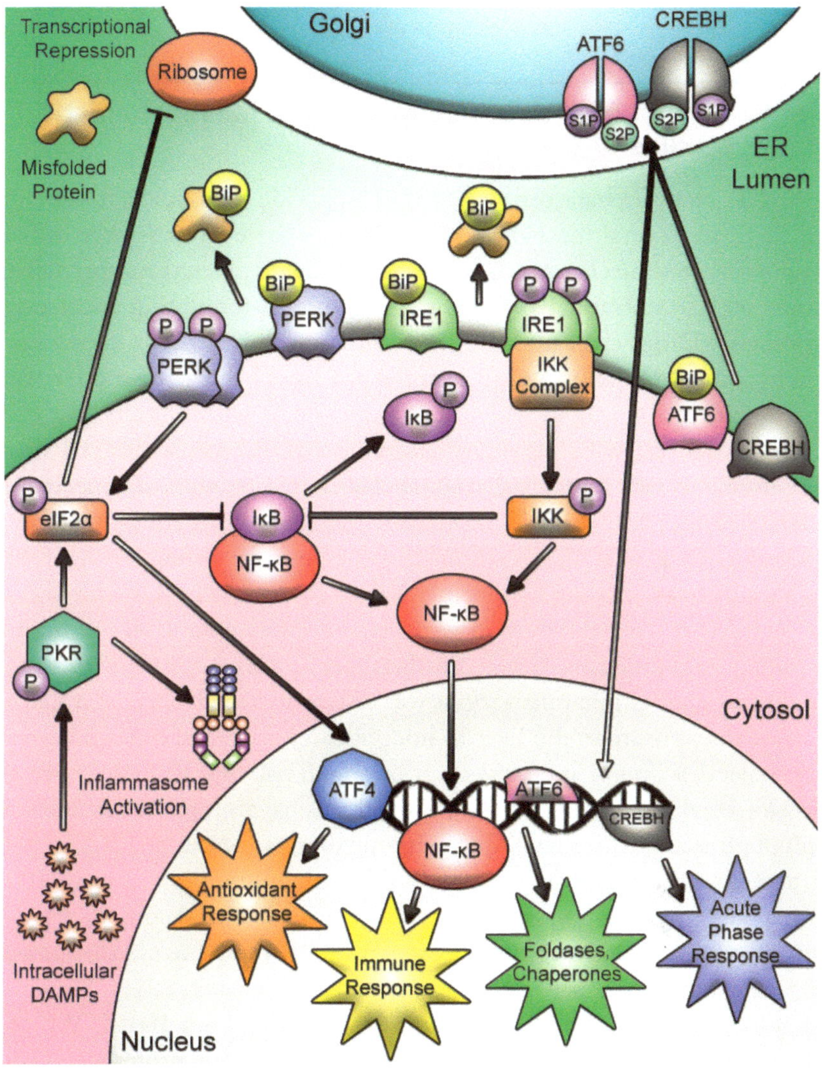

Fig. 3 Reactive metabolites bind to proteins, and this has the potential to lead to an unfolded protein response. The drug-modified proteins likely would not fold properly, and therefore would bind to BiP. This binding releases BiP from binding to PERK, IRE1, and ATF6. This results in the activation of PERK and IRE1 leading to their phosphorylation. Activated PERK phosphorylates eIF2α, which leads to a decrease in the synthesis of most proteins, but an increase in antioxidant proteins and ER chaperones through ATF4. Activation of IRE1 leads to activation of IKK resulting in activation of NF-κB. Dissociation of BiP from ATF6 leads to its movement to the Golgi apparatus where it binds to CREBH ultimately leading to upregulation of acute phase proteins and foldases. Reactive metabolites can also cause cell damage and lead to inflammasome activation through PKR. *Reprinted with permission from Cho, T., & Uetrecht, J. (2017), How reactive metabolites induce an immune response that sometimes leads to an idiosyncratic drug reaction.* Chemical Research and Toxicology, 30, *295–314. Copyright 2017 American Chemical Society.*

5. Animal models that can be used for mechanistic studies of IDILI

The clinical characteristics of IDILI provide vital mechanistic clues, and there are several mechanistic hypotheses. However, it is very difficult to rigorously test mechanistic hypotheses in humans given the unpredictable nature of IDRs. Animal models are very useful for testing mechanistic hypotheses. Drugs can cause IDILI in animals, but it is just as idiosyncratic as in humans. Most animal models in the past have been acute models using very high doses of drug in which the injury occurs within hours (Ng et al., 2012). However, with very few exceptions IDILI has a delayed onset. Therefore, it is very unlikely that acute models involve the same mechanism as IDILI in humans. If IDILI is immune mediated, it might be possible to produce a model of IDILI by stimulating the immune system. Such a model has been developed using lipopolysaccharide co-treatment (Luyendyk et al., 2003); however, it is different in virtually every way from IDILI in humans including an immediate onset. Furthermore, patients with inflammatory conditions such as inflammatory bowel disease in which there is a marked increase in exposure of the liver to lipopolysaccharide and other inflammatory molecules do not appear to be at increased risk of IDILI. We have also tried to develop an animal model of IDILI using multiple drugs and with multiple immune stimulants, but without success (Ng et al., 2012). Most of these studies were never published. Although most drugs that cause IDILI do not cause liver injury in rodents, we found that amodiaquine, which is associated with a relatively high incidence of IDILI in humans, causes a mild delayed-onset liver injury in both mice and rats (Liu et al., 2016). However, it resolves with continued treatment as is common with IDILI. We tried immunizing animals with amodiaquine-modified hepatic proteins and adjuvant to increase the injury, but this led to an increase in T-regulatory cells (Tregs) and paradoxically prevented the mild liver injury that amodiaquine causes in mice (Mak & Uetrecht, 2015a). As mentioned above, although the reactive metabolite of amodiaquine forms a glutathione conjugate, depletion of glutathione did not increase covalent binding, and it paradoxically prevented amodiaquine-induced liver injury (Liu et al., 2016).

The dominant immune response in the liver is immune tolerance (Jenne & Kubes, 2013). Therefore, if immune tolerance could be prevented it might lead to an animal model of IDILI. A major advancement in the treatment of cancer has been the use of immune checkpoint inhibitors that allow the immune system to kill tumors that express antigens not present on normal cells (Pardoll, 2012). The first such treatment was an antibody against cytotoxic T lymphocyte-associated protein 4 (CTLA-4), which binds to CD80 and CD86 on antigen presenting cells thus preventing co-stimulation through CD28 on T cells. Another checkpoint inhibitor is an antibody against programmed cell death protein-1 (PD-1), which is on T cells and prevents T cell activation. Co-treatment of mice with an anti-CTLA-4 antibody led to a small increase in ALT in amodiaquine-treated mice relative to amodiaquine treatment alone; however, the liver injury still resolved with continued treatment (Metushi, Hayes, & Uetrecht, 2015). Treatment of PD-1$^{-/-}$ mice with amodiaquine also led to a small increase in ALT relative to wild-type mice, but again the injury resolved with continued treatment. However, when we treated PD-1$^{-/-}$ mice with both anti-CTLA-4 antibodies and amodiaquine there was a marked increase in the liver injury that did not resolve with continued treatment (Metushi et al., 2015). Histologically, this injury was also characterized by a mononuclear leukocyte infiltrate and piecemeal necrosis that is also characteristic of IDILI in humans. Depletion of CD8 T cells prevented the liver injury in this model (Mak & Uetrecht, 2015b). Together, these data suggest that this impaired immune tolerance model represents a valid animal model of IDILI. It also supports the hypothesis that IDILI is immune mediated, and at least in the case of amodiaquine, involves CD8 cytotoxic T cells.

In addition to our studies, studies in the Lance Pohl lab found that depletion of myeloid-derived suppressor cells in mice treated with halothane led to a much greater immune response and liver injury (Chakraborty et al., 2015). In the case of halothane the effector cells appeared to be cytotoxic CD4 T cells rather than CD8 T cells. We also tested other drugs in the PD-1$^{-/-}$/anti-CTLA-4 impaired immune tolerance model. Other drugs such as nevirapine and isoniazid also produced liver injury in this model, but with other drugs the injury was milder and resolved with continued treatment (Mak & Uetrecht, 2015c). The impaired immune tolerance model also was able to differentiate troglitazone from pioglitazone and tolcapone from entacapone, although again the injury was milder than with amodiaquine (Mak, Kato, Weston, Hayes, & Uetrecht, 2018). These studies also suggest that checkpoint inhibitors would likely increase IDILI risk of co-administered drugs; that appears to be the case (Ribas, Hodi, Callahan, Konto, & Wolchok, 2013).

The results of these studies indicate that by manipulation of the immune system, principally through inhibition of immune tolerance rather than stimulation of the immune system, it is now possible to produce animal models with characteristics very similar to those of IDILI in humans. In turn, these animal models can be used to test mechanistic hypotheses in ways that have not been possible in the past. However, animals are different from humans, and any results in these models should be tested in humans as well.

6. Implications for prevention and treatment

6.1 Prediction of which patients are at increased risk of IDILI

Most patients who are treated with a drug that is associated with a relatively high risk of IDILI will not have an adverse reaction. Therefore, if we could predict who is at increased risk, we could use the drug safely in other patients. In some cases HLA genotyping patients would allow the safe use of such drugs. However, it is likely that most IDILI is not associated with just one HLA genotype, and even when there is an association with one specific genotype, in most cases such as flucloxacillin, the risk is still sufficiently low that HLA genotyping is not a practical solution. In general, strong associations with other genetic factors have not been found.

Given that genetic factors are not sufficient to determine which patients will develop IDILI there must be other risk factors. It has been proposed that an inflammatory environment increases the risk of IDILI (Roth, Luyendyk, Maddox, & Ganey, 2003); however, Hyman Zimmerman famously said that preexisting liver disease does not increase the risk of IDILI (Zimmerman, 1999). As mentioned, inflammatory bowel disease leads to exposure of the liver to a large amount of inflammatory molecules, and yet does not appear to significantly increase the risk of IDILI. It has been proposed that nonalcoholic steatohepatitis (NASH) increases the risk of IDILI (Tarantino et al., 2007), but it is very difficult to produce a valid control group (Massart, Begriche, Moreau, & Fromenty, 2017; Russo & Watkins, 2004). In addition, in our impaired immune tolerance animal model of IDILI, induction of a NASH-like syndrome was not synergistic with the drug-induced liver injury (Mak, Cho, & Uetrecht, 2018). However, it is true that patients with preexisting liver disease have less hepatic reserve and may have altered drug metabolism; therefore, caution is advised. Overall, although it is possible that some preexisting conditions increase the risk of IDILI, the data are not clear, and I think it is fair to say that most patients who develop IDILI do not have some inflammatory condition that augments the immune response to the drug. It appears that impaired immune tolerance significantly increases the risk of IDILI as discussed above; however, it does not appear that most patients who develop IDILI have significantly impaired immune tolerance. If such were the case it would be expected that if a patient developed IDILI to one drug they would have a markedly increased risk of developing IDILI to other drugs. In general, that does not appear to be the case. What then is the missing factor that determines who will develop IDILI to a specific drug? The fact is that the immune system is shaped by everything it has ever been exposed to. Except during an acute immune response, the number of lymphocytes remains the same during a patient's life. Therefore, if a patient develops memory T cells in response to a new antigen, other T cells have to be lost to compensate. The number of possible T cell receptors (TCR) formed by gene recombination is almost unlimited; however, the number of lymphocytes is not. Therefore, in order to be able to deal with the large number of pathogens that we are exposed to, the same lymphocyte must be able to recognize more than one antigen. A peptide from a processed antigen can bind to TCR in multiple ways; therefore, a TCR can recognize several different peptides even if they have significantly different structures. Exposure to one antigen can markedly affect the immune response to other antigens. This is referred to a heterologous immunity (Welsh & Selin, 2002). When it is applied to the mechanism of IDRs, the drug-modified peptide produced by the reactive metabolite of a drug could be recognized by a memory T cell that has primed by a strong immune response to a pathogen (Cho & Uetrecht, 2017; Pavlos, White, Wanjalla, Mallal, & Phillips, 2017). This could lead to an augmented immune response that results in IDILI. This is an attractive hypothesis that could explain the idiosyncratic nature of IDILI, but it is difficult to test. If this is a major mechanism that results in the idiosyncratic nature of these adverse reactions it will also make it difficult to predict who is at risk of developing IDILI to a specific drug. However, the early immune response to a drug may predict who will develop IDILI weeks later. For example, in an animal model of penicillamine-induced autoimmunity, a spike in serum IL-6 at 24h that returns to normal by day 7 predicts which animals will develop autoimmunity 3 weeks later (Zhu, Li, Liu, & Uetrecht, 2011).

Another factor that could influence IDILI risk is the microbiome. There is evidence that the microbiome can affect immune responses (Thaiss, Zmora, Levy, & Elinav, 2016). It is interesting to note that the presence of specific bacteria has a significant effect on the risk of checkpoint inhibitor-induced colitis (Dubin et al., 2016).

6.2 Screening drug candidates for their potential to cause IDILI

If IDILI is immune mediated, then it is likely that the best screening tests for IDILI risk in a drug candidate would be a measure of the immune response to the drug candidate. The impaired immune tolerance model appears to unmask the ability of a drug to cause IDILI; however, it is unlikely to be perfect because there can be species differences such as in metabolic pathways. For example, mice appear to be a better model of isoniazid metabolism than rats, but rats appear to be a better model for nevirapine metabolism than mice. In addition, the pharmaceutical industry prefers in vitro assays because they are quick and are usually amenable to high throughput methods; in contrast, the impaired immune tolerance model is not high throughput and requires approximately 1 month to perform.

One aspect of the working hypothesis for IDILI is that the drug causes the release of DAMPs from hepatocytes that activate APCs. Consistent with this hypothesis, we found that the supernatant from the incubation of amodiaquine or nevirapine with human hepatocyte spheroids activates THP-1 cells (a human monocyte cell line) (Kato & Uetrecht, 2017). We found that amodiaquine is also oxidized by THP-1 cells, which results in covalent binding, and it can directly activate THP-1 cells. In contrast, bioactivation of nevirapine does require bioactivation by hepatocytes, and inhibition of P450s abolished the activation of THP-1 cells by the hepatocyte supernatant. This assay has the potential to represent an in vitro assay to predict IDILI risk, but it is too early to know how accurate this assay may be.

Although most humans do not develop serious IDILI when treated with a drug that can cause IDILI, it is very likely that most patients form what is believed to be the reactive metabolite responsible. Although a specific HLA and memory T cell with a specific T cell receptor may be required for a strong adaptive immune response leading to IDILI, they would not be required for an innate immune response. Therefore, drugs that cause IDILI may induce a subclinical innate immune response in most patients and even most animals. For example, clozapine-induced agranulocytosis is associated with specific HLA genotypes (Chowdhury, Remington, & Kennedy, 2011). However, most patients have an immune response to clozapine, which resolves despite continued treatment. This immune response includes an increase in serum Il-6 and TNF-α, and a paradoxical neutrophilia (Pollmacher, Hinze-Selch, & Mullington, 1996). Rats treated with clozapine have a similar response (Ng, Kennar, & Uetrecht, 2014). Another example is the observation that most patients treated with procainamide develop antinuclear antibodies, but only a few develop a clinically evident lupus-like syndrome (Woosley et al., 1978). One reason that the immune response to clozapine was detected is that patients taking clozapine have their blood drawn every week to determine if they are developing agranulocytosis, and therefore it was relatively easy to do such a study, but such studies have not been performed for other drugs. Therefore, it is plausible that it is very common for a drug that is associated with IDILI to cause an innate immune response in most animals and patients if the appropriate assays were utilized. If that is the case, it may be possible to screen drugs for the potential to cause IDILI. Such studies could first be performed in animals or even in vitro. For example, drugs such as amoxicillin, ofloxacin, and sulfamethoxazole produce an immune response in mice without a clinical adverse reaction (Zhu, Cole, Kawabata, & Whritenour, 2015). But because humans can be different than animals they should be repeated in humans during first-in-human studies. If drugs can cause subtle immune responses in most animals and humans that predict their ability to cause serious IDRs in humans, such studies could add immeasurably to our mechanistic understanding of IDILI.

6.3 Treatment of IDILI

Currently the major treatment of IDILI is to stop the drug. However, in serious cases the injury progresses after the drug is discontinued, and this can ultimately lead to liver failure and death or liver transplantation. Serious cases are often treated with corticosteroids; however, corticosteroids do not appear to decrease mortality (Lee, Lee, et al., 2013). The exceptions are autoimmune IDILI and IDILI associated with checkpoint inhibitors. Other treatments have been tried, but there is little evidence for efficacy (Stine & Lewis, 2016), and controlled studies are lacking.

There may be lessons from other immune-mediated IDRs. Toxic epidermal necrolysis is a very serious skin rash that appears to be mediated by cytotoxic T cells. There have been studies of treatment with corticosteroids, but the studies were not well controlled (Law & Leung, 2015). Cyclosporin appeared to decrease mortality, but again the evidence is not conclusive (Valeyrie-Allanore et al., 2010). Another serious IDR is aplastic anemia, which can be idiopathic, but there are also drugs that cause idiosyncratic aplastic anemia. Whether idiopathic or drug-induced, most cases of aplastic anemia respond to anti-thymocyte globulin or cyclosporin (Young, Calado, & Scheinberg, 2006). At present our mechanistic understanding of IDILI is very superficial.

Mechanistic studies could lead to better treatments of IDILI that would decrease mortality. It will be difficult to perform controlled experiments of IDILI treatments, but such studies are important because it may never be possible to totally prevent IDILI.

7. Conclusion

IDILI remains a significant problem, both for patients and for drug development. Although our mechanistic understanding is superficial, there are multiple lines of evidence to implicate an adaptive immune response as the primary mechanism. However, there may be exceptions, and it is quite plausible that other mechanisms of injury play an important role in the induction of the adaptive immune response. Although the final pathway to serious IDILI appears to be an adaptive immune response, it is unclear what mechanism leads to this adaptive immune response and why it only occurs in the minority of patients. It is likely that it is different for different drugs. Progress in our understanding of IDILI has been slow because of the difficulty in performing rigorous mechanistic studies. The recent ability to manipulate the immune response, principally by inhibition of immune tolerance, holds promise in greatly facilitating mechanistic studies. However, to have full confidence in the findings in such animal models, the results of animal studies should be tested in humans. A better mechanistic understanding of IDILI is likely to lead to better methods to screen drug candidates for IDILI risk and to better treat IDILI when it occurs.

Acknowledgment

The author's research is funded by grants from the Canadian Institutes for Health Research.

Conflict of interest

The author has no conflict of interest to declare.

References

Aleo, M. D., Luo, Y., Swiss, R., Bonin, P. D., Potter, D. M., & Will, Y. (2014). Human drug-induced liver injury severity is highly associated with dual inhibition of liver mitochondrial function and bile salt export pump. *Hepatology*, *60*(3), 1015–1022. https://doi.org/10.1002/hep.27206.

Almanza, A., Carlesso, A., Chintha, C., Creedican, S., Doultsinos, D., Leuzzi, B., et al. (2018). Endoplasmic reticulum stress signalling—From basic mechanisms to clinical applications. *The FEBS Journal*. https://doi.org/10.1111/febs.14608. [Epub ahead of print].

Bettigole, S. E., & Glimcher, L. H. (2015). Endoplasmic reticulum stress in immunity. *Annual Review of Immunology*, *33*, 107–138. https://doi.org/10.1146/annurev-immunol-032414-112116.

Bjornsson, E., & Olsson, R. (2005). Outcome and prognostic markers in severe drug-induced liver disease. *Hepatology*, *42*(2), 481–489. Retrieved from http://www.ncbi.nlm.nih.gov/entrez/query.fcgi?cmd=Retrieve&db=PubMed&dopt=Citation&list_uids=16025496.

Bjornsson, E., Talwalkar, J., Treeprasertsuk, S., Kamath, P. S., Takahashi, N., Sanderson, S., et al. (2010). Drug-induced autoimmune hepatitis: Clinical characteristics and prognosis. *Hepatology*, *51*(6), 2040–2048. https://doi.org/10.1002/hep.23588.

Boelsterli, U. A., & Lim, P. L. (2007). Mitochondrial abnormalities—A link to idiosyncratic drug hepatotoxicity? *Toxicology and Applied Pharmacology*, *220*(1), 92–107. S0041-008X(06)00485-6 [pii]. https://doi.org/10.1016/j.taap.2006.12.013.

Brinkman, K., ter Hofstede, H. J., Burger, D. M., Smeitink, J. A., & Koopmans, P. P. (1998). Adverse effects of reverse transcriptase inhibitors: Mitochondrial toxicity as common pathway. *AIDS*, *12*(14), 1735–1744. Retrieved from http://www.ncbi.nlm.nih.gov/entrez/query.fcgi?cmd=Retrieve&db=PubMed&dopt=Citation&list_uids=9792373.

Bryant, A. E., & Dreifuss, F. E. (1996). Valproic acid hepatic fatalities. III. U.S. experience since 1986. *Neurology*, *46*(2), 465–469. Retrieved from http://www.ncbi.nlm.nih.gov/entrez/query.fcgi?cmd=Retrieve&db=PubMed&dopt=Citation&list_uids=8614514.

Chakraborty, M., Fullerton, A. M., Semple, K., Chea, L. S., Proctor, W. R., Bourdi, M., et al. (2015). Drug-induced allergic hepatitis develops in mice when myeloid-derived suppressor cells are depleted prior to halothane treatment. *Hepatology*, *62*(2), 546–557. https://doi.org/10.1002/hep.27764.

Chan, R., & Benet, L. Z. (2018). Measures of BSEP inhibition in vitro are not useful predictors of DILI. *Toxicological Sciences*, *162*(2), 499–508. https://doi.org/10.1093/toxsci/kfx284.

Chen, J., Mannargudi, B. M., Xu, L., & Uetrecht, J. (2008). Demonstration of the metabolic pathway responsible for nevirapine-induced skin rash. *Chemical Research in Toxicology*, *21*(9), 1862–1870. https://doi.org/10.1021/tx800177k.

Cho, T., & Uetrecht, J. (2017). How reactive metabolites induce an immune response that sometimes leads to an idiosyncratic drug reaction. *Chemical Research in Toxicology*, *30*(1), 295–314. https://doi.org/10.1021/acs.chemrestox.6b00357.

Cho, T. E., & Uetrecht, J. (2018). Testing the mitochondrial dysfunction hypothesis for idiosyncratic drug-induced liver injury (IDILI). *The Toxicologist*, *162*, 23–24.

Chowdhury, N. I., Remington, G., & Kennedy, J. L. (2011). Genetics of antipsychotic-induced side effects and agranulocytosis. *Current Psychiatry Reports*, *13*(2), 156–165. https://doi.org/10.1007/s11920-011-0185-3.

Clay, K. D., Hanson, J. S., Pope, S. D., Rissmiller, R. W., Purdum, P. P., 3rd, & Banks, P. M. (2006). Brief communication: Severe hepatotoxicity of telithromycin: Three case reports and literature review. *Annals of Internal Medicine*, *144*(6), 415–420. Retrieved from http://www.ncbi.nlm.nih.gov/entrez/query.fcgi?cmd=Retrieve&db=PubMed&dopt=Citation&list_uids=16481451.

Czaja, A. J. (2011). Drug-induced autoimmune-like hepatitis. *Digestive Diseases and Sciences*, *56*(4), 958–976. https://doi.org/10.1007/s10620-011-1611-4.

Daly, A. K. (2013). Pharmacogenomics of adverse drug reactions. *Genome Medicine*, *5*(1), 5. https://doi.org/10.1186/gm409.

Daly, A. K., Donaldson, P. T., Bhatnagar, P., Shen, Y., Pe'er, I., Floratos, A., et al. (2009). HLA-B*5701 genotype is a major determinant of drug-induced liver injury due to flucloxacillin. *Nature Genetics*, *41*(7), 816–819. doi:ng.379 [pii]. https://doi.org/10.1038/ng.379.

deLemos, A. S., Foureau, D. M., Jacobs, C., Ahrens, W., Russo, M. W., & Bonkovsky, H. L. (2014). Drug-induced liver injury with autoimmune features. *Seminars in Liver Disease*, *34*(2), 194–204. https://doi.org/10.1055/s-0034-1375959.

Dubin, K., Callahan, M. K., Ren, B., Khanin, R., Viale, A., Ling, L., et al. (2016). Intestinal microbiome analyses identify melanoma patients at risk for checkpoint-blockade-induced colitis. *Nature Communications*, 7, 10391. https://doi.org/10.1038/ncomms10391.

Dykens, J. A., & Will, Y. (2007). The significance of mitochondrial toxicity testing in drug development. *Drug Discovery Today*, *12*(17–18), 777–785. https://doi.org/10.1016/j.drudis.2007.07.013.

Fattinger, K., Funk, C., Pantze, M., Weber, C., Reichen, J., Stieger, B., et al. (2001). The endothelin antagonist bosentan inhibits the canalicular bile salt export pump: A potential mechanism for hepatic adverse reactions. *Clinical Pharmacology and Therapeutics*, *69*(4), 223–231. https://doi.org/10.1067/mcp.2001.114667.

Favalli, E. G., Varenna, M., & Sinigaglia, L. (2005). Drug-induced agranulocytosis during treatment with infliximab in enteropathic spondyloarthropathy. *Clinical and Experimental Rheumatology*, *23*(2), 247–250. Retrieved from http://www.ncbi.nlm.nih.gov/entrez/query.fcgi?cmd=Retrieve&db=PubMed&dopt=Citation&list_uids=15895899.

Feng, S., & He, X. (2013). Mechanism-based inhibition of CYP450: An indicator of drug-induced hepatotoxicity. *Current Drug Metabolism*, *14*(9), 921–945. Retrieved from https://www.ncbi.nlm.nih.gov/pubmed/24016115.

Foureau, D. M., Walling, T. L., Maddukuri, V., Anderson, W., Culbreath, K., Kleiner, D. E., et al. (2015). Comparative analysis of portal hepatic infiltrating leucocytes in acute drug-induced liver injury, idiopathic autoimmune and viral hepatitis. *Clinical and Experimental Immunology*, *180*(1), 40–51. https://doi.org/10.1111/cei.12558.

Giovannoni, G., Gold, R., Selmaj, K., Havrdova, E., Montalban, X., Radue, E. W., et al. (2014). Daclizumab high-yield process in relapsing-remitting multiple sclerosis (SELECTION): A multicentre, randomised, double-blind extension trial. *Lancet Neurology*, *13*(5), 472–481. https://doi.org/10.1016/S1474-4422(14)70039-0.

Hanzlik, R. P., Koen, Y. M., & Fang, J. (2013). Bioinformatic analysis of 302 reactive metabolite target proteins. Which ones are important for cell death. *Toxicological Sciences*, *135*(2), 390–401. https://doi.org/10.1093/toxsci/kft166.

Hayashi, P. H., Rockey, D. C., Fontana, R. J., Tillmann, H. L., Kaplowitz, N., Barnhart, H. X., et al. (2017). Death and liver transplantation within 2 years of onset of drug-induced liver injury. *Hepatology*, *66*(4), 1275–1285. https://doi.org/10.1002/hep.29283.

Hinson, J. A., Roberts, D. W., & James, L. P. (2010). Mechanisms of acetaminophen-induced liver necrosis. *Handbook of Experimental Pharmacology*, *196*, 369–405. https://doi.org/10.1007/978-3-642-00663-0_12.

Jacquemin, E. (2012). Progressive familial intrahepatic cholestasis. *Clinics and Research in Hepatology and Gastroenterology*, *36*(Suppl. 1), S26–S35. https://doi.org/10.1016/S2210-7401(12)70018-9.

Janeway, C. A., Jr. (1989). Approaching the asymptote? Evolution and revolution in immunology. *Cold Spring Harbor Symposia on Quantitative Biology*, *54*(Pt. 1), 1–13. Retrieved from http://www.ncbi.nlm.nih.gov/entrez/query.fcgi?cmd=Retrieve&db=PubMed&dopt=Citation&list_uids=2700931.

Jenne, C. N., & Kubes, P. (2013). Immune surveillance by the liver. *Nature Immunology*, *14*(10), 996–1006. https://doi.org/10.1038/ni.2691.

Kato, R., & Uetrecht, J. (2017). Supernatant from hepatocyte cultures with drugs that cause idiosyncratic liver injury activates macrophage inflammasomes. *Chemical Research in Toxicology*, *30*(6), 1327–1332. https://doi.org/10.1021/acs.chemrestox.7b00065.

Keisu, M., & Andersson, T. B. (2010). Drug-induced liver injury in humans: The case of ximelagatran. In J. P. Uetrecht (Ed.), *Vol. 196. Mechanisms of adverse drug reactions* (pp. 407–418). Heidelberg: Springer-Verlag.

Kim, S. H., & Naisbitt, D. J. (2016). Update on advances in research on idiosyncratic drug-induced liver injury. *Allergy, Asthma & Immunology Research*, *8*(1), 3–11. https://doi.org/10.4168/aair.2016.8.1.3.

Kindmark, A., Jawaid, A., Harbron, C. G., Barratt, B. J., Bengtsson, O. F., Andersson, T. B., et al. (2008). Genome-wide pharmacogenetic investigation of a hepatic adverse event without clinical signs of immunopathology suggests an underlying immune pathogenesis. *The Pharmacogenomics Journal*, *8*(3), 186–195. doi:6500458 [pii]. https://doi.org/10.1038/sj.tpj.6500458.

Kleiner, D. E., Chalasani, N. P., Lee, W. M., Fontana, R. J., Bonkovsky, H. L., Watkins, P. B., et al. (2014). Hepatic histological findings in suspected drug-induced liver injury: Systematic evaluation and clinical associations. *Hepatology*, *59*(2), 661–670. https://doi.org/10.1002/hep.26709.

Köck, K., Ferslew, B. C., Netterberg, I., Yang, K., Urban, T. J., Swaan, P. W., et al. (2014). Risk factors for development of cholestatic drug-induced liver injury: Inhibition of hepatic basolateral bile acid transporters multidrug resistance-associated proteins 3 and 4. *Drug Metabolism and Disposition*, *42*(4), 665–674. https://doi.org/10.1124/dmd.113.054304.

Landsteiner, K., & Jacobs, J. (1935). Studies on the sensitization of animals with simple chemical compounds. *The Journal of Experimental Medicine*, *61*, 643–656.

Law, E. H., & Leung, M. (2015). Corticosteroids in Stevens-Johnson Syndrome/toxic epidermal necrolysis: Current evidence and implications for future research. *The Annals of Pharmacotherapy*, *49*(3), 335–342. https://doi.org/10.1177/1060028014560012.

Lee, K. K., Fujimoto, K., Zhang, C., Schwall, C. T., Alder, N. N., Pinkert, C. A., et al. (2013). Isoniazid-induced cell death is precipitated by underlying mitochondrial complex I dysfunction in mouse hepatocytes. *Free Radical Biology & Medicine*, *65*, 584–594. https://doi.org/10.1016/j.freeradbiomed.2013.07.038.

Lee, T., Lee, Y. S., Yoon, S. Y., Kim, S., Bae, Y. J., Kwon, H. S., et al. (2013). Characteristics of liver injury in drug-induced systemic hypersensitivity reactions. *Journal of the American Academy of Dermatology*, *69*(3), 407–415. https://doi.org/10.1016/j.jaad.2013.03.024.

Leung, L., Kalgutkar, A. S., & Obach, R. S. (2012). Metabolic activation in drug-induced liver injury. *Drug Metabolism Reviews*, *44*(1), 18–33. https://doi.org/10.3109/03602532.2011.605791.

Liu, F., Cai, P., Metushi, I., Li, J., Nakayawa, T., Vega, L., et al. (2016). Exploring an animal model of amodiaquine-induced liver injury in rats and mice. *Journal of Immunotoxicology*, *13*(5), 694–712. https://doi.org/10.3109/1547691X.2016.1166167.

Luyendyk, J. P., Maddox, J. F., Cosma, G. N., Ganey, P. E., Cockerell, G. L., & Roth, R. A. (2003). Ranitidine treatment during a modest inflammatory response precipitates idiosyncrasy-like liver injury in rats. *The Journal of Pharmacology and Experimental Therapeutics*, *307*(1), 9–16. Retrieved from http://www.ncbi.nlm.nih.gov/entrez/query.fcgi?cmd=Retrieve&db=PubMed&dopt=Citation&list_uids=12893837.

Maddrey, W. C., & Boitnott, J. K. (1973). Isoniazid hepatitis. *Annals of Internal Medicine*, *79*(1), 1–12.

Mak, A., Cho, T., & Uetrecht, J. (2018). Use of an animal model to test whether non-alcoholic fatty liver disease increases the risk of idiosyncratic drug-induced liver injury. *Journal of Immunotoxicology*, *15*(1), 90–95. https://doi.org/10.1080/1547691X.2018.1467982.

Mak, A., Kato, R., Weston, K., Hayes, A., & Uetrecht, J. (2018). An impaired immune tolerance animal model distinguishes the potential of troglitazone/pioglitazone and tolcapone/entacapone to cause IDILI. *Toxicological Sciences*, *161*(2), 412–420. https://doi.org/10.1093/toxsci/kfx219.

Mak, A., & Uetrecht, J. (2015a). Immunization with amodiaquine-modified hepatic proteins prevents amodiaquine-induced liver injury. *Journal of Immunotoxicology*, *12*(4), 361–367. https://doi.org/10.3109/1547691X.2014.983660.

Mak, A., & Uetrecht, J. (2015b). The role of CD8 T cells in amodiaquine-induced liver injury in PD1 −/− mice cotreated with anti-CTLA-4. *Chemical Research in Toxicology*, *28*(8), 1567–1573. https://doi.org/10.1021/acs.chemrestox.5b00137.

Mak, A., & Uetrecht, J. (2015c). The combination of anti-CTLA-4 and PD1 −/− mice unmasks the potential of isoniazid and nevirapine to cause liver injury. *Chemical Research in Toxicology*, *28*(12), 2287–2291. https://doi.org/10.1021/acs.chemrestox.5b00305.

Martins, A. S., Alves, I., Helguero, L., Domingues, M. R., & Neves, B. M. (2016). The unfolded protein response in homeostasis and modulation of mammalian immune cells. *International Reviews of Immunology*, *35*(6), 457–476. https://doi.org/10.3109/08830185.2015.1110151.

Massart, J., Begriche, K., Moreau, C., & Fromenty, B. (2017). Role of nonalcoholic fatty liver disease as risk factor for drug-induced hepatotoxicity. *Journal of Clinical and Translational Research*, *3*(Suppl. 1), 212–232. https://doi.org/10.18053/jctres.03.2017S1.006.

Matzinger, P. (1994). Tolerance, danger and the extended family. *Annual Review of Immunology*, *12*, 991–1045.

McKenzie, R., Fried, M. W., Sallie, R., Conjeevaram, H., Di Bisceglie, A. M., Park, Y., et al. (1995). Hepatic failure and lactic acidosis due to fialuridine (FIAU), an investigational nucleoside analogue for chronic hepatitis B. *The New England Journal of Medicine*, *333*(17), 1099–1105. https://doi.org/10.1056/NEJM199510263331702.

Metushi, I. G., Hayes, M. A., & Uetrecht, J. (2015). Treatment of PD-1(−/−) mice with amodiaquine and anti-CTLA4 leads to liver injury similar to idiosyncratic liver injury in patients. *Hepatology*, *61*(4), 1332–1342. https://doi.org/10.1002/hep.27549.

Metushi, I. G., Nakagawa, T., & Uetrecht, J. (2012). Direct oxidation and covalent binding of isoniazid to rodent liver and human hepatic microsomes: Humans are more like mice than rats. *Chemical Research in Toxicology*, *25*(11), 2567–2576. https://doi.org/10.1021/tx300341r.

Metushi, I. G., Sanders, C., Lee, W. M., & Uetrecht, J. (2014). Detection of anti-isoniazid and anti-cytochrome P450 antibodies in patients with isoniazid-induced liver failure. *Hepatology*, *59*(3), 1084–1093. https://doi.org/10.1002/hep.26564.

Morgan, R. E., Trauner, M., van Staden, C. J., Lee, P. H., Ramachandran, B., Eschenberg, M., et al. (2010). Interference with bile salt export pump function is a susceptibility factor for human liver injury in drug development. *Toxicological Sciences*, *118*(2), 485–500. https://doi.org/10.1093/toxsci/kfq269.

Nakayama, S., Atsumi, R., Takakusa, H., Kobayashi, Y., Kurihara, A., Nagai, Y., et al. (2009). A zone classification system for risk assessment of idiosyncratic drug toxicity using daily dose and covalent binding. *Drug Metabolism and Disposition*, *37*(9), 1970–1977. dmd.109.027797 [pii] https://doi.org/10.1124/dmd.109.027797.

Ng, W., Kennar, R., & Uetrecht, J. (2014). Effect of clozapine and olanzapine on neutrophil kinetics: implications for drug-induced agranulocytosis. *Chemical Research in Toxicology*, *27*(7), 1104–1108. https://doi.org/10.1021/tx500183x.

Ng, W., Lobach, A. R., Zhu, X., Chen, X., Liu, F., Metushi, I. G., et al. (2012). Animal models of idiosyncratic drug reactions. *Advances in Pharmacology*, *63*, 81–135. https://doi.org/10.1016/B978-0-12-398339-8.00003-3.

Obach, R. S., Kalgutkar, A. S., Soglia, J. R., & Zhao, S. X. (2008). Can in vitro metabolism-dependent covalent binding data in liver microsomes distinguish hepatotoxic from nonhepatotoxic drugs? An analysis of 18 drugs with consideration of intrinsic clearance and daily dose. *Chemical Research in Toxicology*, *21*(9), 1814–1822. https://doi.org/10.1021/tx800161s.

Osanlou, O., Pirmohamed, M., & Daly, A. K. (2018). Pharmacogenetics of adverse drug reactions. *Advances in Pharmacology*, *83*, 155–190. https://doi.org/10.1016/bs.apha.2018.03.002.

Pardoll, D. M. (2012). The blockade of immune checkpoints in cancer immunotherapy. *Nature Reviews Cancer*, *12*(4), 252–264. https://doi.org/10.1038/nrc3239.

Parker, C. W., & Thiel, J. A. (1963). Studies in human penicillin allergy: A comparison of various penicilloyl-polylysines. *The Journal of Laboratory and Clinical Medicine*, *62*, 482–491.

Retrieved from http://www.ncbi.nlm.nih.gov/entrez/query.fcgi?cmd=Retrieve&db=PubMed&dopt=Citation&list_uids=14061977.

Pavlos, R., White, K. D., Wanjalla, C., Mallal, S. A., & Phillips, E. J. (2017). Severe delayed drug reactions: Role of genetics and viral infections. *Immunology and Allergy Clinics of North America*, *37*(4), 785–815. https://doi.org/10.1016/j.iac.2017.07.007.

Pearce, R. E., Uetrecht, J. P., & Leeder, J. S. (2005). Pathways of carbamazepine bioactivation in vitro. II. The role of human cytochrome P450 enzymes in the formation of 2-hydroxyiminostilbene. *Drug Metabolism and Disposition*, *33*(12), 1819–1826.

Pearce, R. E., Vakkalagadda, G. R., & Leeder, J. S. (2002). Pathways of carbamazepine bioactivation in vitro. I. Characterization of human cytochromes P450 responsible for the formation of 2- and 3-hydroxylated metabolites. *Drug Metabolism and Disposition*, *30*(11), 1170–1179.

Pirmohamed, M., James, S., Meakin, S., Green, C., Scott, A. K., Walley, T. J., et al. (2004). Adverse drug reactions as cause of admission to hospital: Prospective analysis of 18 820 patients. *British Medical Journal*, *329*(7456), 15–19. Retrieved from http://www.ncbi.nlm.nih.gov/entrez/query.fcgi?cmd=Retrieve&db=PubMed&dopt=Citation&list_uids=15231615.

Pollmacher, T., Hinze-Selch, D., & Mullington, J. (1996). Effects of clozapine on plasma cytokine and soluble cytokine receptor levels. *Journal of Clinical Psychopharmacology*, *16*(5), 403–409. Retrieved from http://www.ncbi.nlm.nih.gov/entrez/query.fcgi?cmd=Retrieve&db=PubMed&dopt=Citation&list_uids=8889915.

Ribas, A., Hodi, F. S., Callahan, M., Konto, C., & Wolchok, J. (2013). Hepatotoxicity with combination of vemurafenib and ipilimumab. *The New England Journal of Medicine*, *368*(14), 1365–1366. https://doi.org/10.1056/NEJMc1302338.

Rodrigues, A. D., Lai, Y., Cvijic, M. E., Elkin, L. L., Zvyaga, T., & Soars, M. G. (2014). Drug-induced perturbations of the bile acid pool, cholestasis, and hepatotoxicity: Mechanistic considerations beyond the direct inhibition of the bile salt export pump. *Drug Metabolism and Disposition*, *42*(4), 566–574. https://doi.org/10.1124/dmd.113.054205.

Roth, R. A., Luyendyk, J. P., Maddox, J. F., & Ganey, P. E. (2003). Inflammation and drug idiosyncrasy—Is there a connection? *The Journal of Pharmacology and Experimental Therapeutics*, *307*(1), 1–8. Retrieved from http://www.ncbi.nlm.nih.gov/entrez/query.fcgi?cmd=Retrieve&db=PubMed&dopt=Citation&list_uids=12954806.

Roujeau, J. C. (2005). Clinical heterogeneity of drug hypersensitivity. *Toxicology*, *209*(2), 123–129. S0300-483X(04)00723–1 [pii]. https://doi.org/10.1016/j.tox.2004.12.022.

Russo, M. W., & Watkins, P. B. (2004). Are patients with elevated liver tests at increased risk of drug-induced liver injury? *Gastroenterology*, *126*(5), 1477–1480. Retrieved from http://www.ncbi.nlm.nih.gov/entrez/query.fcgi?cmd=Retrieve&db=PubMed&dopt=Citation&list_uids=15131809.

Senior, J. R. (2006). How can 'Hy's law' help the clinician. *Pharmacoepidemiology and Drug Safety*, *15*(4), 235–239. https://doi.org/10.1002/pds.1210.

Sharma, A. M., Li, Y., Novalen, M., Hayes, M. A., & Uetrecht, J. (2012). Bioactivation of nevirapine to a reactive quinone methide: Implications for liver injury. *Chemical Research in Toxicology*, *25*(8), 1708–1719. https://doi.org/10.1021/tx300172s.

Siddiqui, M. A., Ahmad, J., Farshori, N. N., Saquib, Q., Jahan, S., Kashyap, M. P., et al. (2013). Rotenone-induced oxidative stress and apoptosis in human liver HepG2 cells. *Molecular and Cellular Biochemistry*, *384*(1–2), 59–69. https://doi.org/10.1007/s11010-013-1781-9.

Silva, M. F., Aires, C. C., Luis, P. B., Ruiter, J. P., Ijlst, L., Duran, M., et al. (2008). Valproic acid metabolism and its effects on mitochondrial fatty acid oxidation: A review. *Journal of Inherited Metabolic Disease*, *31*(2), 205–216. https://doi.org/10.1007/s10545-008-0841-x.

Stewart, J. D., Horvath, R., Baruffini, E., Ferrero, I., Bulst, S., Watkins, P. B., et al. (2010). Polymerase gamma gene POLG determines the risk of sodium valproate-induced liver toxicity. *Hepatology, 52*(5), 1791–1796. https://doi.org/10.1002/hep.23891.

Stine, J. G., & Lewis, J. H. (2016). Current and future directions in the treatment and prevention of drug-induced liver injury: A systematic review. *Expert Review of Gastroenterology & Hepatology, 10*(4), 517–536. https://doi.org/10.1586/17474124.2016.1127756.

Tarantino, G., Conca, P., Basile, V., Gentile, A., Capone, D., Polichetti, G., et al. (2007). A prospective study of acute drug-induced liver injury in patients suffering from non-alcoholic fatty liver disease. *Hepatology Research, 37*(6), 410–415. https://doi.org/10.1111/j.1872-034X.2007.00072.x.

Thaiss, C. A., Zmora, N., Levy, M., & Elinav, E. (2016). The microbiome and innate immunity. *Nature, 535*(7610), 65–74. https://doi.org/10.1038/nature18847.

Tirmenstein, M. A., & Nelson, S. D. (1989). Subcellular binding and effects on calcium homeostasis produced by acetaminophen and a nonhepatotoxic regioisomer, 3′-hydroxyacetanilide, in mouse liver. *The Journal of Biological Chemistry, 264*(17), 9814–9819. Retrieved from https://www.ncbi.nlm.nih.gov/pubmed/2524496.

Valeyrie-Allanore, L., Wolkenstein, P., Brochard, L., Ortonne, N., Maître, B., Revuz, J., et al. (2010). Open trial of ciclosporin treatment for Stevens-Johnson syndrome and toxic epidermal necrolysis. *The British Journal of Dermatology, 163*(4), 847–853. https://doi.org/10.1111/j.1365-2133.2010.09863.x.

Vazquez, J. A., Arnold, A. C., Swanson, R. N., Biswas, P., & Bassetti, M. (2016). Safety of long-term use of linezolid: Results of an open-label study. *Therapeutics and Clinical Risk Management, 12*, 1347–1354. https://doi.org/10.2147/TCRM.S109444.

Vergani, D., Mieli-Vergani, G., Alberti, A., Neuberger, J., Eddleston, A., Davis, M., et al. (1980). Antibodies to the surface of halothane-altered rabbit hepatocytes in patients with severe halothane-associated hepatitis. *The New England Journal of Medicine, 303*(2), 66–71.

Warrington, R. J., Tse, K. S., Gorski, B. A., Schwenk, R., & Sehon, A. H. (1978). Evaluation of isoniazid-associated hepatitis by immunological tests. *Clinical and Experimental Immunology, 32*(1), 97–104. Retrieved from http://www.ncbi.nlm.nih.gov/entrez/query.fcgi?cmd=Retrieve&db=PubMed&dopt=Citation&list_uids=668195.

Watkins, P. B., Desai, M., Berkowitz, S. D., Peters, G., Horsmans, Y., Larrey, D., et al. (2011). Evaluation of drug-induced serious hepatotoxicity (eDISH): Application of this data organization approach to phase III clinical trials of rivaroxaban after total hip or knee replacement surgery. *Drug Safety, 34*(3), 243–252. https://doi.org/10.2165/11586600-000000000-00000.

Watkins, P. B., & Whitcomb, R. W. (1998). Hepatic dysfunction associated with troglitazone. *The New England Journal of Medicine, 338*(13), 916–917. Retrieved from http://www.ncbi.nlm.nih.gov/entrez/query.fcgi?cmd=Retrieve&db=PubMed&dopt=Citation&list_uids=9518284.

Welsh, R. M., & Selin, L. K. (2002). No one is naive: The significance of heterologous T-cell immunity. *Nature Reviews Immunology, 2*(6), 417–426. https://doi.org/10.1038/nri820.

Woosley, R. L., Drayer, D. E., Reidenberg, M. M., Nies, A. S., Carr, K., & Oates, J. A. (1978). Effect of acetylator phenotype on the rate at which procainamide induces antinuclear antibodies and the lupus syndrome. *The New England Journal of Medicine, 298*, 1157–1159.

Yip, V. L. M., Meng, X., Maggs, J. L., Jenkins, R. E., Marlot, P. T., Marson, A. G., et al. (2017). Mass spectrometric characterization of circulating covalent protein adducts derived from epoxide metabolites of carbamazepine in patients. *Chemical Research in Toxicology*. https://doi.org/10.1021/acs.chemrestox.7b00063.

Young, N. S., Calado, R. T., & Scheinberg, P. (2006). Current concepts in the pathophysiology and treatment of aplastic anemia. *Blood, 108*(8), 2509–2519. https://doi.org/10.1182/blood-2006-03-010777.

Zhu, X., Cole, S. H., Kawabata, T. T., & Whritenour, J. (2015). Characterization of the draining lymph node response in the mouse drug allergy model: A model for drug hypersensitivity reactions. *Journal of Immunotoxicology*, *12*(4), 376–384. https://doi.org/10.3109/1547691X.2014.988308.

Zhu, X., Li, J., Liu, F., & Uetrecht, J. P. (2011). Involvement of T helper 17 cells in D-penicillamine-induced autoimmune disease in Brown Norway rats. *Toxicological Sciences*, *120*(2), 331–338. kfq392 [pii]. https://doi.org/10.1093/toxsci/kfq392.

Zimmerman, H. (1999). *Hepatotoxicity: The adverse effects of drugs and other chemicals on the liver* (2nd ed.). Philadelphia: Lippincott Williams & Wilkins.

CHAPTER SIX

Idiosyncratic drug-induced liver injury in patients: Detection, severity assessment, and regulatory implications

Paul B. Watkins[1]
Eshelman School of Pharmacy, Institute for Drug Safety Sciences, University of North Carolina, Chapel Hill, NC, United States
[1]Corresponding author: e-mail address: pwatkins@email.unc.edu

Contents

Abstract

Idiosyncratic Drug-Induced Liver Injury (IDILI) is a rare but potentially life-threatening event that is caused by drugs that, at usual therapeutic doses, do not cause any biochemical or clinical evidence of liver injury in the majority of treated patients. The most common clinical phenotypes of IDILI are "acute hepatitis," "mixed hepatocellular-cholestatic hepatitis," and "cholestatic hepatitis" and these are distinguished by clinical, biochemical and histologic characteristics. Anti-microbials, herbals and dietary supplements are now the agents most often implicated in the US Drug-Induced Liver Injury Network registry. There are several scales that have been used to characterize the severity of IDILI events. There are no reliable means to accurately predict the course of an IDILI event at presentation. In clinical trials, the "gold standard" liver safety signal is the occurrence of "Hy's Law Cases." Making the diagnosis of IDILI, and when a patient is taking

Advances in Pharmacology, Volume 85
ISSN 1054-3589
https://doi.org/10.1016/bs.apha.2019.02.004
© 2019 Elsevier Inc.
All rights reserved.

multiple drugs, identifying the most likely culprit can be challenging, but many drugs cause IDILI with characteristic clinical and biochemical presentations, or "signatures." In a clinical trial, it is sometimes possible to identify an overlooked "signature" of IDILI by characterizing more minor, asymptomatic, and transient elevations in liver chemistries. This observation can be helpful in assessing causation in rare serious liver events occurring in the clinical trial, or first recognized post-marketing.

Abbreviations

Alk Phos	Alkaline phosphatase
ALT	Alanine aminotransferase
AST	Aspartate aminotransferase
DILIN	U.S. Drug-Induced Liver Injury Network
eDISH	evaluation of Drug-Induced Serious Hepatoxicity
IDILI	idiosyncratic drug-induced liver injury
MELD	Model for End-stage Liver Disease
NAFLD	Non-alcoholic fatty liver disease
NRH	Nodular Regenerative Hyperplasia
SOS	sinusoidal obstruction syndrome
ULN	upper limits of normal

1. Introduction

There is some controversy regarding the definition of idiosyncratic drug-induced liver injury (referred to simply as "IDILI" in this review). The term "idiosyncratic" derives from the Greek words "idios" meaning "one's own" and "synkrasis" meaning "temperament, mixture of personal characteristics" (https://www.dictionary.com/browse/idiosyncrasy). Few would argue that a mixture of characteristics present in an individual patient can contribute substantially to susceptibility to idiosyncratic DILI, but this is true to greater or lesser extents for all forms of hepatotoxicity. For the purpose of this review, idiosyncratic DILI will be considered to have the following two characteristics: (1) It is a rare and potentially serious event occurring during recommended dosing of the implicated drug and (2) The majority of patients treated at recommended doses with a drug capable of causing idiosyncratic DILI have no clinical or biochemical evidence of liver injury. This review will not be covering hepatotoxicity more frequently caused by drugs in a clear dose-dependent fashion, including acetaminophen overdoses.

This review will also follow international consensus criteria to define an IDILI event (Aithal, Watkins, Andrade, et al., 2011) (Table 1).

Table 1 International consensus criteria for IDILI.

Any of the following peak serum values:
ALT > or = 5 × ULN
Alk phos > or = 2 × ULN in the absence of bone pathology
ALT > or = 3 × ULN and total bilirubin > 2 × ULN

ALT, alanine aminotransferase; Alk phos, alkaline phosphatase; ULN, upper limits of normal for the lab performing the analyses.

Application of these criteria has some caveats. Serum levels of aspartate aminotransferase, although less liver specific than ALT, can replace ALT if ALT values are not available and there is no evidence of muscle injury. In addition, if it is known that chronic liver disease is present before the IDILI event, upper limits of normal (ULN) can be replaced by baseline (pre-IDILI event) values for the each test. Finally, it should be noted that these biochemical thresholds may not be attained with certain phenotypes of IDILI that may still produce significant liver injury, most notably drug-induced chronic hepatitis, nodular regenerative hyperplasia, and hepatic steatosis with lactic acidosis (see IDILI phenotypes listed below).

In the west, the incidence of IDILI was estimated to be 1/100,000–20/100,000 in the general population (Bell & Chalasani, 2009; Bjornsson, 2010; Watkins & Seeff, 2006). Two population-based studies conducted by France and Iceland estimated the annual incidences of IDILI to be approximately 13.9/100,000 and 19.1/100,000, respectively (Bjornsson, Bergmann, Bjornsson, et al., 2013; Sgro, Clinard, Ouazir, et al., 2002). In the United States, the annual incidence of IDILI in the general population has been recently estimated as 2.7 per 100,000 adults, through surveillance in the state of Delaware (Vega, Verma, Beswick, et al., 2017). These figures only capture IDILI events that come to the attention of medical professionals so the true incidence is undoubtedly higher. A recent study examined the most frequent causes of IDILI based on individual case reports in the literature (Teschke, 2018).

2. Clinical phenotypes of IDILI

IDILI can present in many different ways in terms of clinical signs, biochemical abnormalities, and findings on liver biopsy. Indeed, it is often stated that the clinical, biochemical, imaging, and histologic features of

IDILI can mimic every known liver disease (Fontana, 2014). However, the vast majority of IDILI cases fall into three phenotype categories: hepatocellular, cholestatic and mixed (features of both hepatocellular and cholestatic injuries). These three categories are distinguished by the ratio of the alanine aminotransferase (ALT, numerator) and alkaline phosphatase (alk phos, denominator) measured in serum with both values expressed as fold upper limits of normal (ULN) for the laboratory performing the assays. This ratio is termed the "R value" (Danan & Benichou, 1993) and, since the nature of the injury can change over time (as in the case depicted in Fig. 1), the convention is to make this determination with the values obtained at the presentation of the IDILI event. An R value >5.0 signifies a hepatocellular injury, a value <2.0 signifies a cholestatic liver injury, and an R value

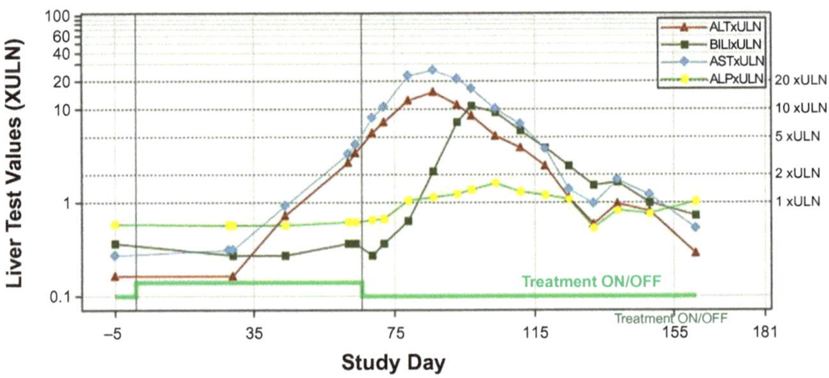

Fig. 1 Typical course of the acute hepatitis phenotype for IDILI. This patient was in a clinical trial and began treatment with the study drug on day 0 (x axis). Liver chemistries shown on the y axis were completely within normal limits (1 × ULN) 1 month on treatment and 45 days on treatment. However, around 2 months on treatment, the liver chemistries started to rise and study drug was discontinued (although neither serum ALT or AST exceeded 3 × ULN at that time). Despite stopping treatment, the AST and ALT values continued to rise for 3 more weeks before beginning to fall. Serum bilirubin was unchanged and within normal limits when the study drug was discontinued, but rose to greater than 10 × ULN before falling. The delayed rise in serum bilirubin relative to the aminotransferases is expected since a large fraction of hepatocytes must die, releasing ALT and AST, before global liver dysfunction occurs sufficient to rise serum bilirubin. It should be noted that alkaline phosphatase also rose but never exceeded 2 × ULN and the R value remained > 5 until very late in the course of the injury. It should also be noted that the greater value for serum AST than ALT throughout most of the course of the injury is unusual for the acute hepatitis phenotype and this patient probably had concomitant muscle injury. *Figure reproduced from Church, R. J., & Watkins, P. B. (2018). In silico modeling to optimize interpretation of liver safety biomarkers in clinical trials.* Experimental Biology and Medicine (Maywood, N.J.), 243, *300–307 with permission.*

between 2.0 and 5.0 signifies a mixed injury (i.e., features of both hepatocellular and cholestatic injuries). It is of note that these three phenotypes of IDILI determined by the R value do not always correlate well with the determination of the three phenotypes by liver biopsy (Kleiner, 2017).

Hepatocellular IDILI results from drug-induced death of hepatocytes, causing release of their contents (including ALT/AST) into blood. Cholestatic liver injury results from interference in the formation and secretion of bile, which typically leads to elevations in serum alkaline phosphatase but little death of hepatocytes. Mixed injuries have features of both types. A detailed listing of drugs that typically cause hepatocellular, cholestatic, or mixed injuries is available (Ortega-Alonso, Stephens, Lucena, et al., 2016).

Drug-induced liver injuries have been further divided into 12 phenotypes (as reviewed in livertox.nih.gov), 8 of which are most applicable to idiosyncratic DILI. The most three common phenotypes of IDILI are acute hepatitis, mixed hepatocellular/cholestatic hepatitis, and cholestatic hepatitis.

1. Acute hepatitis (R value >5)—The clinical course mirrors that of viral hepatitis and typically occurs after 1–6 months of treatment with the offending drug. A typical course is shown in Fig. 1. Symptoms include fatigue, nausea and right upper quadrant pain with progression to jaundice if severe. Symptoms and liver chemistries tend to worsen for 1–3 weeks after stopping the offending drug but then resolve over a month or so. Liver histology looks similar to viral hepatitis with hepatocyte necrosis and lymphocytic infiltration with minimal or no fibrosis. Isoniazid and many other drugs typically cause this phenotype, which is also the most common phenotype for IDILI associated with use of herbal and dietary supplements. This IDILI phenotype generally is of the most concern because symptoms can be unreliable and when jaundice occurs, there has been a potentially life-threatening loss of global hepatic function.
2. Cholestatic hepatitis (R value <2)—The latency and symptoms are similar to those of acute hepatitis, but pruritus (diffuse skin itching) is a typical early and prominent feature and jaundice occurs earlier in the course of the injury. Rash and low-grade fever may be present. Resolution after stopping the offending drug is prolonged, typically taking several months for completion. Histological features include inflammation of bile ducts and the portal tracts and scattered loss of hepatocytes. Examples of drug typically causing this phenotype include amoxicillin-clavulonate, sulfonylureas, and many other drugs.

3. Mixed hepatocellular-cholestatic hepatitis ($2 < R < 5$). This event also generally occurs between 1 and 6 months on drug treatment and has clinical and histological features of both acute hepatitis and cholestatic hepatitis. Recovery after stopping the implicated drug tends to be prolonged, typically taking weeks to months. In the absence of biliary tract disease in an otherwise healthy person, IDILI is the most likely cause for is phenotype of injury.

Other much less frequent phenotypes of IDILI are bland cholestasis, hepatic steatosis with lactic acidosis, nonalcoholic fatty liver, chronic hepatitis, sinusoidal obstruction syndrome and nodular regenerative hyperplasia.

4. Bland cholestasis—($R < 2.0$). This event typically occurs after 2 and 6 months of treatment with the offending drug. Symptoms include itching and jaundice but fatigue, nausea, vomiting and abdominal pain are not typical. Liver biopsies typically reveal generally healthy appearing hepatocytes (hence the generally minimal elevations in serum ALT), dilated bile canaliculi containing "bile plugs," and little or no inflammatory cells. The itching and jaundice often take months to resolve after discontinuing treatment with the offending drug, but full recovery is expected. There are few drugs that typically cause bland cholestasis—most frequently androgenic steroids taken by young body builders.
5. Hepatic steatosis with lactic acidosis (R value variable)—This event typically occurs within 1 month of treatment with the offending drug and typical symptoms are fatigue, nausea, abdominal discomfort, anorexia, and weight loss. Liver chemistries may be only minimally elevated. Liver histology reveals microvesicular steatosis. If the offending drug is not discontinued promptly, the symptoms typically progress to include shortness of breath due to lactic acidosis, and obtundation that progresses to coma and death. The presentation and histology are similar to that observed in Reye' Syndrome (which can be rarely triggered by aspirin use in children). Drugs implicated in causing this type of liver injury include intravenous tetracycline and d-nucleosidase drugs including and zidovudine (AZT). This type of liver injury was also caused by fialuridine (FIAU), a drug targeted for treatment of hepatitis B but abandoned very early in clinical development because liver failure occurred in 7 out of the 15 subjects initially treated with this drug (Institute of Medicine Committee to Review the Fialuridine Clinical T, 1995) (so these events would not be considered IDILI).
6. Nonalcoholic fatty liver (R value variable)—This event typically occurs after 3–12 months of treatment with the offending agent. It is usually

asymptomatic and can be difficult to distinguish from the natural history of non-alcoholic liver disease (NAFLD) unrelated to drug therapy. Liver chemistries are typical of NAFLD with mild to moderate elevations of serum aminotransferases and alkaline phosphatase. Liver histology reveals macrovesicular fat with varying degrees of inflammation, Mallory bodies and pericentral fibrosis that mimics alcoholic hepatitis. Only a few drugs can cause this phenotype, including tamoxifen and methotrexate.

7. Sinusoidal obstruction syndrome (SOS-previously termed veno-occlusive disease)—There are acute and subacute forms of this phenotype. Acute SOS (R value >5.0) presents with abdominal pain and swelling due to the rapid accumulation of ascites. There is also general fluid overload with leg edema and rapid weight gain. Jaundice may signal the onset of liver failure. Subacute and chronic SOS (R value variable) are more subtle events with moderate elevations in liver enzymes with variable R value, and gradual progression of the symptoms of acute SOS. Drugs causing this phenotype are generally chemotherapeutic agents, typically alkylating agents. The onset of SOS is typically within the first month of treatment.
8. Nodular regenerative hyperplasia (NRH) (R value <5)—This phenotype manifests as the development of fatigue, weight loss and ascites with other complications due to portal hypertension. Liver chemistries are usually only mildly abnormal, but a slowly rising serum alkaline phosphatase (over months) is characteristic. Diagnosis can only confidently be made by liver biopsy revealing nodules without much fibrosis. Recognition of this IDILI phenotype is usually delayed well beyond 6 months of treatment with the implicated drug. Drugs implicated as causing this phenotype include azathioprine, mercaptopurine and thioguanine.

3. Immune phenotypes

The most common phenotypes of IDILI (acute hepatitis, mixed hepatocellular/cholestatic hepatitis, and cholestatic hepatitis) and the chronic hepatitis phenotype may be accompanied by clinical, laboratory or histological findings consistent with an immune etiology. Moreover, IDILI due to the same drug typically will have an immune phenotype in some patients but not others. The most common immune phenotypes are "immunoallergic" and "autoimmune."

Fever, skin rash, and eosinophilia are the hallmarks for immunoallergic IDILI. The presence of these features generally makes IDILI a more likely diagnosis, as these are not common features of viral hepatitis or other causes of liver injuries. IDILI with severe rashes, including Stevens Johnson Syndrome (SJS) and Toxic Epidermal Necrolysis (TEN) constitute the DRESS Syndrome (Drug Reaction with Eosinophilia and Systemic Symptoms) (Devarbhavi & Raj, 2018). Liver biopsies characteristically show invasion by eosinophils and this is generally more helpful than peripheral eosinophilia in establishing a diagnosis of IDILI. However, infiltration of the liver with eosinophils can occur in the absence of other immunoallergic features; therefore, the presence of eosinophils in the liver alone is not considered sufficient to qualify as immunoallergic IDILI. Immunoallergic IDILI generally has onset within 1 month of the start of treatment with the implicated drug. Typical drugs causing immunoallergic IDILI are the aromatic anticonvulsants, particularly carbamazepine, and allopurinol.

The second IDILI immune phenotype is autoimmune. Autoimmune IDILI mimics idiopathic autoimmune hepatitis in clinical, biochemical and histologic features (deLemos, Foureau, Jacobs, et al., 2014; Howell et al., 2014; Suzuki, Brunt, Kleiner, et al., 2011). The onset of biochemical abnormalities tends to be months after starting treatment with the offending drug, and the rise in liver enzymes is typically gradual, but can be acute. Recovery after discontinuation of the implicated drug is also typically gradual, often taking many months to complete resolution of the biochemical abnormalities. The drugs most commonly implicated as causing autoimmune IDILI are minocycline, hydralazine nitrofurantoin, and methyldopa. In a recent study (de Boer, Kosinski, Urban, et al., 2017), IDILI events due to these four drugs were categorized as autoimmune or not autoimmune according to a grading system based on multiple autoimmune serologies. The majority of these IDILI cases were classified as autoimmune on this basis, and there was no difference in the average clinical course based on this distinction. It is generally believed that distinction between autoimmune IDILI and idiopathic autoimmune hepatitis can best be made in retrospect. If the injury resolves upon discontinuing treatment with the suspect drug (with or without treatment with immunosuppressive drugs) and does not spontaneously return within 1 year of stopping the drug (and the immune suppression treatment if given), a diagnosis of autoimmune IDILI can be more confidently made, especially if the implicated drug is well-known to cause this type of IDILI (Howell et al., 2014). It has also been reported that autoimmune serologies tend to fall in titer as autoimmune IDILI resolves, and this may also be diagnostically useful (de Boer et al., 2017).

4. Rating severity of IDILI

There are several proposed scales that are used to rate the severity of on IDILI event. For AIDS clinical trials, the Division of AIDS (DAIDS) has a grading scale for all adverse events that includes liver injuries. (https://rsc.niaid.nih.gov/sites/default/files/daidsgradingcorrectedv21.pdf). This scale is based on the peak numerical value of liver chemistries ALT, AST, alk phos and bilirubin observed (expressed as fold upper limits of normal (ULN)) (Table 2).

The Cancer Therapy Evaluation Program of the National Cancer Institute (NCI) has a similar scale referred to as the Common Toxicity Criteria for Adverse Events (CTCAE) (https://ctep.cancer.gov/protocolDevelopment/electronic_applications/docs/CTCAE_v5_Quick_Reference_8.5x11.pdf). There are two differences in the scales. The CTCAE has higher cut offs for the values at each grade, and due to updating in November 2017, has included modifications if the baseline values are abnormal. In this case, the same fold criteria is used, but the baseline value replaces the ULN value.

The criteria in Table 2 were not specifically designed for IDILI and have shortcomings when used in this situation. First, these scales do not take into account how the patient feels (symptoms). The presence of symptoms (fatigue, nausea, vomiting, right upper quadrant pain) support liver inflammation with systemic release of cytokines and are generally ominous signs. Second, the peak values of liver chemistries may not reflect the extent of loss of global liver function. IDILI with rapid onset and resolution can result in

Table 2 Severity of liver injury according to the Division of AIDS (DAIDS) and the National Cancer Institute's Common Toxicity Criteria for Adverse Events (CTCAE).

	DAIDS		CTCAE[a]	
	ALT	Alk phos	ALT	Alk phos
Grade 1 mild	1.25–2	1.1–1.6	1–3	1–3
Grade 2 moderate	2.5–5	1.6–2.6	3–5	3–5
Grade 3 severe	5.0–10	2.5–5.0	5–20	2–5
Grade 4 life-threatening	>10	>5	>20	>5
Grade 5 indicates death				

[a]CTCAE criteria were updated in 11/2017 such that ULN should be replaced by baseline (pre-event) values if these were abnormal.

less percent loss of hepatocytes than an IDILI event with slow progression and slow resolution, yet both may have the same peak liver chemistries (Howell et al., 2014). Third, assessments of liver function such as INR and elevation in serum bilirubin (reflecting global liver function) are not integrated with the criteria to assess severity. Specific criteria have therefore been proposed for assessing severity of IDILI (Table 3).

The first scale proposed was from the U.S Drug-Induced Liver Injury Network (DILIN), which has been creating a registry and tissue bank from patients who experience IDILI in the US (Hoofnagle, 2004). There are five severity categories in the DILIN scale and hospitalization is a key criteria (Fontana, Watkins, Bonkovsky, et al., 2009). The international consensus criteria (Aithal et al., 2011) were proposed after the DILIN criteria were proposed and did not consider hospitalization as a variable, reasoning that the criteria for hospitalization varies substantially across the globe. This resulted in eliminating DILINs Moderate to Severe category. The consensus criteria also proposed that moderate severity include hepatitis symptoms in the absence of elevations in serum bilirubin $>2\times$ ULN. The scales have other more minor differences (Table 3).

5. Outcome of an IDILI event

The majority of IDILI events resolve with full restoration of liver function and liver health. However, the presence of IDILI may result in the discontinuation of important medications, such as interruption of life-saving cancer treatments, with long-term health consequences. Typically, resolution of an IDILI event is the result of stopping treatment with the implicated drug in time to avoid liver failure, but it is interesting that drug-induced liver events qualifying as IDILI also typically resolve with continuation of treatment with the implicated agent (a phenomenon termed "adaptation"). Although these transient treat-though events are typically just asymptomatic elevations in liver chemistries in the absence of jaundice, there is some evidence that even severe IDILI events can sometimes resolve without stopping the implicated drug. For example, in a study conducted in a mental institution, men were treated for latent tuberculosis with isoniazid (INH); serial blood samples were obtained and analyzed retrospectively for liver chemistries (Mitchell, Long, Thorgeirsson, et al., 1975). It was shown that two of the men experienced elevations in both serum AST (ALT was not measured) and serum bilirubin $>2\times$ ULN (qualifying as serious IDILI—i.e., Hy's Law Cases—see section below) but these events went

Table 3 Criteria proposed by the US Drug-Induced Liver Injury Network (DILIN) and international consensus for grading severity of IDILI.[a]

DILIN			**International consensus**[a]		
Category	**Severity**	**Description**	**Category**	**Severity**	**Description**
1	Mild	Increased ALT and/or bilirubin <2.5 mg/dL, INR <1.5	1	Mild	Bilirubin <2× ULN
2	Moderate	Increased ALT and/or bilirubin >2.5 mg/dL or INR <1.5	2	Moderate	Bilirubin >or=2× ULN or symptoms of hepatitis
3	Moderate to severe	Increased ALT and/or bilirubin >2.5 mg/dL and hospitalization[b]			
4	Severe	Increased ALT and/or Alk phos and bilirubin >2.5 mg/dL and Jaundice and symptoms >3 months or INR >1.5 or encephalopathy or other organ failure due to IDILI	3	Severe	Bilirubin > or=2× ULN and INR > or=1.5 or Ascites or encephalopathy[c] or other organ failure due to IDILI
5	Fatal	Death/liver transplant due to IDILI	4	Fatal	Death/liver transplant due to IDILI

[a]All categories must meet the biochemical criteria for IDILI established by international consensus.
[b]Hospitalization or prolongation of hospital stay due to IDILI.
[c]Duration <26 weeks and in the absence of pre-existing cirrhosis.

unrecognized and the liver chemistries returned to normal with continued treatment. The study was conducted prior to availability of hepatitis virus testing so it is not possible to exclude viral hepatitis as the cause of these events. However, the timing of the events was consistent in INH-induced IDILI and similar events did not occur in a men not treated with INH at the same institution and during the same time interval.

6. Death or transplant

International IDILI registries have all reported that about 10% of patients with IDILI have a fatal outcome defined as death or liver transplantation (Andrade, Lucena, Fernandez, et al., 2005; Bjornsson & Bjornsson, 2017; Bjornsson & Olsson, 2005; Chalasani, Bonkovsky, Fontana, et al., 2015). In a recent study (Hayashi, Rockey, Fontana, et al., 2017) of 1089 patients in the registry of the US Drug-Induced Liver Injury Network (DILIN), 107 (9.8%) of the patient died within 2 years of the event. The incidence of fatality was 12% among hepatocellular DILI cases, 6% among mixed cases, and 11% among cholestatic cases (as defined by R value). Each death case was examined to determine the role the IDILI event had played in the fatality. Overall, IDILI was judged to have had a primary role in causing death in 68 (64%), a contributory role in 15 (14%) and no role in 22 (21%). Progression of cancers was the most common cause for death judged to be unrelated to the IDILI event. Among patients with hepatocellular, mixed, and cholestatic IDILI events, the event was considered the primary cause of death in 78%, 26% and 53%, respectively, but to have had contributed to the fatality in 88%, 66%, and 65%, of the cases, respectively. This points out that all three forms of IDILI can have dire health consequences.

7. Chronic DILI

It was traditionally assumed that if they don't have a fatal outcome, patients with acute forms of DILI always recover, although the time to full recovery may vary across and within IDILI phenotypes. However, a study performed in England first suggested that this may not be the case (Aithal & Day, 1999). Thirty-three patients who had experienced an IDILI event based on clinical and liver biopsy criteria were brought back for examination a median of 5 years (range 1–19 years) after the event. Thirteen (40%) of these patients were found to have abnormalities in serum liver chemistries or imaging with no more obvious explanation than a continuation of the IDILI event. Five patients agreed to undergo liver biopsy and histological abnormalities were observed in three of these biopsies. Although there was initial skepticism of this report, persistent liver injury long after stopping treatment with implicated drugs has been supported by the international IDILI registries.

In a report from the US DILIN registry (Fontana, Hayashi, Barnhart, et al., 2015) 19% of patients continue to have abnormal liver chemistries, liver imaging, and/or abnormal liver histology 6 months after the onset of the acute IDILI event. In a follow up report (Fontana, Hayashi, Gu, et al., 2014), 75% of subjects with evidence of ongoing liver injury 6 months after DILI onset continued to have laboratory evidence of persistent liver injury during prolonged follow-up. It was noted that higher serum alkaline phosphatase levels at presentation and older age were independent predictors of persistent liver injury.

8. Predicting IDILI course

It is not currently possible to accurately predict which patients experiencing IDILI will progress to chronic DILI and which will progress to fatality. The ability to make such predictions would obviously be important to physicians caring for IDILI patients, but also would permit identification of a targeted population most ethically appropriate for a therapeutic intervention trial. Dr. Hyman Zimmerman first reported in the 1960s that a patient with drug-induced hepatocellular jaundice (i.e., jaundice due to an hepatocellular injury) has at least a 10% chance of dying from the liver injury, and he noted that that this was true independent of which specific drug caused the IDILI. This was an important observation because the most common cause of hepatocellular jaundice, acute viral hepatitis, rarely has a fatal outcome. The FDA has reinterpreted the observation of Dr. Zimmerman to define a "Hy's Law Case" as a patient with an hepatocellular injury (originally defined as serum ALT $>3\times$ ULN and serum alk phos $<2\times$ ULN) and a concomitant rise in serum bilirubin to greater than $2\times$ ULN (see Table 4 for full criteria for a Hy's Law Case) (https://www.fda.gov/downloads/guidances/UCM174090.pdf). Recently, study of the outcomes of IDILI in the Spanish Network supported a modification of the Hy's Law Case as more predictive of fatal outcome (Robles-Diaz, Lucena, Kaplowitz, et al., 2014). This included defining hepatocellular injury as R value exceeding 5

Table 4 Criteria defining a "Hy' Law Case" observed in a clinical trial.*

1) The serum ALT must exceed 3 × ULN and the serum total bilirubin must simultaneously exceed 2 × ULN
2) The liver injury must be hepatocellular in nature (originally defined as serum Alk Phos <2 × ULN for now typically defined as R value >5)
3) The drug should cause elevations in serum ALT >3 × ULN ("Temples Corollary")
4) There can be no more likely cause of the liver injury than the study drug

*The criteria assume the subject had a healthy liver prior to the event. How to assess subjects with pre-existing liver disease is not resolved.

and replacing serum ALT in the R value equation with the AST value if this results in a higher R value. The superiority of this "nR Hy's Law" vs Hy's Law Case criteria was supported in a recent analysis of the DILIN database (Hayashi et al., 2017).

A recent international collaboration attempted to identify newer biomarkers that could be combined with traditional biomarkers to improve prediction of the outcome of and IDILI event (Church, Kullak-Ublick, Aubrecht, et al., 2019). Serum from 141 patients obtained at entry to the DILIN registry was analyzed and various statistical approaches were used to best identify the 15 of these patients who experienced a fatal outcome (death or liver transplant). It was found that INR was the single best predictor of fatality as might be expected. However, the next most predictive for fatal outcome was osteopontin followed by cytokeratin 18, and then total bilirubin. The Model for End-stage Liver Disease (MELD) score, which is widely used to assign priority to patients awaiting liver transplantation, also had good prediction of fatality in the cohort. However, the investigators observed that the predictive potential of the MELD score was improved when the values for cytokeratin 18 and macrophage colony stimulating factor receptor (MCSFR) were incorporated. Similar studies involving DILIN subjects (Bonkovsky, Barnhart, Foureau, et al., 2018; Steuerwald, Foureau, Norton, et al., 2013), assessed the prognostic value of cytokine profiles assessed in the serum samples obtained within 2 weeks of detection of the IDILI event. The conclusion was that lower levels of RANTES and higher levels of IL-6 and IL8 were associated with fatality. An additional DILIN based study (Russo et al., 2017) examined the profile of micro RNAs in serum as prognostic indicators and found an association between fatal outcome and low levels of miR122. Although each of these studies with non-traditional serum liver biomarkers show some promise as prognostic indicators, the number of fatal outcome cases is relatively small and numerous biomarkers were assessed limiting statistical power of the associations found. These findings must be replicated before they could be considered for prospective clinical use.

9. Diagnosing IDILI

There are as yet no diagnostic tests that can directly make a confident diagnosis of IDILI and it remains a diagnosis of exclusion. Algorithms for employing serological and imaging testing to arrive at the diagnosis of IDILI have been recently published (Avigan, Bjornsson, Pasanen, et al., 2014; Danan & Teschke, 2015; Kullak-Ublick, Andrade, Merz, et al., 2017; Russo et al., 2017). The most universally accepted tool to aid in the diagnosis of DILI is the Roussel Uclaf Causality Assessment Method (RUCAM) (Danan & Teschke, 2015). This tool consists of a series of questions including the start date of drug administration relative the onset of the event, whether the biochemical abnormalities resolved with discontinuation of the implicated drug and how fast did this occur, the results of a series of tests for alternate etiologies (e.g., viral hepatitis serologies), was the patient elderly, pregnant, or consuming alcohol, does the drug have a history of causing IDILI, and was the patient taking other drugs with IDILI liability. The answer to each question scores points and upon completion of the entries, the individual scores are added up to a total which defines likelihood of IDILI due a specific drug. The advantages of the RUCAM tool are that it forces a systematic assessment of the major key factors all would agree are important for assessing the likelihood of a liver injury being do to a drug. Furthermore, you do not need to be an expert in IDILI to appropriately fill out the form and arrive at an assessment. However, there are issues with RUCAM scoring (Garcia-Cortes, Stephens, Lucena, et al., 2011).

One downside of the RUCAM tool is that it only takes two phenotypes of IDILI into consideration—hepatocellular and mixed cases combined with cholestatic cases. The reality is that most drugs that cause IDILI tend to have characteristic presentations, or "signatures" ("although sometimes these signatures are illegible" Willis Maddrey, personal communication). For example, phenytoin characteristically causes a mixed liver injury within 1 month of starting treatment and typically is associated with fever, rash, facial edema and lymphadenopathy. Amoxicillin-clavulonate typically causes liver injury that is first noted 1–3 weeks after stopping treatment, and the injury tends to be hepatocellular in those under 40 years of age and more cholestatic in the elderly. Minocycline and nitrofurantoin typically cause a chronic IDILI after many months of treatment, and often after more than 1 year of treatment. Herbal and dietary supplements tend to cause acute hepatocellular injuries 1–6 months into treatment. As later discussed, tolvaptan can cause an acute hepatitis IDILI after well over one year of treatment. These are just a few of the many instances where knowledge of signature presentations are very helpful in arriving at a diagnosis of IDILI. In fact, most hepatologists experienced with IDILI and who rely on the RUCAM for causality assessment will complement the objective scoring with their knowledge of characteristic IDILI signatures.

The knowledge of IDILI signature is the essence of "Expert Opinion" promoted by the US DILIN (Hayashi, 2016) where three separate hepatologists (experienced with IDILI causality assessment) independently review the relevant data and assign to each case one of five distinct categories of causality likelihood (the first assessment "Is this IDILI?" and the second is individual assessment of the likelihood of up to three different suspect medications taken by the patient). Another often overlooked feature of the DILIN causality process is that the adjudication is not performed until after the subject returns for the 6 month follow up visit, when alternate more likely etiologies have occasionally been revealed. In one publication from this network, there was not a good correlation between the causality assessment as assessed with the RUCAM tool and the causality assessment arrived at by consensus from the DILIN experts (Rockey, Seeff, Rochon, et al., 2010). Of course waiting 6 months to make an IDILI diagnosis is not practical in most clinical settings.

The creation of the Livertox website (livertox.nih.gov) (Hoofnagle, Serrano, Knoben, et al., 2013) has been a great development in terms of allowing open access to signature presentations of IDILI. The site has a structured analysis of the hepatotoxicity potential of virtually all drugs currently on the market in the U.S. and has also begun to include entries for herbal and dietary supplements. Using this website (livertox.nih.gov), non-experts can now add subjective weight to RUCAM causality assessments based on signature presentations where they are known. Investigators within DILIN have been working to incorporate the IDILI signatures into the RUCAM, or a RUCAM-like instrument. The plan is to create a web-based tool where the investigator fills in the relevant information on smart e-forms, and a signature phenotype is automatically determined. The selected signature is then factored into the scoring to improve identification of an IDILI event and, if the patient is taking more than one suspect drug, identify which is most likely the culprit.

It should be noted that there has been some progress in identifying genetic risk factors for IDILI, although the associations have been largely drug-specific (Daly, 2017; Urban, Daly, & Aithal, 2014). Moreover, none of the associations have been sufficiently predictive to recommend genotyping prior to dosing a drug capable of IDILI. However, in some instances, genotyping if available would probably be useful in causality assessment (Aithal, 2015).

Liver biopsies are not usually obtained during an acute IDILI event or considered to be important in diagnostic assessment. This is because most IDILI events resolve off treatment. Further, IDILI can cause very diverse histological abnormalities on liver biopsy and for this reason, it has been widely assumed that liver biopsy is generally not very helpful in causality assessment. However, the presence of eosinophils or granuloma are well known to suggest IDILI and observations from the US DILIN has identified other biopsy features that can help establish or refute an IDILI diagnosis (Kleiner, Chalasani, Lee, et al., 2014). The US DILIN attempts to collect liver biopsy slides including unstained slides and the paraffin-embedded tissue when a liver biopsy has been performed. This has permitted histology and immunochemistry-based studies of DILI (Foureau, Walling, Maddukuri, et al., 2015). The data collected suggest that liver biopsy can actually be quite helpful to identify or exclude IDILI. DILIN investigators are now systematically evaluating whether knowledge of liver biopsy findings would have altered the causality assessments that were made without knowledge of these findings.

10. Detecting IDILI potential of new drugs in clinical trials

Although all phenotypes of IDILI can have serious health consequences, the acute hepatitis phenotype has been of most serious concern for drug developers and regulators (Avigan, 2014). This is because these events tend to be asymptomatic early in the course and can therefore only be detected by routine liver chemistry monitoring. Furthermore, once jaundice occurs during this IDILI phenotype, there is substantial loss of global liver function and, as discussed earlier, the patient has at least a 10% chance of liver failure. With mixed and cholestatic liver injuries, jaundice occurs earlier in the course of the injury. The patient in effect, becomes their own "color indicator" of the problem before there is crucial loss of global liver function. Routine liver monitoring therefore is rarely recommended for drugs with only cholestatic IDILI liability.

The challenge in detecting a new drug candidate's potential for IDILI is that the most sensitive serum test for hepatocellular injury, ALT, can be elevated substantially by drugs that have little or no potential to cause clinically important liver injury (Senior, 2012). For example, in the clinical trials of tacrine for the treatment of Alzheimer's Disease, asymptomatic ALT alterations $> 3\times$ ULN were observed in 25% of treated patients, with elevations exceeding $20\times$ ULN in 40 patients (2%) (Watkins, Zimmerman, Knapp, et al., 1994). Yet, patients who experienced tacrine-related elevations in serum ALT, even elevations exceeding $20\times$ ULN, were generally able to continue uninterrupted treatment with the drug with complete resolution of the biochemical abnormalities (Watkins, 2009). Although this "adaptation" (Dara, Liu, & Kaplowitz, 2016) in itself does not exclude the possibility that tacrine could cause clinically significant IDILI in rare patients, clinically important liver injuries have not been reported in association with tacrine treatment. It has also been noted that recurrent treatment with heparins and cholestyramine also cause relatively frequent ALT elevations (some $> 10\times$ ULN) (Harrill, Roach, Fier, et al., 2012; Singhal, Harrill, Menguy-Vacheron, et al., 2014), but these drugs have not been associated with a serious DILI liability. Finally, serum ALT elevations are also surprisingly frequent in healthy adults receiving recurrent therapeutic doses of acetaminophen (APAP) (Watkins, Kaplowitz, Slattery, et al., 2006). Although overdose of APAP is the most common cause of drug-induced liver failure in the western world, significant liver injury among those taking this drug as directed is extraordinarily rare, if it occurs at all. The "benign" ALT elevations observed with these and other drugs are sometimes referred to as "transaminitis." Although the mechanisms underlying these elevations are often unclear, it is interesting that biomarker studies involving dosing of heparins (Harrill et al., 2012) and cholestyramine (Singhal et al., 2014) indicate that they result from hepatocyte injury or death (and not passive leakage, increased synthesis, or decreased clearance from the blood). The resolution of these injuries despite continued dosing presumably reflects engagement of compensatory mechanisms, and this has been shown with APAP in rodent studies (O'Connor, Koza-Taylor, Campion, et al., 2014).

Dr. Robert Temple at the FDA has stated that drugs that are capable of causing IDILI also cause typically transient elevations in serum ALT >3 × ULN in a small subset of treated patients (Temple, 2006). This is typically identified as an incidence in the range of 1–5% above that observed in patients treated in the trial with placebo or a drug known not to cause ALT elevations. This observation has been termed "Temple's Corollary" by John Senior (i.e., as in a corollary to "Hy's Law"). Hence, the ideal situation in clinical drug development is for a new drug candidate to not satisfy Temple's Corollary. Once it is clear that a new drug causes ALT elevations >3 × ULN, the challenge is find out whether this is "transaminitis" or signals that portend the occurrence IDILI.

11. The FDA approach to assess liver safety in clinical trials

There are currently no serum biomarkers that can accurately predict the outcome of an IDILI event when the only abnormalities are asymptomatic elevations in the serum aminotransferases. The most recent FDA guidance on assessing liver safety in clinical trials (https://www.fda.gov/downloads/guidances/UCM174090.pdf) therefore recommends continuing treatment with a new drug candidate when a clinical trial patient experiences a moderate rise in serum ALT (<8 × ULN or 5–8 × ULN less than 2 weeks) and symptoms of hepatitis are not present. The goal is to see whether the patient remains asymptomatic and recovers, or progresses to develop early signs of global liver dysfunction (as assessed by elevations in serum total bilirubin). As discussed above, the prognostic importance of a rise in serum TBIL in a patient with the acute hepatitis phenotype of IDILI was first appreciated by Dr. Hyman ("Hy") Zimmerman (Zimmerman, 1968). Based on this observation, FDA has defined criteria for a "Hy's Law Case" (Table 4). Hepatocellular injury was originally defined as a concomitant serum alkaline phosphatase (alk phos) rise >2 × ULN but now is typically defined by the initial R value (i.e., $R \geq 5$). The 2009 FDA guidance is currently being re-written and it is likely that R-value criteria will replace alk phos >2 × ULN in defining an hepatocellular injury.

A standard way the FDA assesses liver safely in large clinical trial databases is with the use of "eDISH" (evaluation of Drug-Induced Serious Hepatotoxicity) software developed by John Senior and Ted Guo at the FDA (Watkins, Desai, Berkowitz, et al., 2011). This software creates a graphical display of the peak serum ALT levels (x axis) and peak serum TBIL levels (y axis) observed in each subject in a clinical trial. Vertical and horizontal lines are inserted on the graph to indicate 3× ULN for ALT and 2× ULN for TBIL, respectively (Fig. 2). The lower right quadrant therefore identifies subjects experiencing ALT elevations >3× ULN and this has been termed the "Temple's Corollary" quadrant after Bob Temple's

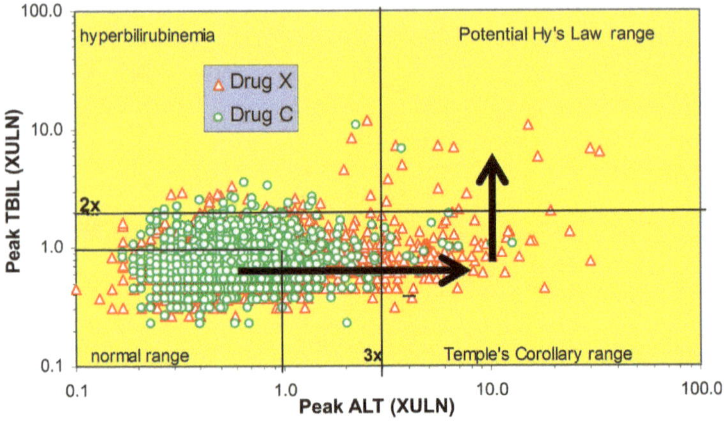

Fig. 2 Analysis of liver safety in a large clinical trial using eDISH (evaluation of Drug-Induced Serious Hepatoxicity). In the graph, each subject in the clinical trial is represented by a single symbol—red triangles are subjects treated with the study drug and the green circles are subjects treated with a comparator drug that does not cause ALT elevations. The position of each subject corresponds to the peak serum ALT value observed (x axis) and the peak serum total bilirubin observed (y axis) in that subject. A vertical line is drawn corresponding to a value for serum ALT equal to 3× ULN and a horizontal line is drawn corresponding to a serum bilirubin value of 2× ULN. It can be observed many more study drug- treated subjects than comparator treated subjects experienced elevations in serum ALT >3× ULN and serum bilirubin >2× ULN (i.e., the imbalance in the right upper quadrant). Since in this case treatment randomization was 1:1, this observation strongly suggests that the study drug caused Hy's Law Cases and therefore can cause potentially fatal IDILI. However, it is still important to examine each of these cases in this quadrant to determine if the qualifying elevations were concurrent and that the liver injury was hepatocellular in nature, and that there was no more obvious cause for the liver injuries (Table 4). Since death of hepatocytes precedes loss of global liver function sufficient to cause an elevation in serum bilirubin, subjects who end up in the right upper quadrant will drift following the arrows (see case in Fig. 1). Most of the subjects that enter the right lower quadrant will return to the normal range quadrant, either due to stopping study drug, or often due to adaptation to the injury. This is the basis for the observation by Bob Temple that drugs that cause serious IDILI are expected to cause ALT elevations >3× ULN in a larger population of treated subjects. *Figure reproduced from Church, R. J., & Watkins, P. B. (2018). In silico modeling to optimize interpretation of liver safety biomarkers in clinical trials. Experimental Biology and Medicine (Maywood, N.J.), 243, 300–307 with permission.*

previously mentioned observation. The upper right quadrant of the eDISH plot, in which both ALT and TBIL are elevated above these "Hy's Law" thresholds, contains potential Hy's Law cases. Consistent with Bob Temple's observation, Hy's Law Cases are characteristically associated with a much larger population of treated patients appearing in the Temple's Corollary quadrant. This is because isolated elevations in serum ALT due to drugs generally resolve either because treatment with the study drug is discontinued per protocol, or due to adaptation with continued study drug treatment. As shown by the typical case of the IDILI with the acute hepatitis phenotype (Fig. 1), the rise in serum bilirubin should lag behind the rise is serum ALT reflecting ongoing liver cell death prior to loss of global liver function. Concern therefore is raised if a clinical trial subject first drifts into the Temple's Corollary quadrant (i.e., has a rise in serum ALT $>3\times$ ULN but not a concurrent rise in serum TBIL $>2\times$ ULN) and does not fall back into the left lower quadrant, but drifts up into the Hy's Law quadrant (the trajectory shown with the arrows in Fig. 2). Of course, a clinical trial subject could show a trajectory to the Hy's Law quadrant due to contracting viral hepatitis or other acute liver diseases, and the injury may not be hepatocellular in nature (serum alk phos values are not displayed on the graph). It is therefore essential to look at all the relevant data and perform a thorough diagnostic assessment of each case that appears in this quadrant (Senior, 2014). The eDISH software that the FDA uses is not currently available outside the agency, but there are commercially available software packages that provide similar analyses, including more relevant data (like color coding sex, BMI, alk phos or R values) (Merz, Lee, Kullak-Ublick, et al., 2014). These packages permit examination of the eDISH plot in near real-time during a clinical trial and permit quick access to relevant data. This includes graphs of serial liver chemistries as a function of time on treatment (as shown in Fig. 1), for each patient visualized by mouse clicking on each subject symbol on the eDISH graph.

The presence of a single Hy's Law case in clinical trials is considered very concerning and may prevent FDA approval a drug that does not have an unmet medical need (Temple, 2006). Two Hy's Law cases is considered highly predictive of acute liver failure potential and few development programs outside of oncology would survive this clinical trial finding. With a new drug candidate that causes serum ALT elevations $>3\times$ ULN, and if the FDA guidelines concerning treatment modification are followed, the absence of Hy's Law Cases is reassuring. However, depending on unmet medical need, drug developers may still face the challenge of "proving a negative." This is because as discussed, most serum ALT elevations caused by IDILI drugs resolve with continued treatment, appearing like "transaminitis." The issue then becomes how many patients are needed in the clinical trial to reduce the risk of IDILI so that the perceived benefit outweighs the estimated risk. A recent case in point involves the new antibiotic solithromycin (Owens, 2017). In the phase three clinical trials for treatment of community acquired pneumonia (CAP), solithromycin was associated with a higher incidence of elevations in serum ALT than was observed with the comparator (moxifloxacin). No Hy's Law cases were observed in this trial where about 900 patients received solithromycin. According to the "rule of three" commonly used by the FDA in assessing safety of new drug candidates, the available data in the 900 solithromycin treated patients only excluded the ability of solithromycin to cause a Hy's Law case in about 1 in 300 treated patients. Assuming a 10% estimate of liver failure among Hy's Law Cases, the current clinical trial data was interpreted as excluding a liver failure risk of only 1 in 3000 treated patients. The FDA did not feel the unmet medical need for solithromycin outweighed this estimate of potential risk and requested a new clinical trial with 9000 solithromcyin-treated patients before consideration of marketing approval. If no Hy's Law Cases were identified in this large trial, the risk of fatal IDILI would be reduced to less than 1:30,000 treated patients, which evidently was considered an appropriate level of safety for this drug. The necessity for such large clinical trials to assess safety of course delays delivery to patients of new drugs and drives up their costs. Furthermore, there have been IDILI related fatalities in clinical trials even though the current dose modification recommendations were followed (Watkins, 2011). This is because in the acute hepatitis phenotype of IDILI, the injury typically progresses up to weeks after stopping treatment the implicated drug (Fig. 1). There is a clear need for new biomarkers, or combinations of biomarkers to replace the Hy's Law case and enable detection of a drug's IDILI potential long before serious liver IDILI occurs.

12. Causality assessment in clinical trials

Assessing causality of liver events during clinical trials of new drug candidates is similar to assessing causality in the post-marketing setting with one exception. The characteristic clinical presentation(s) for IDILI due to the new drug candidate is usually unknown and hence expert opinion has little advantage over RUCAM assessment by non-experts. However, when a potentially serious liver event occurs, there are often clues in the clinical trial database that are helpful in defining a signature. Specifically, it is important to examine closely the transient, asymptomatic and "treat through" elevations in liver chemistries that may have occurred to see if the timing of onset, rate of rise and resolution, and calculated R values are similar to what is observed in the more severe liver events. There is now ample data to support the idea that these transient and mild events are often mechanistically linked to more clinically important IDILI events. For example, the genetic associations with risk of clinically important IDILI caused by xymelagatran (Kindmark, Jawaid, Harbron, et al., 2008), lapatinib (Spraggs, Parham, Briley, et al., 2018) and lumiracoxib (Singer, Lewitzky, Leroy, et al., 2010) were not identified by studying the few patients with severe liver injury. They were discovered by examining the genetic data from the much larger number of patients who experienced clinically insignificant ALT elevations compared to those treated with these drugs but did not experience enzyme elevations.

One interesting example of assessing liver safety concerns the drug troglitazone. This drug was withdrawn from worldwide markets several years after its commercial introduction due to acute hepatitis IDILI resulting in multiple deaths and transplants. This liability was not recognized prior to marketing, in part because in the clinical trials, the incidence of serum ALT elevations $>1\times$ ULN was actually lower in the troglitazone-treated patients than in the placebo-treated patients (Watkins & Whitcomb, 1998). We now know that this was likely because troglitazone had a beneficial effect on fatty liver disease resulting in a fall in mean serum ALT in the patients receiving this drug (relative to placebo). However, the incidence of elevations in serum ALT $>3\times$ ULN was greater in the troglitazone-treated patients (1.9%) vs those receiving (0.5%) (Watkins & Whitcomb, 1998). The pattern of these asymptomatic events was hepatocellular, and the majority of these events occurred between 3 and 7 months on treatment. The majority of the serious liver injuries attributed to troglitazone once it was on the market also occurred between 3 and 7 months and the characteristics of the serious events were qualitatively very similar to the minor events observed in the clinical trials. Interestingly, two patients treated with troglitazone in the clinical trials experienced hepatocellular jaundice that in retrospect was probably due to troglitazone (Watkins & Whitcomb, 1998). Since roughly 2000 patients received troglitazone in the clinical trials, the incidence of Hy's Law Cases (1:1000) would predict an incidence of liver failure of about 1:10,000 treated patients, which may be near the actual incidence observed post-marketing (Graham, Drinkard, & Shatin, 2003).

A recommended way to assess the timing of ALT elevations is to plot the frequency of initial elevations as a function of time on drug (Fig. 3). This can typically define the "susceptibility window" for the elevations, and if routine liver chemistry monitoring is employed post-marketing, this analysis can define the interval where monitoring can be best justified. In some cases, this analysis has forced a reassessment of causality and an example is tolvaptan. This drug was the first to show efficacy in delaying growth of kidney cysts in patients with autosomal dominant polycystic kidney disease, but approval in the US was delayed due to concern regarding liver safety (two probable Hy's Law Cases were observed in the clinical trials (Watkins, Lewis, Kaplowitz, et al., 2015)). During the clinical trials, a group of hepatologists had analyzed each liver event to arrive at consensus regarding

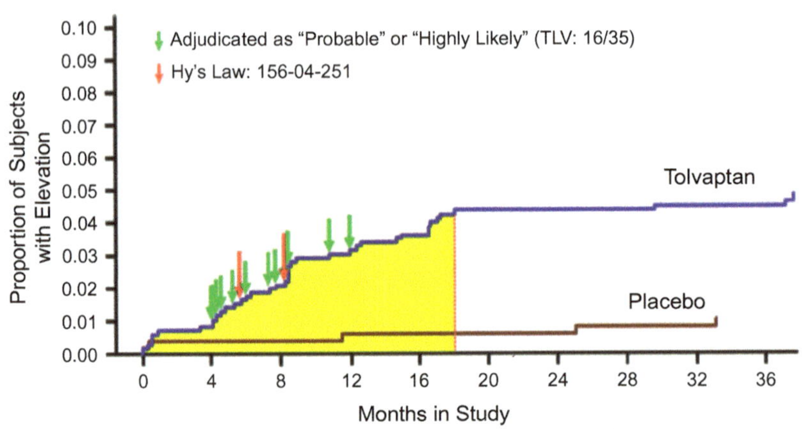

Days in Study	0	100	200	300	400	500	600	700	800	900	1000	1100
Tolvaptan N=	961	884	836	812	796	774	765	751	740	734	726	268
Placebo N=	483	476	468	459	452	445	442	433	425	422	415	147

Fig. 3 Kaplan–Meyer type analysis of the incidence of initial elevations in serum ALT $>3\times$ ULN as a function of time. The total number of patients receiving tolvaptan or placebo at each time point is shown. The total number of patients treated at each time point is shown in the box. It can be seen that the "window of susceptibility" (shaded area) extends beyond 12 months, which is unusual for IDILI. The cases adjudicated as probably related to tolvaptan (as judged by hepatologists experienced with IDILI) are shown by the arrows. The two red arrows indicate cases adjudicated to be Hy's Law Cases. The typical, or "signature" clinical presentation of tolvaptan IDILI is an acute hepatocellular injury occurring between 4 and 18 months on treatment. If a serious event occurred outside this interval, it would argue against a role for tolvaptan. *Reproduced from Watkins, P. B., Lewis, J. H., Kaplowitz, N., et al. (2015). Clinical pattern of tolvaptan-associated liver injury in subjects with autosomal dominant polycystic kidney disease: Analysis of clinical trials database.* Drug Safety, 38, *1103–1113 with permission.*

a role of tolvaptan. Because acute liver events due to drugs is quite unusual after 1 year of continuous treatment, all events occurring after 1 year were judged as unlikely due to tolvaptan. However, after the analysis shown in Fig. 3, it was clear that the "window of susceptibility" for tolvaptan-related events extended beyond 1 year. In retrospect, it seems likely that some of the events occurring after 12 months of treatment with tolvaptan were due to the drug. Note that the increased incidence of liver events in the tolvaptan vs placebo treatment did not clearly begin until after the second month of treatment. Had a Hy's Law Case (red arrows, Fig. 3) occurred prior to 2 months on treatment, this observation would have argued against a causal role for the drug (i.e., the serious case was not consistent with the "signature" indicated by the more minor events). The long latency to the acute liver events in this case likely relates to progression of the ADPKD, which somehow lowers the threshold for the acute toxicity.

13. Conclusion

The diagnosis of IDILI remains a challenge in the clinic and in clinical trials. Creation of international registries of IDILI cases has permitted the identification of characteristic or "signature" presentations for IDILI that aid in causality assessment. These signatures can sometimes be detected in clinical trials by examining the characteristics of asymptomatic and transient abnormalities in liver chemistries. Although it is well known that an acute IDILI event can progress to liver failure and death, it has been more recently appreciated that an acute IDILI event can lead to chronic liver injury. It is not generally possible to accurately predict the outcome when an IDILI event is first recognized. Continued search of genetic and non-genetic biomarkers that can aid the diagnosis of IDILI, identify which drug is responsible, and accurately predict the outcome is a high priority.

References

Aithal, G. P. (2015). Pharmacogenetic testing in idiosyncratic drug-induced liver injury: Current role in clinical practice. *Liver International*, *35*, 1801–1808.

Aithal, P. G., & Day, C. P. (1999). The natural history of histologically proved drug induced liver disease. *Gut*, *44*, 731–735.

Aithal, G. P., Watkins, P. B., Andrade, R. J., et al. (2011). Case definition and phenotype standardization in drug-induced liver injury. *Clinical Pharmacology and Therapeutics*, *89*, 806–815.

Andrade, R. J., Lucena, M. I., Fernandez, M. C., et al. (2005). Drug-induced liver injury: An analysis of 461 incidences submitted to the Spanish registry over a 10-year period. *Gastroenterology*, *129*, 512–521.

Avigan, M. I. (2014). DILI and drug development: A regulatory perspective. *Seminars in Liver Disease*, *34*, 215–226.
Avigan, M. I., Bjornsson, E. S., Pasanen, M., et al. (2014). Liver safety assessment: Required data elements and best practices for data collection and standardization in clinical trials. *Drug Safety*, *37*(Suppl. 1), S19–S31.
Bell, L. N., & Chalasani, N. (2009). Epidemiology of idiosyncratic drug-induced liver injury. *Seminars in Liver Disease*, *29*, 337–347.
Bjornsson, E. (2010). Review article: Drug-induced liver injury in clinical practice. *Alimentary Pharmacology & Therapeutics*, *32*, 3–13.
Bjornsson, E. S., Bergmann, O. M., Bjornsson, H. K., et al. (2013). Incidence, presentation, and outcomes in patients with drug-induced liver injury in the general population of Iceland. *Gastroenterology*, *144*, 1419–1425, 1425.e1–3; quiz e19–20.
Bjornsson, E. S., & Bjornsson, H. K. (2017). Mortality associated with drug-induced liver injury (DILI). *Translational Gastroenterology and Hepatology*, *2*, 114.
Bjornsson, E., & Olsson, R. (2005). Outcome and prognostic markers in severe drug-induced liver disease. *Hepatology*, *42*, 481–489.
Bonkovsky, H. L., Barnhart, H. X., Foureau, D. M., et al. (2018). Cytokine profiles in acute liver injury-results from the US drug-induced liver injury network (DILIN) and the acute liver failure study group. *PLoS One*, *13*, e0206389.
Chalasani, N., Bonkovsky, H. L., Fontana, R., et al. (2015). Features and outcomes of 899 patients with drug-induced liver injury: The DILIN prospective study. *Gastroenterology*, *148*, 1340–1352.e7.
Church, R. J., Kullak-Ublick, G. A., Aubrecht, J., et al. (2019). Candidate biomarkers for the diagnosis and prognosis of drug-induced liver injury: An international collaborative effort. *Hepatology*, *69*(2), 760–773.
Daly, A. K. (2017). Are polymorphisms in genes relevant to drug disposition predictors of susceptibility to drug-induced liver injury? *Pharmaceutical Research*, *34*, 1564–1569.
Danan, G., & Benichou, C. (1993). Causality assessment of adverse reactions to drugs—1. A novel method based on the conclusions of international consensus meetings: Application to drug-induced liver injuries. *Journal of Clinical Epidemiology*, *46*, 1323–1330.
Danan, G., & Teschke, R. (2015). RUCAM in drug and herb induced liver injury: The update. *International Journal of Molecular Sciences*, *17*, 1–33.
Dara, L., Liu, Z. X., & Kaplowitz, N. (2016). Mechanisms of adaptation and progression in idiosyncratic drug induced liver injury, clinical implications. *Liver International*, *36*, 158–165.
de Boer, Y. S., Kosinski, A. S., Urban, T. J., et al. (2017). Features of autoimmune hepatitis in patients with drug-induced liver injury. *Clinical Gastroenterology and Hepatology*, *15*, 103–112.e2.
deLemos, A. S., Foureau, D. M., Jacobs, C., et al. (2014). Drug-induced liver injury with autoimmune features. *Seminars in Liver Disease*, *34*, 194–204.
Devarbhavi, H., & Raj, S. (2018). Drug-induced liver injury with skin reactions: Drugs and host risk factors, clinical phenotypes and prognosis. *Liver International*.
Fontana, R. J. (2014). Pathogenesis of idiosyncratic drug-induced liver injury and clinical perspectives. *Gastroenterology*, *146*, 914–928.
Fontana, R. J., Hayashi, P. H., Barnhart, H., et al. (2015). Persistent liver biochemistry abnormalities are more common in older patients and those with cholestatic drug induced liver injury. *The American Journal of Gastroenterology*, *110*, 1450–1459.
Fontana, R. J., Hayashi, P. H., Gu, J., et al. (2014). Idiosyncratic drug-induced liver injury is associated with substantial morbidity and mortality within 6 months from onset. *Gastroenterology*, *147*, 96–108.e4.
Fontana, R. J., Watkins, P. B., Bonkovsky, H. L., et al. (2009). Drug-induced liver injury network (DILIN) prospective study rationale: Design and conduct. *Drug Safety*, *32*, 55–68.

Foureau, D. M., Walling, T. L., Maddukuri, V., et al. (2015). Comparative analysis of portal hepatic infiltrating leucocytes in acute drug-induced liver injury, idiopathic autoimmune and viral hepatitis. *Clinical and Experimental Immunology, 180*, 40–51.
Garcia-Cortes, M., Stephens, C., Lucena, M. I., et al. (2011). Causality assessment methods in drug induced liver injury: Strengths and weaknesses. *Journal of Hepatology, 55*, 683–691.
Graham, D. J., Drinkard, C. R., & Shatin, D. (2003). Incidence of idiopathic acute liver failure and hospitalized liver injury in patients treated with troglitazone. *The American Journal of Gastroenterology, 98*, 175–179.
Harrill, A. H., Roach, J., Fier, I., et al. (2012). The effects of heparins on the liver: Application of mechanistic serum biomarkers in a randomized study in healthy volunteers. *Clinical Pharmacology and Therapeutics, 92*, 214–220.
Hayashi, P. H. (2016). Drug-induced liver injury network causality assessment: Criteria and experience in the united states. *International Journal of Molecular Sciences, 17*, 201.
Hayashi, P. H., Rockey, D. C., Fontana, R. J., et al. (2017). Death and liver transplantation within 2 years of onset of drug-induced liver injury. *Hepatology, 66*, 1275–1285.
Hoofnagle, J. H. (2004). Drug-induced liver injury network (DILIN). *Hepatology, 40*, 773.
Hoofnagle, J. H., Serrano, J., Knoben, J. E., et al. (2013). LiverTox: A website on drug-induced liver injury. *Hepatology, 57*, 873–874.
Howell, B. A., Siler, S. Q., Shoda, L. K., Yang, Y., Woodhead, J. L., & Watkins, P. B. (2014). A mechanistic model of drug-induced liver injury aids the interpretation of elevated liver transaminase levels in a phase I clinical trial. *CPT: Pharmacometrics & Systems Pharmacology, 3*(e98), PMID: 24500662, PMCID: PMC3944113.
Institute of Medicine Committee to Review the Fialuridine Clinical T. (1995). In F. J. Manning & M. Swartz (Eds.), *Review of the fialuridine (FIAU) clinical trials*. Washington, DC: National Academies Press (US). Copyright 1995 by the National Academy of Sciences. All rights reserved.
Kindmark, A., Jawaid, A., Harbron, C. G., et al. (2008). Genome-wide pharmacogenetic investigation of a hepatic adverse event without clinical signs of immunopathology suggests an underlying immune pathogenesis. *The Pharmacogenomics Journal, 8*, 186–195.
Kleiner, D. E. (2017). The histopathological evaluation of drug-induced liver injury. *Histopathology, 70*, 81–93.
Kleiner, D. E., Chalasani, N. P., Lee, W. M., et al. (2014). Hepatic histological findings in suspected drug-induced liver injury: Systematic evaluation and clinical associations. *Hepatology, 59*, 661–670.
Kullak-Ublick, G. A., Andrade, R. J., Merz, M., et al. (2017). Drug-induced liver injury: Recent advances in diagnosis and risk assessment. *Gut, 66*, 1154–1164.
Merz, M., Lee, K. R., Kullak-Ublick, G. A., et al. (2014). Methodology to assess clinical liver safety data. *Drug Safety, 37*(Suppl. 1), S33–S45.
Mitchell, J. R., Long, M. W., Thorgeirsson, U. P., et al. (1975). Acetylation rates and monthly liver function tests during one year of isoniazid preventive therapy. *Chest, 68*, 181–190.
O'Connor, M. A., Koza-Taylor, P., Campion, S. N., et al. (2014). Analysis of changes in hepatic gene expression in a murine model of tolerance to acetaminophen hepatotoxicity (autoprotection). *Toxicology and Applied Pharmacology, 274*, 156–167.
Ortega-Alonso, A., Stephens, C., Lucena, M. I., et al. (2016). Case characterization, clinical features and risk factors in drug-induced liver injury. *International Journal of Molecular Sciences, 17*, 715–723.
Owens, B. (2017). Solithromycin rejection chills antibiotic sector. *Nature Biotechnology, 35*, 187–188.
Robles-Diaz, M., Lucena, M. I., Kaplowitz, N., et al. (2014). Use of Hy's law and a new composite algorithm to predict acute liver failure in patients with drug-induced liver injury. *Gastroenterology, 147*, 109–118.e5.

Rockey, D. C., Seeff, L. B., Rochon, J., et al. (2010). Causality assessment in drug-induced liver injury using a structured expert opinion process: Comparison to the roussel-uclaf causality assessment method. *Hepatology*, *51*, 2117–2126.

Russo, M. W., Steuerwald, N., Norton, H. J., Anderson, W. E., Foureau, D., Chalasani, N., et al. (2017). Profiles of miRNAs in serum in severe acute drug induced liver injury and their prognostic significance. *Liver International*, *37*(5), 757–764. https://doi.org/10.1111/liv.13312. Epub 2016 Nov 29, PMID: 27860186.

Senior, J. R. (2012). Alanine aminotransferase: A clinical and regulatory tool for detecting liver injury-past, present, and future. *Clinical Pharmacology and Therapeutics*, *92*, 332–339.

Senior, J. R. (2014). Evolution of the food and drug administration approach to liver safety assessment for new drugs: Current status and challenges. *Drug Safety*, *37*(Suppl. 1), S9–S17.

Sgro, C., Clinard, F., Ouazir, K., et al. (2002). Incidence of drug-induced hepatic injuries: A French population-based study. *Hepatology*, *36*, 451–455.

Singer, J. B., Lewitzky, S., Leroy, E., et al. (2010). A genome-wide study identifies HLA alleles associated with lumiracoxib-related liver injury. *Nature Genetics*, *42*, 711–714.

Singhal, R., Harrill, A. H., Menguy-Vacheron, F., et al. (2014). Benign elevations in serum aminotransferases and biomarkers of hepatotoxicity in healthy volunteers treated with cholestyramine. *BMC Pharmacology and Toxicology*, *15*, 1–7.

Spraggs, C. F., Parham, L. R., Briley, L. P., et al. (2018). Characterisation of the HLA-DRB1*07:01 biomarker for lapatinib-induced liver toxicity during treatment of early-stage breast cancer patients with lapatinib in combination with trastuzumab and/or taxanes. *The Pharmacogenomics Journal*, *18*, 480–486.

Steuerwald, N. M., Foureau, D. M., Norton, H. J., et al. (2013). Profiles of serum cytokines in acute drug-induced liver injury and their prognostic significance. *PLoS One*, *8*, e81974.

Suzuki, A., Brunt, E. M., Kleiner, D. E., et al. (2011). The use of liver biopsy evaluation in discrimination of idiopathic autoimmune hepatitis versus drug-induced liver injury. *Hepatology*, *54*, 931–939.

Temple, R. R. (2006). Hy's law: Predicting serious hepatotoxicity. *Pharmacoepidemiology and Drug Safety*, *15*, 241–243.

Teschke, R. (2018). Top-ranking drugs out of3312 drug-induced liver injury cases evaluated by the roussel uclaf causality assessment method. *Expert Opinion on Drug Metabolism & Toxicology*, *14*, 1169–1187.

Urban, T. J., Daly, A. K., & Aithal, G. P. (2014). Genetic basis of drug-induced liver injury: Present and future. *Seminars in Liver Disease*, *34*, 123–133.

Vega, M., Verma, M., Beswick, D., et al. (2017). The incidence of drug- and herbal and dietary supplement-induced liver injury: Preliminary findings from gastroenterologist-based surveillance in the population of the state of Delaware. *Drug Safety*, *40*, 783–787.

Watkins, P. B. (2009). Biomarkers for the diagnosis and management of drug-induced liver injury. *Seminars in Liver Disease*, *29*, 393–399.

Watkins, P. B. (2011). Drug safety sciences and the bottleneck in drug development. *Clinical Pharmacology and Therapeutics*, *89*, 788–790.

Watkins, P. B., Desai, M., Berkowitz, S. D., et al. (2011). Evaluation of drug-induced serious hepatotoxicity (eDISH): Application of this data organization approach to phase III clinical trials of rivaroxaban after total hip or knee replacement surgery. *Drug Safety*, *34*, 243–252.

Watkins, P. B., Kaplowitz, N., Slattery, J. T., et al. (2006). Aminotransferase elevations in healthy adults receiving 4 grams of acetaminophen daily: A randomized controlled trial. *JAMA*, *296*, 87–93.

Watkins, P. B., Lewis, J. H., Kaplowitz, N., et al. (2015). Clinical pattern of tolvaptan-associated liver injury in subjects with autosomal dominant polycystic kidney disease: Analysis of clinical trials database. *Drug Safety*, *38*, 1103–1113.

Watkins, P. B., & Seeff, L. B. (2006). Drug-induced liver injury: Summary of a single topic clinical research conference. *Hepatology*, *43*, 618–631.
Watkins, P. B., & Whitcomb, R. W. (1998). Hepatic dysfunction associated with troglitazone. *New England Journal of Medicine*, *338*, 916–917.
Watkins, P. B., Zimmerman, H. J., Knapp, M. J., et al. (1994). Hepatotoxic effects of tacrine administration in patients with alzheimer's disease. *JAMA*, *271*, 992–998.
Zimmerman, H. J. (1968). The spectrum of hepatotoxicity. *Perspectives in Biology and Medicine*, *12*, 135–161.

CHAPTER SEVEN

Acetaminophen hepatotoxicity: A mitochondrial perspective

Anup Ramachandran*, Hartmut Jaeschke
Department of Pharmacology, Toxicology, and Therapeutics, University of Kansas Medical Center, Kansas City, KS, United States
*Corresponding author: e-mail address: aramachandran@kumc.edu

Contents

Abstract

Acetaminophen (APAP) is a highly effective analgesic, which is safe at therapeutic doses. However, an overdose can cause hepatotoxicity and even liver failure. APAP toxicity is currently the most common cause of acute liver failure in the United States. Decades of research on mechanisms of liver injury have established the role of mitochondria as central players in APAP-induced hepatocyte necrosis and this chapter examines the various facets of the organelle's involvement in the process of injury as well as in resolution of damage. The injury process is initiated by formation of a reactive metabolite, which binds to sulfhydryl groups of cellular proteins including mitochondrial proteins. This inhibits the electron transport chain and leads to formation of reactive oxygen species, which induce the activation of redox-sensitive members of the MAP kinase family ultimately causing activation of c-Jun N terminal kinase, JNK. Translocation of JNK to the mitochondria then amplifies mitochondrial dysfunction, ultimately resulting in mitochondrial permeability transition and release of mitochondrial intermembrane proteins,

Advances in Pharmacology, Volume 85
ISSN 1054-3589
https://doi.org/10.1016/bs.apha.2019.01.007
© 2019 Elsevier Inc. All rights reserved.

which trigger nuclear DNA fragmentation. Together, these events result in hepatocyte necrosis, while adaptive mechanisms such as mitophagy remove damaged mitochondria and minimize the extent of the injury. This oscillation between recovery and necrosis is predominant in cells at the edge of the necrotic area in the liver, where induction of mitochondrial biogenesis is important for liver regeneration. All these aspects of mitochondria in APAP hepatotoxicity, as well as their relevance to humans with APAP overdose and development of therapeutic approaches will be examined in detail in this chapter.

Abbreviations

AIF apoptosis inducing factor
AMAP 3′-hydroxyacetanilide
APAP acetaminophen
ASK1 apoptosis signaling kinase 1.
CuZnSOD copper zinc superoxide dismutase.
DAMP damage associated molecular pattern.
eNOS endothelial nitric oxide synthase.
ER endoplasmic reticulum.
ERK extracellular signal regulated kinase.
ETC electron transport chain.
GLDH glutamate dehydrogenase.
GSK-3β glycogen synthase kinase-3β.
JNK c-jun N-terminal kinase.
MAP mitogen activated protein.
MKK4 mitogen-activated protein kinase kinase 4.
MLK3 mixed-lineage kinase 3.
MnSOD manganese superoxide dismutase.
MPTP mitochondrial permeability transition pore.
NAC *N*-acetyl cysteine.
NAPQI *N*-acetyl-*p*-benzoquinone imine.
nNOS neuronal nitric oxide synthase.
NO nitric oxide.
NOS nitric oxide synthase.
PARK7 parkinsonism associated deglycase.
ROS reactive oxygen species
SEC sinusoidal endothelial cell
VDAC voltage dependent anion channel

1. Introduction

Acetaminophen (APAP) is the most consumed drug for pain and fever in the United States and Europe and is very effective at therapeutic doses. In addition to its availability as a single drug, APAP is also extensively marketed in combination with a wide variety of other drugs, increasing its consumption in the general population. While very safe at therapeutic doses, APAP unfortunately can produce severe hepatotoxicity as an overdose and is the most common cause of acute liver failure in the United States. In addition to the instances of attempted self-harm with APAP, an unintentional overdose is also common due to the plethora of combination products containing APAP. Decades of research have provided significant insight into the mechanisms of APAP-induced hepatotoxicity, which is initiated by its cytochrome P450 mediated metabolism into a reactive metabolite *N*-acetyl-*p*-benzoquinone imine (NAPQI). Hepatic glutathione depletion and subsequent mitochondrial dysfunction then sets the stage for induction of a characteristic centrilobular hepatocyte necrosis, which ultimately can lead to acute liver failure in the absence of supportive treatment. The standard of care currently for an APAP overdose is administration of *N*-acetylcysteine (NAC), which replenishes hepatic glutathione stores and supports recovery of mitochondrial function. However, NAC has a short therapeutic window for maximum benefit and there is an ongoing search for additional therapeutics with alternate targets, which could complement NAC and increase the therapeutic window. The central role of mitochondria in APAP-induced liver injury make this an attractive target and this review will focus on the organelle and delve into the various facets of mitochondrial biology in the context of APAP-induced cell signaling.

2. Mitochondria in APAP overdose

As mentioned earlier, APAP-induced cell death is initiated by the cytochrome P450-mediated generation of NAPQI. While the role of the reactive metabolite NAPQI in mediating APAP-induced liver injury was recognized relatively early, with identification of protein adducts within various cellular compartments, the recognition of the important role of the mitochondria came later. Since cytochrome P450 is localized to the endoplasmic reticulum (ER), studies using radioactive APAP demonstrated highest levels of covalent binding of radioactive material to the ER and cytosolic fractions, with smaller amounts in the mitochondria (Jollow et al., 1973). Subsequently, changes in mitochondrial ultrastructure after APAP were appreciated on electron microscopy in the late 1970s (Petersen & Vilstrup, 1979) and further studies on mitochondrial respiration and ultrastructure after APAP indicated the organelle's role in APAP-induced cell signaling (Myers, Beierschmitt, Khairallah, & Cohen, 1986; Placke, Ginsberg, Wyand, & Cohen, 1987). Functional deficits in mitochondria were also recognized (Andersson, Rundgren, Nelson, & Harder, 1990; Donnelly, Walker, & Racz, 1994), though whether these were causes or consequence of the APAP-induced injury was not very clear. The role of mitochondrial free radicals as well as oxidative stress in mediating APAP-induced injury *in vivo* was first described in the early 1990s (Jaeschke, 1990) and subsequently confirmed by others *in vitro* (Burcham & Harman, 1991). Further studies reported evidence for peroxynitrite formation during APAP hepatotoxicity (Hinson, Pike, Pumford, & Mayeux, 1998), which was also located inside of mitochondria (Cover et al., 2005). The importance of mitochondrial peroxynitrite over general oxidant stress was also documented (Knight, Ho, Farhood, & Jaeschke, 2002). Further studies in the mid to late 2000s uncovered the role of translocation of cytosolic proteins such as Bax (Bajt, Farhood, Lemasters, & Jaeschke, 2008) and the MAP kinase JNK (Gunawan et al., 2006) onto mitochondria, which amplifies the oxidant stress and ultimately induces the mitochondrial permeability transition pore opening. These various aspects will be examined in detail in the subsequent sections.

3. Mitochondrial protein adducts in APAP hepatotoxicity

Studies using the regioisomer of APAP, 3′-hydroxyacetanilide (AMAP), which has been shown to be non-toxic in mice, hamsters and several cell lines, indicated that the main difference between the two was formation of mitochondrial protein adducts with APAP but not AMAP (Matthews, Hinson, Roberts, & Pumford, 1997; Myers et al., 1995; Tirmenstein & Nelson, 1989). Interestingly it was found that AMAP was actually toxic in human hepatocytes, where it did induce the formation of mitochondrial protein adducts (Xie, McGill, et al., 2015), again confirming the importance of these mitochondrial adducts in APAP-induced liver injury. Mitochondrial protein adducts also seem to be responsible for the APAP-induced mitochondrial dysfunction (Hu, Ramshesh, McGill, Jaeschke, & Lemasters, 2016). But why is it that these comparatively lower amounts of mitochondrial protein adducts are directly involved in mediating downstream effects rather than the more abundant adducts in ER and microsomes? While a definitive answer is still lacking, several inferences can be made based on the information from proteomic studies examining specific mitochondrial targets, as well as the functions of the mitochondria. The mitochondrial electron transport chain (ETC) normally transfers electrons to cytochrome *c* oxidase (Complex IV) to generate the proton gradient used by ATP synthase (Complex V) for ATP synthesis. However, even during physiological respiration, leakage of electrons from the ETC results in generation of free radicals such as the superoxide anion. Thus, any alteration in ETC components, which increase leak of electrons could presumably elevate generation of superoxide and result in oxidant stress. This does not occur physiologically since the robust anti-oxidant systems within the mitochondria, including manganese superoxide dismutase (MnSOD), copper zinc superoxide dismutase (CuZnSOD) within the intermembrane space (Okado-Matsumoto & Fridovich, 2001), glutathione peroxidase and thioredoxin function to scavenge these radicals and keep oxidant stress under control. This is all the more important with the presence of nitric oxide (NO) generating systems within the mitochondria, since reaction of superoxide with NO can generate the potent oxidant peroxynitrite. While the source of NO within the mitochondria is not well characterized, it seems that one possibility could be the presence of the alpha isoform of neuronal NOS within mitochondria (Lacza, Pankotai, & Busija, 2009). Additionally, it has also been shown that endothelial NOS (eNOS) could be associated with VDAC2 (Alvira et al., 2012), an outer mitochondrial membrane protein, and could thus produce NO close to the mitochondria. Thus, formation of APAP adducts on mitochondrial proteins would need to hit multiple targets, including components of the ETC, mitochondrial anti-oxidants and modulate nitric oxide to ultimately result in mitochondrial oxidative and nitrosative stress.

Though the direct connections between formation of NAPQI-mitochondrial protein adducts and increased superoxide and peroxynitrite formation within the mitochondria are still nebulous, a number of proteomic analysis examining adducted proteins within mitochondria enable the generation of hypotheses which could be tested. Proteomic analysis of whole liver homogenates after exposure of mice to APAP *in vivo* have identified a number of mitochondrial proteins which were adducted, including the α-subunit of ATP synthetetase (Qiu, Benet, & Burlingame, 1998). Since ATP synthase is central for mitochondrial ATP generation, formation of APAP adducts on the protein could be expected to prevent ATP synthesis, which had been shown very early in studies on APAP hepatotoxicity (Andersson et al., 1990; Jaeschke, 1990) and decreases in ATP synthase enzyme activity have also been demonstrated (Parmar, Ahmed, Khandkar, & Katyare, 1995), albeit in a rat model. The other prominent target identified was glutathione peroxidase, which would again be relevant since this is an important mitochondrial anti-oxidant enzyme and its inactivation by APAP-adduct formation could compromise free radical scavenging within mitochondria and aggravate mitochondrial oxidant stress. Interestingly however, deficiency of glutathione peroxidase did not make mice more sensitive to APAP compared to wild type mice (Knight et al., 2002), indicating that adducts on glutathione peroxidase are probably a general effect rather than causative of downstream events. Another recent proteomic study identified additional mitochondrial proteins modified by NAPQI in 3D cultures of human hepatocytes and nonparenchymal cells (Bruderer et al., 2015). These included antioxidant enzymes such as peroxiredoxin 6 and the redox sensitive chaperone PARK7, as well as the voltage gated ion channel VDAC2 present on the mitochondrial outer membrane (Bruderer et al., 2015). Since it has been shown that NAPQI binding to mitochondrial proteins correlates with APAP toxicity (Jaeschke, Knight, & Bajt, 2003) the finding of APAP-adducts on ATP synthase, coupled with the preponderance of anti-oxidant targets being adducted after an APAP overdose lends credence to the hypothesis that the initial source of enhanced superoxide within mitochondria after an APAP overdose is the *ETC*. This probably occurs due to the over-reduction of the coenzyme Q pool and the higher membrane potential due to block of ATP synthase, which results in reverse electron transport and enhanced generation of superoxide. Coupled with the compromised anti-oxidant systems, this would then result in the subsequent mitochondrial oxidant stress (Fig. 1).

4. APAP induced mitochondrial oxidative and nitrosative stress

Whether mitochondrial adduct formation is directly responsible for it or not, APAP overdose causes substantial elevations in mitochondrial superoxide levels (Yan, Ramachandran, Bajt, Lemasters, & Jaeschke, 2010), as well as peroxynitrite (Cover et al., 2005). As alluded to earlier, the scavenging capacity of the mitochondria for these free radicals seems to be a critical feature of the injury process, since mice with a partial deficiency of the main superoxide scavenging mitochondrial enzyme, manganese superoxide dismutase show significant exacerbation of APAP induced liver injury

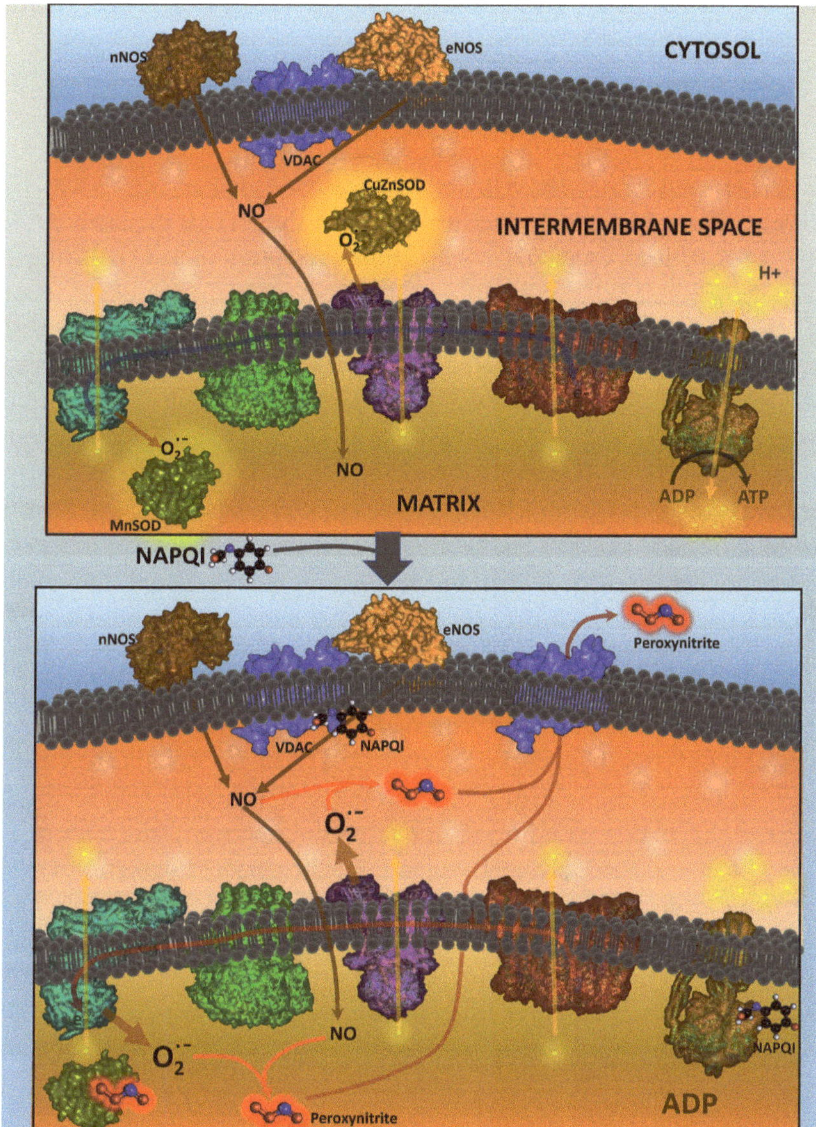

Fig. 1 Peroxynitrite formation is critical for initial mitochondrial dysfunction and signaling to the cytosol: The mitochondrial electron transport chain (ETC) comprised of 4 proteins transfer electrons from complex I to complex IV, while pumping protons to generate a proton gradient which is utilized by ATP synthase (complex V) to generate ATP. Though free radicals such as superoxide are generated during electron transport, superoxide dismutases (SOD) within the mitochondria scavenge them efficiently. Thus, reaction of superoxide with nitric oxide (NO) generated from neuronal NOS and probably eNOS on mitochondria is minimal. When mitochondria are exposed to NAPQI, adduct formation on mitochondrial proteins such as ATP synthase could result in reverse electron transport within the ETC, which elevates superoxide generation. Protein adduct formation on anti-oxidant enzymes prevents efficient scavenging of superoxide, which enables its reaction with nitric oxide to form peroxynitrite radicals. These in turn can modify enzymes such as SOD as well as spill out of the mitochondria into the cytosol, probably through outer membrane protein such as VDAC.

(Fujimoto et al., 2009; Ramachandran, Lebofsky, Weinman, & Jaeschke, 2011). This is further corroborated by the protective effect of the mitochondria-targeted SOD-mimetic—Mito-Tempo, which provides significant protection against APAP hepatotoxicity (Du et al., 2019; Du, Farhood, & Jaeschke, 2017). Further proof that the ETC is the likely source of these free radicals comes from early studies on permeabilized hepatocytes, which demonstrated that exposure to APAP resulted in the loss of mitochondrial respiratory function, accompanied by a decrease in ATP levels, which was preceded by a loss of reduced glutathione (Burcham & Harman, 1991). Complex II in particular was found to be more sensitive to inhibition by direct exposure to NAPQI, when compared to complex I (Burcham & Harman, 1991; Lee, Imaizumi, Chamberland, Alder, & Boelsterli, 2015; Ramsay, Rashed, & Nelson, 1989). However, these direct effects of NAPQI were demonstrated *in vitro* and hence their relevance *in vivo* is not known. Acetaminophen overdose *in vivo* in mice was shown to significantly inhibit complex I activity, which may contribute to the oxidative stress (Du et al., 2016). It was also demonstrated that APAP interferes with the formation of mitochondrial respiratory super complexes *via* the mitochondrial negative regulator MCJ, which leads to decreased production of ATP and increased generation of ROS (Barbier-Torres et al., 2017). In any case, in the context of APAP-induced mitochondrial oxidant stress, it seems that reaction of the generated superoxide with nitric oxide to produce peroxynitrite is more relevant (Cover et al., 2005; Knight, Kurtz, Bajt, Hinson, & Jaeschke, 2001) than superoxide generation *per se*. Interestingly, nitro-tyrosine staining used as a marker of protein modification induced by peroxynitrite revealed early staining in sinusoidal endothelial cells prior to hepatocytes after APAP (Knight et al., 2001). Endothelial cell staining was evident at 1 h post APAP, and staining in hepatocytes was only visible by 4 h, the next time point tested (Knight et al., 2001). This time course tallies with scanning electron microscopy studies which showed morphological changes in the sinusoidal endothelium prior to alterations in hepatocytes. One of the earliest changes appreciated was formation of large pores of 0.5–3 μm diameter in the sinusoidal endothelial cell lining at 1.5 h after APAP (Walker, Racz, & McElligott, 1983). Since this occurs subsequent to peroxynitrite staining in endothelial cells, it is possible that APAP initially causes sinusoidal endothelial cell (SEC) dysfunction prior to affecting hepatocytes. In fact, SEC have been shown to be susceptible to APAP-induced injury *in vitro* (DeLeve et al., 1997). SEC damage during APAP hepatotoxicity varies among mouse strains depending on the P450 content of the SEC (Yin et al., 2010). Thus, the evidence of early peroxynitrite formation, coupled with morphological changes suggest that the earliest target of APAP-induced injury are SEC (Ito, Bethea, Abril, & McCuskey, 2003) and it is likely that endothelial mitochondrial oxidant stress and peroxynitrite formation play a critical role in this process (Knight & Jaeschke, 2004). However, the role SEC mitochondrial dysfunction plays in subsequent hepatocyte injury is not well characterized and needs further study. This is all the more relevant considering the role of nitric oxide in the process. While studies have been conducted on the role of NO in mediating APAP induced SEC damage (Ito, Abril, Bethea, & McCuskey, 2004), they lacked a mitochondrial focus. This is relevant since nitric oxide would have to be produced close to the location where superoxide is being produced for efficient reaction to peroxynitrite. It has been shown that pharmacological inhibition of nNOS, the putative mitochondrial NOS, protects hepatocytes against APAP-induced injury *in vitro* (Banerjee et al., 2015). This was corroborated *in vivo* too, where nNOS deficient mice were protected against APAP-induced hepatotoxicity (Agarwal et al., 2012). Interestingly, one of the targets for modification by peroxynitrite is mitochondrial manganese superoxide dismutase (Agarwal et al., 2011), which would further corrode the cells superoxide scavenging ability. The elevated peroxynitrite also contributes to mitochondrial DNA damage and loss after APAP (Cover et al., 2005), which has significant consequences later during resolution and recovery from APAP induced injury, which will be discussed in the last paragraph. The important role of peroxynitrite in mediating APAP-induced liver injury is clear by the fact that its direct scavenging either by mitochondrial glutathione (Knight et al., 2002; Saito, Zwingmann, & Jaeschke, 2010) or resveratrol (Du, McGill, Xie, Bajt, & Jaeschke, 2015), prevented APAP hepatotoxicity. Since most recent studies on APAP hepatotoxicity focus on hepatocytes, the role played by nitric oxide in modulation of mitochondrial function in sinusoidal endothelial cells is not well understood. This is relevant since NO can have significant effects on endothelial mitochondrial function (Ramachandran, Ceaser, & Darley-Usmar, 2004) and one study has shown endothelial-derived NO affecting APAP hepatotoxicity *in vivo* (Salhanick et al., 2006). However, SEC damage appears to be mouse strain-dependent and may not be particularly relevant for the human pathophysiology (Maes, Vinken, & Jaeschke, 2016). Even if the SEC are the primary target for induction of mitochondrial oxidative and nitrosative stress, the functional consequences of APAP overdose are mediated by mitochondrial dysfunction in hepatocytes and this will be elaborated next.

5. Consequences of mitochondrial oxidative/nitrosative stress in the cytosol

It could be argued that a cell such as the hepatocyte, with large number of mitochondria, would be expected to have significant reserve mitochondrial capacity to overcome dysfunction of few mitochondria due to oxidative damage. This could be the case if the consequences of NAPQI adduct formation and subsequent steps were restricted to only the organelle. In APAP overdose however, hepatocyte mitochondrial oxidative/nitrosative stress initiates signaling events within the cytosol, which subsequently amplify the mitochondrial damage and perpetuate the injury process. Though the half-life of peroxynitrite is short, in the range of 10–20ms, this is sufficient to cross biological membranes, and diffuse one to two cell diameters (Pacher, Beckman, & Liaudet, 2007) and it has been shown that peroxynitrite can cross erythrocyte membranes either through an anion channel in its anionic form or by passive diffusion in the protonated form (Denicola, Souza, & Radi, 1998). This could mean that APAP-induced peroxynitrite generated within mitochondria could either passively diffuse out or be transported through mitochondrial anion channels such as VDAC, which have been shown to control the release of the superoxide anion from mitochondria to cytosol (Han, Antunes, Canali, Rettori, & Cadenas, 2003). The presence of peroxynitrite in the cytosol then enables activation of an MAP kinase cascade resulting in activation of the c-Jun N-terminal kinase (JNK), which ultimately amplifies the mitochondrial dysfunction.

Though the exact stepwise mechanism of JNK activation by mitochondrial peroxynitrite is not well characterized, the process is likely initiated by oxidation of the protein thioredoxin, which has been shown to be a target both within the mitochondria as well as in the cytosol. Oxidation of thioredoxin 2 within mitochondria has been shown after APAP overdose (Ramachandran, Lebofsky, Yan, Weinman, & Jaeschke, 2015) and both mitochondrial thioredoxin 2 as well as cytosolic thioredoxin 1 are susceptible to direct modification by NAPQI (Jan et al., 2014). Administration of recombinant thioredoxin-1 fused to albumin in a delayed fashion, 4h after APAP was also shown to be protective in mice (Tanaka et al., 2014). Thioredoxin 1 in the cytosol is typically associated with its binding partner apoptosis signal-regulating kinase 1 (ASK1) and oxidation of thioredoxin 1 after APAP results in its dissociation from ASK1, and activation of ASK1 by phosphorylation (Nakagawa et al., 2008). The role of peroxynitrite in this process of activation of JNK is all the more probable since it has been shown that peroxynitrite can induce ASK1-thioredoxin dissociation in post ischemic myocardial infarction (Tao et al., 2006), which could also be occurring in the liver after APAP overdose. Other components of the APAP induced MAP kinase cascade include Mixed-lineage kinase 3 (MLK3), which is a ubiquitously expressed mammalian mitogen-activated protein kinase kinase kinase (MAP3K), which is suggested to control a positive feedback loop titrating proliferative or cell death signaling in response to ROS (Lee, Hwang, Shin, Kwon, & Cho, 2014). It was found that low concentrations of ROS induced activating phosphorylation of ERKs and proliferation, whereas high concentrations of ROS activated phosphorylation of JNKs and cell death (Lee et al., 2014). These studies suggested that ASK1 may be involved in the ROS-induced activation of the MLK3-mediated positive feedback loop (Lee et al., 2014). MLK3 has also been shown to be activated during APAP hepatotoxicity (Sharma, Gadang, & Jaeschke, 2012), and ultimately, activated ASK1 and MLK3 phosphorylate MKK4 (Zhang et al., 2017), which then phosphorylates JNK (Hanawa et al., 2008; Saito, Lemasters, & Jaeschke, 2010). The role of ASK1 in the process is further illustrated by the protection against APAP induced liver injury afforded by pharmacological inhibition of ASK1 (Xie, Ramachandran, et al., 2015) or inhibition of JNK activation in mice lacking ASK1 (Nakagawa et al., 2008).

While activated JNK translocates to the mitochondria to amplify mitochondrial dysfunction, it also facilitates movement of other proteins such as Bax to the mitochondria (Bajt et al., 2008; El-Hassan et al., 2003). Bax is typically tethered to the 14-3-3 protein in the cytosol and JNK has bene shown to promote Bax translocation to mitochondria through phosphorylation of 14-3-3 proteins (Tsuruta et al., 2004). Bax can also be phosphorylated by activated glycogen synthase kinase-3β (GSK-3β), which also induces its translocation to the mitochondria, at least in cancer cells (Chiara & Rasola, 2013). However, silencing of GSK-3β did not have any effect on Bax translocation in the liver (Shinohara et al., 2010), rendering this connection tenuous. However, APAP treatment in mice was shown to cause GSK-3β activation and translocation to mitochondria during the initial phase of APAP-induced liver, and animals lacking GSK-3β showed significant protection against APAP hepatotoxicity (Shinohara et al., 2010). Thus, GSK-3β does play a role in the early activation of mitochondrial dysfunction after APAP, though the exact mechanisms behind its role are not very clear. Subsequent to these changes in the cytosol, which result in JNK, Bax and GSK-3β activation, all three proteins translocate to the mitochondria to amplify organelle dysfunction.

6. Mitochondrial amplification of injury

APAP-induced phosphorylation of JNK in the cytosol results in its translocation to the mitochondria (Hanawa et al., 2008), where it binds to the scaffold protein Sab on the outer mitochondrial membrane (Win, Than, Han, Petrovic, & Kaplowitz, 2011). In case of GSK-3β, though direct evidence after APAP overdose is lacking, experiments in cardiomyoblasts have indicated that GSK-3β translocation to the mitochondria occurs in a kinase activity dependent manner where the N-terminal domain of GSK-3β may function as a mitochondrial targeting sequence, with the protein binding to VDAC2 on the mitochondrial outer membrane (Tanno et al., 2014). Though the exact mechanism of activated Bax translocation is still being worked out, there is a consensus that the protein directly inserts into the membrane (Westphal, Dewson, Czabotar, & Kluck, 2011) rather than requiring a ligand to dock unlike the case for JNK. While it is known that mitochondrial membrane lipids such as cardiolipin are susceptible to oxidation in various pathologies (Yin & Zhu, 2012), and APAP has been shown to remodel cardiolipin in mitochondria to affect mitochondrial respiration (Vergeade et al., 2016), those studies were unfortunately carried out in myeloma cells, and their relevance to hepatocytes is unknown. Binding of JNK to Sab on the mitochondrial outer membrane initiates inhibition of the mitochondrial electron transport chain in a Src dependent manner, resulting in amplification of oxidative stress (Win et al., 2011) and peroxynitrite generation (Saito, Lemasters, & Jaeschke, 2010). The critical role of phospho-JNK translocation to the mitochondria in mediating APAP induced hepatotoxicity is illustrated by the protection afforded when JNK translocation to mitochondria is blocked (Huo et al., 2017). The effect of Bax translocation to mitochondria after APAP is a bit more ambiguous, since it was found that while mice deficient in Bax were protected initially against APAP hepatotoxicity, they showed both liver necrosis as well as peroxynitrite generation similar to wild type mice at later time periods (Bajt et al., 2008), suggesting that cells could adapt to the lack of Bax and pursue alternate necrotic signaling in response to APAP. However, Bax, along with its homolog Bak have been suggested to form pores on the mitochondrial outer membrane to facilitate mitochondrial membrane permeability, which will be the focus of the next section.

7. The end game: Mitochondrial permeability transition and subsequent cellular necrosis

The above mentioned translocation of JNK and Bax to the mitochondria further compromises mitochondrial function through inhibition of the mitochondrial ETC and subsequent amplification of superoxide and peroxynitrite production (Fig. 2). Though this ultimately results in activation of the mitochondrial permeability transition pore and collapse of

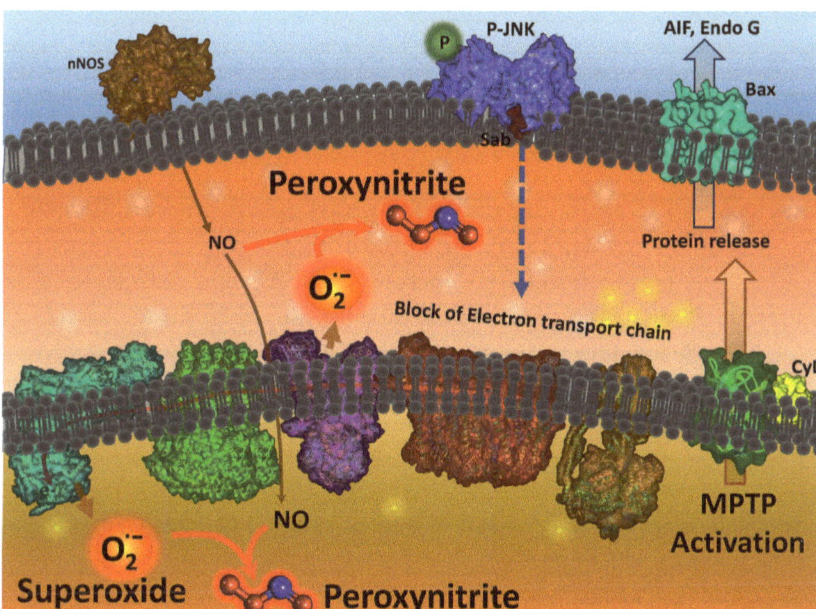

Fig. 2 JNK and Bax translocation to mitochondria amplify mitochondrial dysfunction: Phosphorylated JNK as well as Bax translocate to the mitochondria and JNK binds to its ligand Sab, on the outer mitochondrial membrane. This binding initiates a signaling cascade which inhibits the ETC and further amplifies superoxide and peroxynitrite generation. This in turn activates the mitochondrial permeability transition pore on the inner membrane, of which cyclophilin D is a component. This, along with the formation of Bax pores on the outer membrane allow release of mitochondrial proteins such as endonuclease G and apoptosis inducing factor (AIF) into the cytosol.

mitochondrial membrane potential (Kon, Kim, Jaeschke, & Lemasters, 2004; Masubuchi, Suda, & Horie, 2005; Ramachandran, Lebofsky, Baines, Lemasters, & Jaeschke, 2011), these events are titrated to the dose of APAP and are reversible at lower doses of APAP as will be elaborated below. The mitochondrial permeability transition pore (MPTP) forms within the inner membrane allowing movement of molecules of less than 1.5 kDa (Halestrap, 2009), and while its exact molecular composition is still being determined, one of its well defined components is cyclophilin D, which regulates it from within the mitochondrial matrix (Baines et al., 2005; Karch & Molkentin, 2015). Thus, the role of the mitochondrial MPTP in APAP hepatotoxicity was implicated by protection offered by pharmacological blockade of cyclophilin D *in vitro* (Kon et al., 2004). However, this protection was transient, and lost at later time points similar to the effect seen *in vivo* with Bax deficient mice. Interestingly a dose-dependent effect was seen *in vivo*, where mice deficient in cyclophilin D were protected against APAP-induced liver injury at a dose of 200 mg/kg (Ramachandran, Lebofsky, Baines, et al., 2011), while animals subjected to a higher 600 mg/kg dose showed no protection (LoGuidice & Boelsterli, 2011). Also, animals treated with APAP doses of 150 mg/kg showed reversible induction of MPTP accompanied by transient JNK activation, while those receiving 300 mg/kg had irreversible MPTP (Hu, Ramshesh, et al., 2016). In addition to the various proteins translocating to the mitochondria in response to APAP-induced cytosolic oxidant stress, translocation of lysosomal iron has also been shown to occur in mouse hepatocytes after treatment with APAP, with induction of the MPTP (Kon, Kim, Uchiyama, Jaeschke, & Lemasters, 2010). This translocation of iron occurs through the calcium uniporter (Hu, Kholmukhamedov, et al., 2016) and is probably due to lysosomal instability, which has also been demonstrated after APAP overdose (Woolbright et al., 2012).

While the components of the MPTP on the inner membrane other than cyclophilin D are still being characterized, it is well recognized that the outer membrane components are composed of Bax, along with the protein Bak on the mitochondrial outer membrane (Karch et al., 2013; Karch & Molkentin, 2014). Though these outer membrane components function during the MPTP, they are not essential for loss of mitochondrial membrane potential since it has been shown that the inner membrane portion of the MPTP was functional even in the absence of Bax and Bak, and able to induce opening that resulted in loss of membrane potential (Karch et al., 2013). This could be another explanation for lack of protection in Bax deficient mice, where the sustained production of peroxynitrite by upstream events would ultimately cause activation of the inner membrane components of the MPTP, loss of mitochondrial membrane potential and subsequent dysfunction. Another layer of complexity is added to this process by the fact that mitochondria are dynamic organelles undergoing continuous fusion and fission reactions for maintenance of cellular homeostasis. The fact that APAP overdose affects mitochondrial dynamics was first recognized by the identification of significant elevations in the mitochondrial fission protein Drp1 and its translocation to mitochondria after APAP overdose (Ramachandran et al., 2013), which was subsequently confirmed by independent studies (Dara et al., 2015), indicating that mitochondrial dynamics could influence cellular signaling after APAP overdose. This is relevant for induction of the MPTP, since spatial and temporal interactions between Drp1 and Bax have been identified (Karbowski et al., 2002), and Bax and Drp1 have both been shown to regulate each other in a reciprocal manner (Wang et al., 2015; Wu, Zhou, Zhang, & Xing, 2011). Thus, these interactions between Bax and Drp1, could influence activation of the MPTP after APAP and subsequent mitochondrial dysfunction.

Ultimately as a consequence of the MPTP, critical mitochondrial proteins such as cytochrome *c*, endonuclease G, apoptosis inducing factor and Smac are released into the cytosol to initiate DNA fragmentation and cell necrosis. While loss of cytochrome *c* compromises mitochondrial electron transport and shuts down ATP synthesis, apoptosis inducing factor and endonuclease G have nuclear localization signals (Norberg, Orrenius, & Zhivotovsky, 2010), which allow their translocation to the nucleus (Bajt, Cover, Lemasters, & Jaeschke, 2006). The importance of AIF in APAP induced hepatotoxicity is indicated by protection offered in mice with a partial deficiency of AIF (Bajt et al., 2011). In the nucleus, AIF causes chromatin condensation and DNA fragmentation (Boujrad, Gubkina, Robert, Krantic, & Susin, 2007), while endonuclease G cleaves nuclear DNA resulting in DNA fragmentation (Cover et al., 2005).

8. Mitochondria in adaptation and recovery after APAP overdose

In addition to the well characterized role of mitochondria in APAP-induced injury detailed above, more recent studies highlight the role of the organelle in adaptive responses to APAP as well as in recovery after

APAP-induced injury. An important adaptive feature within the liver after APAP-induced formation of protein adducts is induction of a form of autophagy, called mitophagy, which enables removal of damaged mitochondria (Ni, Bockus, Boggess, Jaeschke, & Ding, 2012; Ni, Williams, Jaeschke, & Ding, 2013). The importance of this is illustrated by the aggravation of APAP hepatotoxicity by prevention of mitophagy by cholesterol accumulation (Baulies et al., 2015). Mitophagy would also be beneficial from a spatial perspective, where cells at the border of the necrotic area may be spared induction of cell death by timely removal of damaged mitochondria (Ni et al., 2013). The cells at the border of the necrotic area are also important from the perspective of recovery after an APAP overdose and recent evidence shows spatially defined activation of mitochondrial biogenesis in these cell populations, which plays a critical role in recovery (Du, Ramachandran, et al., 2017). Induction of mitochondrial biogenesis was also shown to facilitate recovery and regeneration after APAP-induced liver injury (Du, Ramachandran, et al., 2017).

9. Role of mitochondria-derived damage-associated molecular patterns in injury and recovery

Because of the extensive mitochondrial damage and the resulting severe necrosis after APAP overdose, mitochondrial components are released into the cytosol and ultimately into the circulation. Some of the macromolecules detected in plasma include mtDNA, the matrix enzymes glutamate dehydrogenase (GLDH) and carbamoyl phosphate synthetase-1 and long-chain acylcarnitines (Bhattacharyya et al., 2014; Chen, Krausz, Shah, Idle, & Gonzalez, 2009; McGill et al., 2012; McGill, Li, et al., 2014; Weerasinghe, Jang, Fontana, & Omary, 2014). All these compounds can be used as mechanistic biomarkers to detect mitochondrial damage in the pathophysiology of APAP hepatotoxicity and potentially predict outcome in patients (McGill & Jaeschke, 2018). However, some of these mitochondria-derived molecules, *e.g.,* mtDNA, are potent damage-associated molecular patterns (DAMPs), which bind to toll like receptors on macrophages, *e.g.,* TLR9, and transcriptionally activate cytokine and chemokine formation (Kubes & Mehal, 2012; Woolbright & Jaeschke, 2017). The resulting activation and hepatic recruitment of neutrophils and monocyte-derived macrophages has the potential to further aggravate the injury (Kubes & Mehal, 2012). However, the preponderance of experimental evidence suggest that these inflammatory cells are mainly recruited to clear necrotic cell debris and promote regeneration (Woolbright & Jaeschke, 2017). Importantly, the pro-regenerative function of neutrophils and monocytes is also supported by human studies (Antoniades et al., 2012; Williams et al., 2014). Thus, mitochondria-derived and other DAMPs prepare the damaged tissue for recovery.

10. Relevance of APAP-induced mitochondrial dysfunction to humans

While most findings on mitochondrial involvement in APAP-induced hepatotoxicity has been determined by investigations in the mouse model, the organelle's involvement in APAP induced hepatotoxicity in humans has also been extensively documented. As mentioned earlier, formation of mitochondrial protein adducts have been recognized in human hepatocytes treated with AMAP (Xie, McGill, et al., 2015) and studies on freshly isolated human hepatocytes exposed to APAP overdose demonstrated formation of mitochondrial protein adducts as well as a time dependent activation and mitochondrial translocation of phospho-JNK to the mitochondria, followed by loss of mitochondrial membrane potential (Xie et al., 2014). A number of mitochondrial proteins modified by NAPQI have also been identified in 3D cultures of human hepatocytes and nonparenchymal cells (Bruderer et al., 2015). Human HepaRG cells exposed to APAP show mitochondrial oxidant stress and peroxynitrite formation (McGill et al., 2011) as in the mouse, indicating that similar mechanisms are operative in human hepatocytes subsequent to APAP overdose. This is corroborated by direct evidence from human patients, where biomarkers of mitochondrial damage such as circulating mitochondrial DNA and glutamate dehydrogenase were also elevated in APAP overdose patients with liver injury (McGill et al., 2012). Patients with more mitochondrial damage are also less likely to survive, since the levels of these mitochondrial biomarkers were also found to be significantly higher in non-surviving patients when compared to survivors (McGill, Staggs, et al., 2014). The relevance of APAP-induced mitochondrial dysfunction in human patients with APAP overdose is further re-iterated by the introduction into clinical trials of a SOD mimetic, which will be discussed below.

11. Conclusion

While the mitochondria are a critical target during APAP-induced hepatotoxicity and act as an integration center for various cellular signaling components of necrotic cell death, the organelle also plays very important roles in adaptation and regeneration in a spatially defined manner to enable robust recovery of cells further away from the necrotic area. While extensive experimentation has provided significant mechanistic insight into the role of hepatocyte mitochondria in APAP-induced liver injury, they have also uncovered tantalizing clues toward the other roles the organelle plays, especially in recovery and regeneration after APAP overdose. Studies to better understand these roles, such as the influence of mitochondrial dynamics and biogenesis in mediating recovery and regeneration are ongoing with the ultimate hope to develop mitochondrial targeted therapeutics to prevent APAP-induced acute liver failure. Our unpublished data indicate that drugs such as 4-methylpyrazole, which provides protection against APAP-induced injury (Akakpo et al., 2018), inhibits not only cytochrome P450 enzymes but also prevents JNK activation and its mitochondrial translocation and could thus be a useful therapeutic with similar potency as the current standard of care *N*-acetylcysteine. The SOD mimetics Calmangafodipir and Mito-TEMPO were also shown to have beneficial effects in APAP overdose in mice (Bedda et al., 2003; Du et al., 2019; Du, Farhood, & Jaeschke, 2017) and Calmangafodipir is currently in clinical trials (Dear, Morrison, Henriksen, & Näsström, 2017). Methylene blue, a redox-active compound used clinically to treat methemoglobinemia has also been shown to protect against APAP-induced mitochondrial injury by circumventing the compromised complexes I/II of the electron transport chain (Lee et al., 2015). In addition, inducers of mitochondrial biogenesis such as SRT1720 have also been shown to be beneficial (Du, Ramachandran, et al., 2017) and could be developed as therapeutics. Overall, while research over the previous decades have provided significant insight into the role of mitochondria in APAP-induced injury, the various facets of the organelle in recovery and regeneration, which probably have more therapeutic potential, are poised to be discovered in the future.

Acknowledgments

Work in the authors' laboratory was supported by a grant from McNeil Consumer Health Care, Inc., the National Institutes of Health grant R01 DK102142, and the National Institute of General Medical Sciences (P20 GM103549 and P30 GM118247) from the National Institutes of Health.

Conflict of interest statement

The authors have no conflict.

References

Agarwal, R., Hennings, L., Rafferty, T. M., Letzig, L. G., McCullough, S., James, L. P., et al. (2012). Acetaminophen-induced hepatotoxicity and protein nitration in neuronal nitric-oxide synthase knockout mice. *The Journal of Pharmacology and Experimental Therapeutics*, *340*(1), 134–142.

Agarwal, R., MacMillan-Crow, L. A., Rafferty, T. M., Saba, H., Roberts, D. W., Fifer, E. K., et al. (2011). Acetaminophen-induced hepatotoxicity in mice occurs with inhibition of activity and nitration of mitochondrial manganese superoxide dismutase. *The Journal of Pharmacology and Experimental Therapeutics*, *337*(1), 110–116.

Akakpo, J. Y., Ramachandran, A., Kandel, S. E., Ni, H. M., Kumer, S. C., Rumack, B. H., et al. (2018). 4-Methylpyrazole protects against acetaminophen hepatotoxicity in mice and in primary human hepatocytes. *Human & Experimental Toxicology*, *37*(12), 1310–1322.

Alvira, C. M., Umesh, A., Husted, C., Ying, L., Hou, Y., Lyu, S. C., et al. (2012). Voltage-dependent anion channel-2 interaction with nitric oxide synthase enhances pulmonary artery endothelial cell nitric oxide production. *American Journal of Respiratory Cell and Molecular Biology*, *47*(5), 669–678.

Andersson, B. S., Rundgren, M., Nelson, S. D., & Harder, S. (1990). N-acetyl-p-benzoquinone imine-induced changes in the energy metabolism in hepatocytes. *Chemico-Biological Interactions*, *75*(2), 201–211.

Antoniades, C. G., Quaglia, A., Taams, L. S., Mitry, R. R., Hussain, M., Abeles, R., et al. (2012). Source and characterization of hepatic macrophages in acetaminophen-induced acute liver failure in humans. *Hepatology*, *56*(2), 735–746.

Baines, C. P., Kaiser, R. A., Purcell, N. H., Blair, N. S., Osinska, H., Hambleton, M. A., et al. (2005). Loss of cyclophilin D reveals a critical role for mitochondrial permeability transition in cell death. *Nature*, *434*(7033), 658–662.

Bajt, M. L., Cover, C., Lemasters, J. J., & Jaeschke, H. (2006). Nuclear translocation of endonuclease G and apoptosis-inducing factor during acetaminophen-induced liver cell injury. *Toxicological Sciences*, *94*(1), 217–225.

Bajt, M. L., Farhood, A., Lemasters, J. J., & Jaeschke, H. (2008). Mitochondrial bax translocation accelerates DNA fragmentation and cell necrosis in a murine model of acetaminophen hepatotoxicity. *The Journal of Pharmacology and Experimental Therapeutics*, *324*(1), 8–14.

Bajt, M. L., Ramachandran, A., Yan, H. M., Lebofsky, M., Farhood, A., Lemasters, J. J., et al. (2011). Apoptosis-inducing factor modulates mitochondrial oxidant stress in acetaminophen hepatotoxicity. *Toxicological Sciences*, *122*(2), 598–605.

Banerjee, S., Melnyk, S. B., Krager, K. J., Aykin-Burns, N., Letzig, L. G., James, L. P., et al. (2015). The neuronal nitric oxide synthase inhibitor NANT blocks acetaminophen toxicity and protein nitration in freshly isolated hepatocytes. *Free Radical Biology & Medicine*, *89*, 750–757.

Barbier-Torres, L., Iruzubieta, P., Fernandez-Ramos, D., Delgado, T. C., Taibo, D., Guitierrez-de-Juan, V., et al. (2017). The mitochondrial negative regulator MCJ is a therapeutic target for acetaminophen-induced liver injury. *Nature Communications*, *8*(1), 2068.

Baulies, A., Ribas, V., Nunez, S., Torres, S., Alarcon-Vila, C., Martinez, L., et al. (2015). Lysosomal cholesterol accumulation sensitizes to acetaminophen hepatotoxicity by impairing mitophagy. *Scientific Reports*, *5*, 18017.

Bedda, S., Laurent, A., Conti, F., Chereau, C., Tran, A., Tran-Van Nhieu, J., et al. (2003). Mangafodipir prevents liver injury induced by acetaminophen in the mouse. *Journal of Hepatology*, *39*(5), 765–772.

Bhattacharyya, S., Yan, K., Pence, L., Simpson, P. M., Gill, P., Letzig, L. G., et al. (2014). Targeted liquid chromatography-mass spectrometry analysis of serum acylcarnitines in acetaminophen toxicity in children. *Biomarkers in Medicine*, *8*(2), 147–159.

Boujrad, H., Gubkina, O., Robert, N., Krantic, S., & Susin, S. A. (2007). AIF-mediated programmed necrosis: A highly regulated way to die. *Cell Cycle*, *6*(21), 2612–2619.

Bruderer, R., Bernhardt, O. M., Gandhi, T., Miladinovic, S. M., Cheng, L. Y., Messner, S., et al. (2015). Extending the limits of quantitative proteome profiling with data-independent acquisition and application to acetaminophen-treated three-dimensional liver microtissues. *Molecular & Cellular Proteomics*, *14*(5), 1400–1410.

Burcham, P. C., & Harman, A. W. (1991). Acetaminophen toxicity results in site-specific mitochondrial damage in isolated mouse hepatocytes. *The Journal of Biological Chemistry*, *266*(8), 5049–5054.

Chen, C., Krausz, K. W., Shah, Y. M., Idle, J. R., & Gonzalez, F. J. (2009). Serum metabolomics reveals irreversible inhibition of fatty acid beta-oxidation through the suppression of PPARalpha activation as a contributing mechanism of acetaminophen-induced hepatotoxicity. *Chemical Research in Toxicology*, *22*(4), 699–707.

Chiara, F., & Rasola, A. (2013). GSK-3 and mitochondria in cancer cells. *Frontiers in Oncology*, *3*, 16.

Cover, C., Mansouri, A., Knight, T. R., Bajt, M. L., Lemasters, J. J., Pessayre, D., et al. (2005). Peroxynitrite-induced mitochondrial and endonuclease-mediated nuclear DNA damage in acetaminophen hepatotoxicity. *The Journal of Pharmacology and Experimental Therapeutics*, *315*(2), 879–887.

Dara, L., Johnson, H., Suda, J., Win, S., Gaarde, W., Han, D., et al. (2015). Receptor interacting protein kinase 1 mediates murine acetaminophen toxicity independent of the necrosome and not through necroptosis. *Hepatology*, *62*(6), 1847–1857.

Dear, J. W., Morrison, E., Henriksen, D., & Näsström, J. (2017). Calmangafodipir is a new treatment for late stage liver toxicity after acetaminophen overdose. *Hepatology*, *66*(S1), 4A.

DeLeve, L. D., Wang, X., Kaplowitz, N., Shulman, H. M., Bart, J. A., & van der Hoek, A. (1997). Sinusoidal endothelial cells as a target for acetaminophen toxicity. Direct action versus requirement for hepatocyte activation in different mouse strains. *Biochemical Pharmacology*, *53*(9), 1339–1345.

Denicola, A., Souza, J. M., & Radi, R. (1998). Diffusion of peroxynitrite across erythrocyte membranes. *Proceedings of the National Academy of Sciences of the United States of America*, *95*(7), 3566–3571.

Donnelly, P. J., Walker, R. M., & Racz, W. J. (1994). Inhibition of mitochondrial respiration in vivo is an early event in acetaminophen-induced hepatotoxicity. *Archives of Toxicology*, *68*(2), 110–118.

Du, K., Farhood, A., & Jaeschke, H. (2017). Mitochondria-targeted antioxidant Mito-tempo protects against acetaminophen hepatotoxicity. *Archives of Toxicology*, *91*(2), 761–773.

Du, K., McGill, M. R., Xie, Y., Bajt, M. L., & Jaeschke, H. (2015). Resveratrol prevents protein nitration and release of endonucleases from mitochondria during acetaminophen hepatotoxicity. *Food and Chemical Toxicology*, *81*, 62–70.

Du, K., Ramachandran, A., McGill, M. R., Mansouri, A., Asselah, T., Farhood, A., et al. (2017). Induction of mitochondrial biogenesis protects against acetaminophen hepatotoxicity. *Food and Chemical Toxicology*, *108*(Pt A), 339–350.

Du, K., Ramachandran, A., Weemhoff, J. L., Chavan, H., Xie, Y., Krishnamurthy, P., et al. (2016). Editor's highlight: Metformin protects against acetaminophen hepatotoxicity by attenuation of mitochondrial oxidant stress and dysfunction. *Toxicological Sciences*, *154*(2), 214–226.

Du, K., Ramachandran, A., Weemhoff, J. L., Woolbright, B. L., Jaeschke, A. H., Chao, X., et al. (2019). Mito-tempo protects against acute liver injury but induces limited secondary apoptosis during the late phase of acetaminophen hepatotoxicity. *Archives of Toxicology*, *93*, 163–178.

El-Hassan, H., Anwar, K., Macanas-Pirard, P., Crabtree, M., Chow, S. C., Johnson, V. L., et al. (2003). Involvement of mitochondria in acetaminophen-induced apoptosis and hepatic injury: Roles of cytochrome c, Bax, bid, and caspases. *Toxicology and Applied Pharmacology*, *191*(2), 118–129.
Fujimoto, K., Kumagai, K., Ito, K., Arakawa, S., Ando, Y., Oda, S., et al. (2009). Sensitivity of liver injury in heterozygous Sod2 knockout mice treated with troglitazone or acetaminophen. *Toxicologic Pathology*, *37*(2), 193–200.
Gunawan, B. K., Liu, Z. X., Han, D., Hanawa, N., Gaarde, W. A., & Kaplowitz, N. (2006). C-Jun N-terminal kinase plays a major role in murine acetaminophen hepatotoxicity. *Gastroenterology*, *131*(1), 165–178.
Halestrap, A. P. (2009). What is the mitochondrial permeability transition pore? *Journal of Molecular and Cellular Cardiology*, *46*(6), 821–831.
Han, D., Antunes, F., Canali, R., Rettori, D., & Cadenas, E. (2003). Voltage-dependent anion channels control the release of the superoxide anion from mitochondria to cytosol. *The Journal of Biological Chemistry*, *278*(8), 5557–5563.
Hanawa, N., Shinohara, M., Saberi, B., Gaarde, W. A., Han, D., & Kaplowitz, N. (2008). Role of JNK translocation to mitochondria leading to inhibition of mitochondria bioenergetics in acetaminophen-induced liver injury. *The Journal of Biological Chemistry*, *283*(20), 13565–13577.
Hinson, J. A., Pike, S. L., Pumford, N. R., & Mayeux, P. R. (1998). Nitrotyrosine-protein adducts in hepatic centrilobular areas following toxic doses of acetaminophen in mice. *Chemical Research in Toxicology*, *11*(6), 604–607.
Hu, J., Kholmukhamedov, A., Lindsey, C. C., Beeson, C. C., Jaeschke, H., & Lemasters, J. J. (2016). Translocation of iron from lysosomes to mitochondria during acetaminophen-induced hepatocellular injury: Protection by starch-desferal and minocycline. *Free Radical Biology & Medicine*, *97*, 418–426.
Hu, J., Ramshesh, V. K., McGill, M. R., Jaeschke, H., & Lemasters, J. J. (2016). Low dose acetaminophen induces reversible mitochondrial dysfunction associated with transient c-Jun N-terminal kinase activation in mouse liver. *Toxicological Sciences*, *150*(1), 204–215.
Huo, Y., Win, S., Than, T. A., Yin, S., Ye, M., Hu, H., et al. (2017). Antcin H protects against acute liver injury through disruption of the interaction of c-Jun-N-terminal kinase with mitochondria. *Antioxidants & Redox Signaling*, *26*(5), 207–220.
Ito, Y., Abril, E. R., Bethea, N. W., & McCuskey, R. S. (2004). Role of nitric oxide in hepatic microvascular injury elicited by acetaminophen in mice. *American Journal of Physiology. Gastrointestinal and Liver Physiology*, *286*(1), G60–G67.
Ito, Y., Bethea, N. W., Abril, E. R., & McCuskey, R. S. (2003). Early hepatic microvascular injury in response to acetaminophen toxicity. *Microcirculation*, *10*(5), 391–400.
Jaeschke, H. (1990). Glutathione disulfide formation and oxidant stress during acetaminophen-induced hepatotoxicity in mice in vivo: The protective effect of allopurinol. *The Journal of Pharmacology and Experimental Therapeutics*, *255*(3), 935–941.
Jaeschke, H., Knight, T. R., & Bajt, M. L. (2003). The role of oxidant stress and reactive nitrogen species in acetaminophen hepatotoxicity. *Toxicology Letters*, *144*(3), 279–288.
Jan, Y. H., Heck, D. E., Dragomir, A. C., Gardner, C. R., Laskin, D. L., & Laskin, J. D. (2014). Acetaminophen reactive intermediates target hepatic thioredoxin reductase. *Chemical Research in Toxicology*, *27*(5), 882–894.
Jollow, D. J., Mitchell, J. R., Potter, W. Z., Davis, D. C., Gillette, J. R., & Brodie, B. B. (1973). Acetaminophen-induced hepatic necrosis. II. Role of covalent binding in vivo. *The Journal of Pharmacology and Experimental Therapeutics*, *187*(1), 195–202.
Karbowski, M., Lee, Y. J., Gaume, B., Jeong, S. Y., Frank, S., Nechushtan, A., et al. (2002). Spatial and temporal association of Bax with mitochondrial fission sites, Drp1, and Mfn2 during apoptosis. *The Journal of Cell Biology*, *159*(6), 931–938.

Karch, J., Kwong, J. Q., Burr, A. R., Sargent, M. A., Elrod, J. W., Peixoto, P. M., et al. (2013). Bax and Bak function as the outer membrane component of the mitochondrial permeability pore in regulating necrotic cell death in mice. *eLife*, *2*, e00772.

Karch, J., & Molkentin, J. D. (2014). Identifying the components of the elusive mitochondrial permeability transition pore. *Proceedings of the National Academy of Sciences of the United States of America*, *111*(29), 10396–10397.

Karch, J., & Molkentin, J. D. (2015). Regulated necrotic cell death: The passive aggressive side of Bax and Bak. *Circulation Research*, *116*(11), 1800–1809.

Knight, T. R., Ho, Y. S., Farhood, A., & Jaeschke, H. (2002). Peroxynitrite is a critical mediator of acetaminophen hepatotoxicity in murine livers: Protection by glutathione. *The Journal of Pharmacology and Experimental Therapeutics*, *303*(2), 468–475.

Knight, T. R., & Jaeschke, H. (2004). Peroxynitrite formation and sinusoidal endothelial cell injury during acetaminophen-induced hepatotoxicity in mice. *Comparative Hepatology*, *3*(Suppl 1), S46.

Knight, T. R., Kurtz, A., Bajt, M. L., Hinson, J. A., & Jaeschke, H. (2001). Vascular and hepatocellular peroxynitrite formation during acetaminophen toxicity: Role of mitochondrial oxidant stress. *Toxicological Sciences*, *62*(2), 212–220.

Kon, K., Kim, J. S., Jaeschke, H., & Lemasters, J. J. (2004). Mitochondrial permeability transition in acetaminophen-induced necrosis and apoptosis of cultured mouse hepatocytes. *Hepatology*, *40*(5), 1170–1179.

Kon, K., Kim, J. S., Uchiyama, A., Jaeschke, H., & Lemasters, J. J. (2010). Lysosomal iron mobilization and induction of the mitochondrial permeability transition in acetaminophen-induced toxicity to mouse hepatocytes. *Toxicological Sciences*, *117*(1), 101–108.

Kubes, P., & Mehal, W. Z. (2012). Sterile inflammation in the liver. *Gastroenterology*, *143*(5), 1158–1172.

Lacza, Z., Pankotai, E., & Busija, D. W. (2009). Mitochondrial nitric oxide synthase: Current concepts and controversies. *Frontiers in Bioscience*, *14*, 4436–4443.

Lee, H. S., Hwang, C. Y., Shin, S. Y., Kwon, K. S., & Cho, K. H. (2014). MLK3 is part of a feedback mechanism that regulates different cellular responses to reactive oxygen species. *Science Signaling*, 7(328), ra52.

Lee, K. K., Imaizumi, N., Chamberland, S. R., Alder, N. N., & Boelsterli, U. A. (2015). Targeting mitochondria with methylene blue protects mice against acetaminophen-induced liver injury. *Hepatology*, *61*(1), 326–336.

LoGuidice, A., & Boelsterli, U. A. (2011). Acetaminophen overdose-induced liver injury in mice is mediated by peroxynitrite independently of the cyclophilin D-regulated permeability transition. *Hepatology*, *54*(3), 969–978.

Maes, M., Vinken, M., & Jaeschke, H. (2016). Experimental models of hepatotoxicity related to acute liver failure. *Toxicology and Applied Pharmacology*, *290*, 86–97.

Masubuchi, Y., Suda, C., & Horie, T. (2005). Involvement of mitochondrial permeability transition in acetaminophen-induced liver injury in mice. *Journal of Hepatology*, *42*(1), 110–116.

Matthews, A. M., Hinson, J. A., Roberts, D. W., & Pumford, N. R. (1997). Comparison of covalent binding of acetaminophen and the regioisomer 3′-hydroxyacetanilide to mouse liver protein. *Toxicology Letters*, *90*(1), 77–82.

McGill, M. R., & Jaeschke, H. (2018). Biomarkers of drug-induced liver injury: Progress and utility in research, medicine, and regulation. *Expert Review of Molecular Diagnostics*, *18*(9), 797–807.

McGill, M. R., Li, F., Sharpe, M. R., Williams, C. D., Curry, S. C., Ma, X., et al. (2014). Circulating acylcarnitines as biomarkers of mitochondrial dysfunction after acetaminophen overdose in mice and humans. *Archives of Toxicology*, *88*(2), 391–401.

McGill, M. R., Sharpe, M. R., Williams, C. D., Taha, M., Curry, S. C., & Jaeschke, H. (2012). The mechanism underlying acetaminophen-induced hepatotoxicity in humans and mice involves mitochondrial damage and nuclear DNA fragmentation. *The Journal of Clinical Investigation*, *122*(4), 1574–1583.

McGill, M. R., Staggs, V. S., Sharpe, M. R., Lee, W. M., Jaeschke, H., & Acute Liver Failure Study, G (2014). Serum mitochondrial biomarkers and damage-associated molecular patterns are higher in acetaminophen overdose patients with poor outcome. *Hepatology*, *60*(4), 1336–1345.

McGill, M. R., Yan, H. M., Ramachandran, A., Murray, G. J., Rollins, D. E., & Jaeschke, H. (2011). HepaRG cells: A human model to study mechanisms of acetaminophen hepatotoxicity. *Hepatology*, *53*(3), 974–982.

Myers, L., Beierschmitt, W., Khairallah, E., & Cohen, S. (1986). In vivo and in vitro inhibition of hepatic mitochondria1 respiration by acetaminophen. *The Pharmacologist*, *28*, 125.

Myers, T. G., Dietz, E. C., Anderson, N. L., Khairallah, E. A., Cohen, S. D., & Nelson, S. D (1995). A comparative study of mouse liver proteins arylated by reactive metabolites of acetaminophen and its nonhepatotoxic regioisomer, 3′-hydroxyacetanilide. *Chemical Research in Toxicology*, *8*(3), 403–413.

Nakagawa, H., Maeda, S., Hikiba, Y., Ohmae, T., Shibata, W., Yanai, A., et al. (2008). Deletion of apoptosis signal-regulating kinase 1 attenuates acetaminophen-induced liver injury by inhibiting c-Jun N-terminal kinase activation. *Gastroenterology*, *135*(4), 1311–1321.

Ni, H. M., Bockus, A., Boggess, N., Jaeschke, H., & Ding, W. X. (2012). Activation of autophagy protects against acetaminophen-induced hepatotoxicity. *Hepatology*, *55*(1), 222–232.

Ni, H. M., Williams, J. A., Jaeschke, H., & Ding, W. X. (2013). Zonated induction of autophagy and mitochondrial spheroids limits acetaminophen-induced necrosis in the liver. *Redox Biology*, *1*, 427–432.

Norberg, E., Orrenius, S., & Zhivotovsky, B. (2010). Mitochondrial regulation of cell death: Processing of apoptosis-inducing factor (AIF). *Biochemical and Biophysical Research Communications*, *396*(1), 95–100.

Okado-Matsumoto, A., & Fridovich, I. (2001). Subcellular distribution of superoxide dismutases (SOD) in rat liver: Cu,Zn-SOD in mitochondria. *The Journal of Biological Chemistry*, *276*(42), 38388–38393.

Pacher, P., Beckman, J. S., & Liaudet, L. (2007). Nitric oxide and peroxynitrite in health and disease. *Physiological Reviews*, *87*(1), 315–424.

Parmar, D. V., Ahmed, G., Khandkar, M. A., & Katyare, S. S. (1995). Mitochondrial ATPase: A target for paracetamol-induced hepatotoxicity. *European Journal of Pharmacology*, *293*(3), 225–229.

Petersen, P., & Vilstrup, H. (1979). Relation between liver function and hepatocyte ultrastructure in a case of paracetamol intoxication. *Digestion*, *19*(6), 415–419.

Placke, M. E., Ginsberg, G. L., Wyand, D. S., & Cohen, S. D. (1987). Ultrastructural changes during acute acetaminophen-induced hepatotoxicity in the mouse: A time and dose study. *Toxicologic Pathology*, *15*(4), 431–438.

Qiu, Y., Benet, L. Z., & Burlingame, A. L. (1998). Identification of the hepatic protein targets of reactive metabolites of acetaminophen in vivo in mice using two-dimensional gel electrophoresis and mass spectrometry. *The Journal of Biological Chemistry*, *273*(28), 17940–17953.

Ramachandran, A., Ceaser, E., & Darley-Usmar, V. M. (2004). Chronic exposure to nitric oxide alters the free iron pool in endothelial cells: Role of mitochondrial respiratory complexes and heat shock proteins. *Proceedings of the National Academy of Sciences of the United States of America*, *101*(1), 384–389.

Ramachandran, A., Lebofsky, M., Baines, C. P., Lemasters, J. J., & Jaeschke, H. (2011). Cyclophilin D deficiency protects against acetaminophen-induced oxidant stress and liver injury. *Free Radical Research*, *45*(2), 156–164.

Ramachandran, A., Lebofsky, M., Weinman, S. A., & Jaeschke, H. (2011). The impact of partial manganese superoxide dismutase (SOD2)-deficiency on mitochondrial oxidant stress, DNA fragmentation and liver injury during acetaminophen hepatotoxicity. *Toxicology and Applied Pharmacology*, *251*(3), 226–233.

Ramachandran, A., Lebofsky, M., Yan, H. M., Weinman, S. A., & Jaeschke, H. (2015). Hepatitis C virus structural proteins can exacerbate or ameliorate acetaminophen-induced liver injury in mice. *Archives of Toxicology*, *89*(5), 773–783.

Ramachandran, A., McGill, M. R., Xie, Y., Ni, H. M., Ding, W. X., & Jaeschke, H. (2013). Receptor interacting protein kinase 3 is a critical early mediator of acetaminophen-induced hepatocyte necrosis in mice. *Hepatology*, *58*(6), 2099–2108.

Ramsay, R. R., Rashed, M. S., & Nelson, S. D. (1989). In vitro effects of acetaminophen metabolites and analogs on the respiration of mouse liver mitochondria. *Archives of Biochemistry and Biophysics*, *273*(2), 449–457.

Saito, C., Lemasters, J. J., & Jaeschke, H. (2010). C-Jun N-terminal kinase modulates oxidant stress and peroxynitrite formation independent of inducible nitric oxide synthase in acetaminophen hepatotoxicity. *Toxicology and Applied Pharmacology*, *246*(1–2), 8–17.

Saito, C., Zwingmann, C., & Jaeschke, H. (2010). Novel mechanisms of protection against acetaminophen hepatotoxicity in mice by glutathione and N-acetylcysteine. *Hepatology*, *51*(1), 246–254.

Salhanick, S. D., Orlow, D., Holt, D. E., Pavlides, S., Reenstra, W., & Buras, J. A. (2006). Endothelially derived nitric oxide affects the severity of early acetaminophen-induced hepatic injury in mice. *Academic Emergency Medicine*, *13*(5), 479–485.

Sharma, M., Gadang, V., & Jaeschke, A. (2012). Critical role for mixed-lineage kinase 3 in acetaminophen-induced hepatotoxicity. *Molecular Pharmacology*, *82*(5), 1001–1007.

Shinohara, M., Ybanez, M. D., Win, S., Than, T. A., Jain, S., Gaarde, W. A., et al. (2010). Silencing glycogen synthase kinase-3beta inhibits acetaminophen hepatotoxicity and attenuates JNK activation and loss of glutamate cysteine ligase and myeloid cell leukemia sequence 1. *The Journal of Biological Chemistry*, *285*(11), 8244–8255.

Tanaka, R., Ishima, Y., Maeda, H., Kodama, A., Nagao, S., Watanabe, H., et al. (2014). Albumin fusion prolongs the antioxidant and anti-inflammatory activities of thioredoxin in mice with acetaminophen-induced hepatitis. *Molecular Pharmaceutics*, *11*(4), 1228–1238.

Tanno, M., Kuno, A., Ishikawa, S., Miki, T., Kouzu, H., Yano, T., et al. (2014). Translocation of glycogen synthase kinase-3beta (GSK-3beta), a trigger of permeability transition, is kinase activity-dependent and mediated by interaction with voltage-dependent anion channel 2 (VDAC2). *The Journal of Biological Chemistry*, *289*(42), 29285–29296.

Tao, L., Jiao, X., Gao, E., Lau, W. B., Yuan, Y., Lopez, B., et al. (2006). Nitrative inactivation of thioredoxin-1 and its role in postischemic myocardial apoptosis. *Circulation*, *114*(13), 1395–1402.

Tirmenstein, M. A., & Nelson, S. D. (1989). Subcellular binding and effects on calcium homeostasis produced by acetaminophen and a nonhepatotoxic regioisomer, 3′-hydroxyacetanilide, in mouse liver. *The Journal of Biological Chemistry*, *264*(17), 9814–9819.

Tsuruta, F., Sunayama, J., Mori, Y., Hattori, S., Shimizu, S., Tsujimoto, Y., et al. (2004). JNK promotes Bax translocation to mitochondria through phosphorylation of 14-3-3 proteins. *The EMBO Journal*, *23*(8), 1889–1899.

Vergeade, A., Bertram, C. C., Bikineyeva, A. T., Zackert, W. E., Zinkel, S. S., May, J. M., et al. (2016). Cardiolipin fatty acid remodeling regulates mitochondrial function by modifying the electron entry point in the respiratory chain. *Mitochondrion*, *28*, 88–95.

Walker, R. M., Racz, W. J., & McElligott, T. F. (1983). Scanning electron microscopic examination of acetaminophen-induced hepatotoxicity and congestion in mice. *The American Journal of Pathology*, *113*(3), 321–330.

Wang, P., Wang, P., Liu, B., Zhao, J., Pang, Q., Agrawal, S. G., et al. (2015). Dynamin-related protein Drp1 is required for Bax translocation to mitochondria in response to irradiation-induced apoptosis. *Oncotarget*, *6*(26), 22598–22612.

Weerasinghe, S. V., Jang, Y. J., Fontana, R. J., & Omary, M. B. (2014). Carbamoyl phosphate synthetase-1 is a rapid turnover biomarker in mouse and human acute liver injury. *American Journal of Physiology. Gastrointestinal and Liver Physiology*, *307*(3), G355–G364.

Westphal, D., Dewson, G., Czabotar, P. E., & Kluck, R. M. (2011). Molecular biology of Bax and Bak activation and action. *Biochimica et Biophysica Acta*, *1813*(4), 521–531.

Williams, C. D., Bajt, M. L., Sharpe, M. R., McGill, M. R., Farhood, A., & Jaeschke, H. (2014). Neutrophil activation during acetaminophen hepatotoxicity and repair in mice and humans. *Toxicology and Applied Pharmacology*, *275*(2), 122–133.

Win, S., Than, T. A., Han, D., Petrovic, L. M., & Kaplowitz, N. (2011). C-Jun N-terminal kinase (JNK)-dependent acute liver injury from acetaminophen or tumor necrosis factor (TNF) requires mitochondrial sab protein expression in mice. *The Journal of Biological Chemistry*, *286*(40), 35071–35078.

Woolbright, B. L., & Jaeschke, H. (2017). Role of the inflammasome in acetaminophen-induced liver injury and acute liver failure. *Journal of Hepatology*, *66*(4), 836–848.

Woolbright, B. L., Ramachandran, A., McGill, M. R., Yan, H. M., Bajt, M. L., Sharpe, M. R., et al. (2012). Lysosomal instability and cathepsin B release during acetaminophen hepatotoxicity. *Basic & Clinical Pharmacology & Toxicology*, *111*(6), 417–425.

Wu, S., Zhou, F., Zhang, Z., & Xing, D. (2011). Bax is essential for Drp1-mediated mitochondrial fission but not for mitochondrial outer membrane permeabilization caused by photodynamic therapy. *Journal of Cellular Physiology*, *226*(2), 530–541.

Xie, Y., McGill, M. R., Dorko, K., Kumer, S. C., Schmitt, T. M., Forster, J., et al. (2014). Mechanisms of acetaminophen-induced cell death in primary human hepatocytes. *Toxicology and Applied Pharmacology*, *279*(3), 266–274.

Xie, Y., McGill, M. R., Du, K., Dorko, K., Kumer, S. C., Schmitt, T. M., et al. (2015). Mitochondrial protein adducts formation and mitochondrial dysfunction during N-acetyl-m-aminophenol (AMAP)-induced hepatotoxicity in primary human hepatocytes. *Toxicology and Applied Pharmacology*, *289*(2), 213–222.

Xie, Y., Ramachandran, A., Breckenridge, D. G., Liles, J. T., Lebofsky, M., Farhood, A., et al. (2015). Inhibitor of apoptosis signal-regulating kinase 1 protects against acetaminophen-induced liver injury. *Toxicology and Applied Pharmacology*, *286*(1), 1–9.

Yan, H. M., Ramachandran, A., Bajt, M. L., Lemasters, J. J., & Jaeschke, H. (2010). The oxygen tension modulates acetaminophen-induced mitochondrial oxidant stress and cell injury in cultured hepatocytes. *Toxicological Sciences*, *117*(2), 515–523.

Yin, H., Cheng, L., Holt, M., Hail, N., Jr., Maclaren, R., & Ju, C. (2010). Lactoferrin protects against acetaminophen-induced liver injury in mice. *Hepatology*, *51*(3), 1007–1016.

Yin, H., & Zhu, M. (2012). Free radical oxidation of cardiolipin: Chemical mechanisms, detection and implication in apoptosis, mitochondrial dysfunction and human diseases. *Free Radical Research*, *46*(8), 959–974.

Zhang, J., Min, R. W. M., Le, K., Zhou, S., Aghajan, M., Than, T. A., et al. (2017). The role of MAP2 kinases and p38 kinase in acute murine liver injury models. *Cell Death & Disease*, *8*(6), e2903.

CHAPTER EIGHT

Biomarkers of drug-induced liver injury

Mitchell R. McGill*[,†,1], Hartmut Jaeschke[‡]

*Department of Environmental and Occupational Health, Fay W. Boozman College of Public Health, University of Arkansas for Medical Sciences, Little Rock, AR, United States

[†]Department of Pharmacology and Toxicology, University of Arkansas for Medical Sciences, Little Rock, AR, United States

[‡]Department of Pharmacology, Toxicology, and Therapeutics, University of Kansas Medical Center, Kansas City, KS, United States

[1]Corresponding author: e-mail address: mmcgill@uams.edu

Contents

Abstract

Drug-induced liver injury (DILI) is a major clinical and regulatory challenge. As a result, interest in DILI biomarkers is growing. So far, considerable progress has been made in identification of biomarkers for diagnosis (acetaminophen-cysteine protein adducts), prediction (genetic biomarkers), and prognosis (microRNA-122, high mobility group box 1 protein, keratin-18, glutamate dehydrogenase, mitochondrial DNA). Many of those biomarkers also provide mechanistic insight. The purpose of this chapter is to review major advances in DILI biomarker research over the last decade, and to highlight some of the challenges involved in implementation. Although much work has been done, more liver-specific biomarkers, more DILI-specific biomarkers, and better prognostic biomarkers for survival are all still needed. Furthermore, more work is needed to define reference intervals and medical decision limits.

Advances in Pharmacology, Volume 85
ISSN 1054-3589
https://doi.org/10.1016/bs.apha.2019.02.001

© 2019 Elsevier Inc.
All rights reserved.

Abbreviations

AFP α-fetoprotein
ALF acute liver failure
ALT alanine aminotransferase
APAP acetaminophen
APAP-CYS acetaminophen-cysteine
AST aspartate aminotransferase
DIALF drug-induced acute liver failure
DILI drug-induced liver injury
GLDH glutamate dehydrogenase
HMGB1 high mobility group box 1 protein
IDILI idiosyncratic drug-induced liver injury
K18 keratin-18
mtDNA mitochondrial DNA
NPV negative predictive value
PCNA proliferating cell nuclear antigen
PPV positive predictive value

1. Introduction

Drug-induced liver injury (DILI) can be a problem at any point in the life cycle of a drug. It is commonly encountered during testing of new drugs, and roughly half with early clinical evidence of hepatotoxicity are terminated before reaching the market (Olson et al., 2000). Postapproval, it is a common reason for black box warnings and other packaging modifications (Issa et al., 2007; Solotke, Dhruva, Downing, Shah, & Ross, 2018) and for drug withdrawals (Onakpoya, Heneghan, & Aronson, 2016). It is also the chief cause of acute liver failure (ALF) in the United States, the United Kingdom, Australia and some European countries (Lee, 2008). Though approximately 50% of drug-induced ALF cases in the United States are due to acetaminophen (APAP) overdose (Lee, 2008), many other drugs on the market can also cause hepatotoxicity, including the relatively new class of drugs known as immune checkpoint inhibitors. Clearly, DILI is a serious obstacle in both drug development and patient care.

DILI is often grouped into two classes: (1) intrinsic and (2) idiosyncratic. Intrinsic DILI is hepatotoxicity due to natural properties of a drug or its metabolite(s). It usually involves overdose, and it is highly reproducible. On the other hand, idiosyncratic DILI (IDILI), a subset of the broader category of idiosyncratic adverse drug reactions, occurs at recommended therapeutic doses, and is relatively rare. Some drugs cause IDILI in

<0.01% of consumers, though the prevalence of IDILI varies greatly (McGill & Jaeschke, 2018).

Decades after the introduction of alkaline phosphatase and aminotransferases (ALT, AST) as the first biomarkers of liver injury, interest in identification of novel DILI biomarkers has been growing (McGill, 2016). Although current clinical laboratory tests are helpful for detection of liver injury or dysfunction in many cases, they are not useful for diagnosis of etiology or for prognosis (Antoine et al., 2013; Dear et al., 2018; Levine, O'Connor, Padilla-Jones, & Gerkin, 2016; McGill, Li et al., 2014; McGill, Staggs, et al., 2014; Senior, 2014). The US National Institutes of Health and US Food and Drug Administration Biomarker Working Group has defined a biomarker as a "characteristic that is measured as an indicator of normal biological processes, pathogenic processes, or responses to an exposure or intervention" (US FDA, 2016). They further divided biomarkers into seven categories: biomarkers of risk/susceptibility, diagnosis, monitoring, prediction, prognosis, pharmacodynamics, and safety. DILI biomarkers have potential for use in three of those categories: diagnosis, prediction (or risk), and prognosis. Additionally, several biomarkers have been introduced that provide insight into pathophysiological mechanisms, commonly referred to as mechanistic biomarkers. Here, we discuss important recent advances in the DILI biomarker field in each of those categories. Table 1 is a summary of the most promising current DILI biomarkers for these major uses, but we will begin with a discussion of the issue of prevalence, which affects both clinical and regulatory biomarker utility.

2. The problem of low prevalence in DILI biomarker development

A critical concept in development of serum or plasma biomarkers for DILI is the effect of prevalence on utility. Curiously, although the challenge of low prevalence has been extensively discussed in publications on the subject of genetic biomarkers of IDILI (Alfirevic & Pirmohamed, 2012), it is rarely mentioned with regard to serum DILI biomarkers. It is occasionally proposed that serum or genetic biomarkers could be used to predict IDILI in patients before treatment with a drug known to cause it (Chen, Borlak, & Tong, 2014). However, the real-world utility of a biomarker depends in part upon the prevalence of the disease or outcome of interest (Fig. 1) (McGill & Jaeschke, 2018), and IDILI is rare. Due to the low prevalence of IDILI among patients taking almost any given IDILI-associated

Table 1 Most promising DILI biomarkers.

Diagnostic biomarkers
Protein-derived APAP-CYS
Predictive biomarkers
Genetic associations (e.g., HLA B*5701)
Prognostic biomarkers
miR-122
HMGB1
K18
Mechanistic biomarkers
HMGB1
K18
GLDH
mtDNA
Nuclear DNA fragments

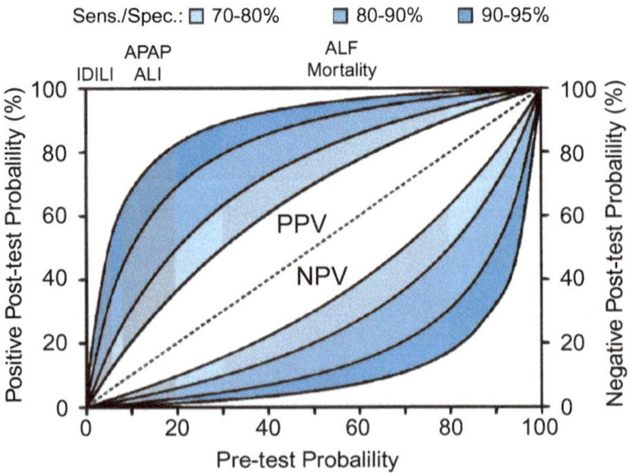

Fig. 1 Relationship between prevalence and predictive values. Positive posttest probability (left upper portion), a surrogate of PPV when pretest probability or prevalence is estimated, increases with increasing prevalence, while negative posttest probability (right lower portion), a surrogate for negative predictive value (NPV), decreases. Blue-shaded areas show different levels sensitivity and specificity. For the different levels, both sensitivity and specificity were set at either 70, 80, 90, or 95%. Vertical, gray-shaded areas show the approximate ranges of prevalence for idiosyncratic drug-induced liver injury (IDILI) among users of a given IDILI-associated drug, for acute liver injury (ALI) among early-presenting acetaminophen (APAP) overdose patients, and for mortality among acute liver failure (ALF) patients.

drug, it would be difficult, nearly impossible, to develop a biomarker with sufficient positive predictive value (PPV) to predict it (Fig. 1) (McGill & Jaeschke, 2018; Senior, 2014). Although it has been argued that biomarkers with high negative predictive value (NPV) could be used to rule-out risk of IDILI, the pretest probability is typically <1%. That is, you can be at least 99% certain in most cases that IDILI will not occur before administering the drug without the help of a biomarker. So the value added by a high NPV biomarker in that context is questionable.

Nevertheless, there are clear uses of biomarkers in DILI that are not as limited by prevalence. Estimates of the prevalence of all-cause DILI among patients presenting with evidence of acute liver injury range from 10 to 15% (Björnsson, Olafsson, Bermann, & Björnsson, 2016; Breu et al., 2018; Galvin, McDonaugh, Ryan, & Stewart, 2015). Thus, it is theoretically possible to develop a useful biomarker to diagnose DILI in general, though it will have to have high sensitivity and specificity (>90%) in order to achieve moderately high PPV and NPV (70–80%). It will also need to be specific for DILI, but not specific for the particular drug that is the cause; as mentioned, the prevalence of DILI due to any single drug would be too low. As we will see, the single exception to the latter is serum APAP-protein adducts to diagnose APAP overdose. Together, those requirements set a very high bar, but not necessarily prohibitively high as long as we understand that the predictive values will be modest. Furthermore, biomarkers may aid prognosis. Approximately 15% of patients who present early after APAP overdose with normal-to-low ALT values go on to develop hepatotoxicity despite *N*-acetylcysteine treatment (Antoine et al., 2013; Rumack & Peterson, 1978; Rumack, Peterson, Koch, & Amara, 1981; Smilkstein et al., 1991). Hence, it is also possible to predict hepatotoxicity in asymptomatic early-presenters with moderate-to-high predictive values. Indeed, some biomarkers already show promise for that purpose, and are probably approaching the limits of what is possible. More importantly, biomarkers could be developed for prognosis in drug-induced acute liver failure (DIALF), or ALF in general. ALF and DIALF have very high mortality (Devarbhavi et al., 2018; Lee, 2012; Reddy et al., 2016), so biomarkers with high PPV and NPV for poor outcome could easily be developed (Fig. 1). A biomarker with sensitivity and specificity as low as 80% could be useful in that context, and considerable research should be focused in that area. Finally, biomarkers could be developed to distinguish between dangerous and innocuous changes in liver function tests, such as the transient ALT elevations that have been reported in patients taking therapeutic doses of APAP (Watkins et al., 2006).

3. Biomarkers of DILI diagnosis

The only major biomarker that has been proposed for diagnosis of DILI so far is protein-derived APAP-cysteine (APAP-CYS). As mentioned above and described in detail elsewhere (McGill & Jaeschke, 2018; Senior, 2014), it would be extremely difficult to develop biomarkers of DILI for most individual drugs. However, APAP overdose accounts for approximately half or more of all DILI cases in many Western countries (Breu et al., 2018; Galvin et al., 2015; Lee, 2008). As a result, it is possible to develop diagnostics specifically for APAP overdose, like APAP-CYS. Such diagnostics could be used to confirm a diagnosis of APAP overdose when multiple etiologies are suspected, or to direct a patient for psychotherapy in cases of APAP overdose with suicidal intent. Three approaches have been used to measure APAP-CYS. The first is an immunoassay using antibodies developed against a conjugate of APAP and *N*-acetylcysteine coupled to keyhole limpet hemocyanin (Roberts, Pumford, Potter, Benson, & Hinson, 1987). Using an ELISA format, APAP-CYS was measured in liver homogenates and serum from APAP-treated mice (Pumford et al., 1989), and later in serum from pediatric APAP overdose patients (James et al., 2001). A method based on high pressure liquid chromatography and electrochemical detection (HPLC-EC) improved sensitivity, making it possible to measure protein-derived APAP-CYS in serum in the absence of ALT elevation and even after low doses of APAP (Heard et al., 2011; McGill et al., 2013; Muldrew et al., 2002). More recent methods have been based on HPLC with mass spectrometry (Cook et al., 2015; McGill et al., 2011), with similar results to HPLC-EC. Together, data from studies of protein-derived APAP-CYS in APAP overdose patients have demonstrated that a cutoff of 1 nmol/mL is sensitive and specific for severe hepatotoxicity (ALT $\geq$1000 U/L) after APAP overdose (Alonso, James, Zhang, Squires, & Pediatric Acute Liver Failure Study Group, 2015; Heard et al., 2011; James et al., 2009; Khandelwal et al., 2011). More recently, a prospective study across seven sites in the United States revealed that a novel point-of-care (POC) lateral flow immunoassay had both PPV and NPV $\geq$90% for APAP diagnosis among patients registered in an ALF study (Roberts et al., 2017). Importantly, APAP-protein adducts appear to circulate freely, and therefore are readily detectable by a POC immunoassay (Duan et al., 2019). Overall, available data strongly support the utility of protein-derived APAP-CYS for diagnosis of APAP-induced liver injury.

Although many other biomarkers have been tested for ability to detect DILI, they are not specific for DILI, nor even for the liver in most cases, and therefore cannot diagnose it. For example, circulating keratin 18 (K18) has an area under the receiver operating characteristic (ROC) curve of 0.947, indicating high sensitivity and specificity for detection of liver injury among patients with a DILI diagnosis (Church & Watkins, 2018). However, K18 is also dramatically increased in plasma from patients with hypoxic hepatitis (Weemhoff et al., 2017), alcohol-associated liver disease (Gonzalez-Quintela et al., 2006; Woolbright et al., 2017), non-alcoholic steatohepatitis (Yilmaz et al., 2007), and other diseases. One exception may be microRNA profiles. There is limited evidence that microRNA profiles can be used to differentiate between causes of acute liver injury (Ward et al., 2014), but that requires further investigation.

4. Biomarkers of DILI prediction

It has been proposed that genetic biomarkers could be developed to predict IDILI, or to manage risk of IDILI, in patients before treatment with an IDILI-associated drug as part of the personalized medicine approach (Mosedale & Watkins, 2017; Urban, Daly, & Aithal, 2014). Dozens of gene variants have been identified that are associated with susceptibility to DILI (McGill & Jaeschke, 2018; Urban et al., 2014). Many are variants of human leukocyte antigen (HLA) genes (McGill & Jaeschke, 2018; Urban et al., 2014). The only gene variant associated with IDILI for which clinical laboratories currently test is HLA B*5701 in candidates for abacavir treatment (Mallal et al., 2002). However, the utility of HLA B*5701 testing is due to the cumulative prevalence of all immunoallergic reactions to the drug. Approximately 5% of patients treated with abacavir develop an adverse reaction, but only a fraction of those reactions include liver injury (Hetherington et al., 2001). Other gene variants associated with DILI affect drug metabolizing enzymes (Daly et al., 2007; Huang et al., 2003; Markova et al., 2013; Urban et al., 2014; Yimer et al., 2012), transporters (Daly et al., 2007; Haas et al., 2006), and antioxidant defense systems (Huang et al., 2007; Lucena et al., 2010).

It is unlikely that many gene variants will be adopted for routine prediction of IDILI among drug treatment candidates. As mentioned, the prevalence of IDILI among users of a given drug is typically very low (Fig. 1). In addition, others have pointed out that nearly all genetic associations with IDILI so far are weak (Mosedale & Watkins, 2017). Still, predictive biomarkers may be useful in some cases. For example, ximelagatran, for which IDILI prevalence is relatively high and there is a fairly robust genetic association with DRB*0701, the probability of toxicity with a positive test result is roughly 20–60% (Alfirevic & Pirmohamed, 2012). For drugs that have many alternatives or that treat relatively minor conditions, any probability above 10% or so may be sufficient to compel a clinician not to prescribe it. In the case of a life-saving drug, a clinician may decide to prescribe it despite the risk, but closely monitor liver function tests for evidence of hepatotoxicity.

One application for which genetic biomarkers may be more useful is in the case of patients taking known DILI-causing drug who develop liver test abnormalities. In such cases, a clinician may wish to determine if the drug is likely to be responsible for the abnormal liver test results. Testing the patient for a gene variant that is strongly associated with DILI for that particular drug may help the clinician to decide if the drug should be discontinued (Mosedale & Watkins, 2017).

5. Biomarkers of DILI prognosis

DILI biomarkers appear to have greater potential for prognosis than for almost any other purpose. Many biomarkers have been tested for prognosis, and a few show promise. In particular, several biomarkers may be useful to determine (1) likelihood of toxicity in early-presenting APAP overdose patients, and (2) likelihood of mortality in DIALF patients. It should be noted that most of these biomarkers have been primarily tested in APAP overdose patients, due to the greater availability of samples from that population, but we will also discuss evidence from non-APAP DILI studies wherever possible.

One of the most promising prognostic biomarkers is the microRNA miR-122. It has been demonstrated that miR-122 is elevated in circulation in humans after APAP overdose (Krauskopf et al., 2015; Starkey Lewis et al., 2011; Ward et al., 2014; Yang et al., 2015), acute non-APAP DILI (Russo et al., 2017; Thulin et al., 2014), ischemic hepatitis (Weemhoff et al., 2017), and alcohol ingestion (McCrae, Sharkey, Webb, Vliegenthart, & Dear, 2016). It is also somewhat elevated in patients who develop transient ALT elevations after therapeutic doses of APAP or antitubercular drugs (Thulin et al., 2014). Most prospective studies so far have demonstrated that admission miR-122 values in early presenters and patients with normal to low-elevated ALT have predictive values in the range of 70–90% for development of later injury (defined as ALT above a predetermined value) (Antoine et al., 2013; Dear et al., 2018); likely approaching the limit of what is possible based on prevalence (Fig. 1) (McGill & Jaeschke, 2018). The utility of miR-122 to predict mortality after APAP overdose has not been tested, but it has been tested in non-APAP DILI with surprising results (Russo et al., 2017). Values for miR-122 were actually lower in samples from non-survivors compared to survivors, though both groups appeared to have higher values than controls (Russo et al., 2017). It is not yet clear if the difference between survivors and non-survivors is sufficient to determine likelihood of mortality. It should be noted that two major problems with miR-122 measurement have been described. First, there is controversy surrounding the correct way to measure and normalize miR-122 values (Qi, Weiland, Gao, Zhou, & Mi, 2012), though novel and rapid point-of-care methods may help to overcome that issue (Vliegenthart, Berends, Potter, Kersaudy-Kerhoas, & Dear, 2017). Second, miR-122 displays high between- and within-subject variability (Church et al., 2018). It has been pointed out that the high biological variation may not matter when applying miR-122 to APAP overdose patients because patients with APAP toxicity have very high values (Church et al., 2018), around two orders of magnitude higher than controls (Starkey Lewis et al., 2011; Yang et al., 2015). But the difference seems to be smaller in non-APAP DILI, which may prohibit its use in that patient population. Indeed, some organizations have already abandoned miR-122 as a serious biomarker for IDILI (Church et al., 2018).

High mobility group box 1 (HMGB1) protein is another promising biomarker of prognosis in DILI. Normally, HMGB1 is physically associated with DNA, but values for total HMGB1 in circulation are also elevated in DILI patients (Basta, Del Turco, Navarra, Lee, & Acute Liver Failure Study Group, 2015; Craig et al., 2011). Despite variation between cohorts, HMGB1 values have performed similarly overall to miR-122 to forecast hepatotoxicity in early-presenting APAP overdose patients (Antoine et al., 2013; Dear et al., 2018). Antoine et al. (2012) also reported evidence that indicates that total HMGB1 values can be used to determine likelihood of mortality after APAP overdose, though the results of that study are currently in question and two other studies found no evidence for higher values in patients with poor outcome after either APAP or non-APAP acute liver injury (Basta et al., 2015; Craig et al., 2011). Overall, HMGB1 values may be useful to predict toxicity in early-presenting APAP overdose patients, but it probably cannot be used to determine mortality. As of yet, no studies have been conducted to test the prognostic value of HMGB1 in non-APAP DILI.

Keratin-18 (K18) is a cytoskeletal protein, but circulating levels are elevated in APAP DILI (Antoine et al., 2013; Craig et al., 2011) and in patients with transient ALT elevations after therapeutic doses of either APAP or antitubercular drugs (Thulin et al., 2014). Two forms of K18 have been detected in circulation after DILI (Dear et al., 2018), full-length and caspase-cleaved and both forms have potential for prognostic use (Dear et al., 2018). In particular, full-length or total K18 has high sensitivity and specificity for liver injury in early-presenting APAP overdose patients, though only modest positive predictive value (Dear et al., 2018). Although it was significantly elevated in patients with transaminitis due to antitubercular drugs early after initiation of therapy, ALT was also elevated at that time point so it did not add to the value of traditional clinical laboratory tests (Thulin et al., 2014). However, a more recent study revealed that K18 may be useful to determine likelihood of poor outcomes in patients with both APAP and non-APAP DILI (Dear et al., 2018).

At least two mitochondrial macromolecules are also elevated in DILI. Glutamate dehydrogenase (GLDH) is an enzyme that is elevated in circulation during DILI, as well as other forms of acute liver injury (McGill, Li, et al., 2014; McGill, Staggs, et al., 2014; McGill et al., 2012; Schomaker et al., 2013). Mitochondrial DNA (mtDNA) is also elevated (Marques et al., 2012; McGill et al., 2012). However, although it was once thought that GLDH and mtDNA may be useful for prognosis in APAP overdose patients, they have poor sensitivity and poor predictive values for prediction of both later injury and mortality (Dear et al., 2018; McGill, Li, et al., 2014; McGill, Staggs, et al., 2014). However, GLDH may be useful to distinguish between liver injury and muscle damage in some cases because GLDH is more liver specific than ALT or AST (Church et al., 2018).

Finally, liver regeneration biomarkers are in development. Liver regeneration appears to be critical for survival of acute liver injury and ALF. Kayano et al. (1992) reported that proliferating cell nuclear antigen (PCNA) staining is greater in liver tissue from survivors of liver failure than from non-survivors. Furthermore, traditional clinical laboratory markers of liver function that can reflect regeneration and recovery, such as bilirubin and prothrombin time, are associated with mortality (Church et al., 2018; Lee, 2005; O'Grady, Alexander, Hayllar, & Williams, 1989). Unfortunately, those traditional test values increase late in the disease progression, often after injury is complete and treatment becomes more difficult. That late increase limits their utility. Nevertheless, available data indicate that biomarkers of liver regeneration may be useful for prognosis. Indeed, α-fetoprotein (AFP) increases more in survivors of ALF, including APAP-induced ALF, than non-survivors or others with poor outcome (Schmidt & Dalhoff, 2005). However, a problem with AFP is that it does not increase until late in the course of injury. In addition, it is higher in ALF patients compared to non-ALF patients with liver injury (Church et al., 2018) which could make interpretation difficult in a clinical setting. Other regeneration biomarkers that have been proposed include leukocyte cell derived chemotaxin 2 (LECT2) (Sato et al., 2004), butyric acid (Rudnick et al., 2009), and phosphatidic acid (Lutkewitte et al., 2018), but considerably more work is needed to validate them. Research should be focused in development of these regeneration biomarkers because it is clear that markers with high prognostic utility for patient outcome could be developed.

6. Mechanistic biomarkers

Several biomarkers of cell death mechanisms and inflammation have been measured in DILI. HMGB1 in circulation can be a biomarker of oncotic necrosis, inflammation, or both. Cells undergoing apoptosis do not release HMGB1, but necrotic cells and cells undergoing necroptosis do release it (Scaffidi, Mistelli, & Bianchi, 2002; Tang et al., 2016). HMGB1 acts as a damage-associated molecular pattern (DAMP) and induces inflammation via receptors on macrophages and other inflammatory cells (Andersson, Yang, & Harris, 2018). Normally, HMGB1 is sequestered in the nucleus in most cells. However, when inflammation begins, it will be hyperacetylated in inflammatory cells, which causes it to shift out of the nucleus and ultimately targets it for release into the extracellular space (Andersson et al., 2018; McGill & Jaeschke, 2014). Thus, acetylated HMGB1 is considered a biomarker of macrophage activation and inflammation (Bonaldi et al., 2003). Total HMGB1 is elevated in circulation after APAP overdose (Antoine et al., 2013), indicating that the primary mode of cell death in humans with APAP hepatotoxicity is necrosis. Measurements of the caspase-cleaved form of K18 have confirmed that hypothesis. Caspases are zymogens that are activated during apoptosis, among other phenomena (Ramirez & Salveson, 2018). Cleavage of K18 by certain caspases during apoptosis reveals a unique epitope on K18 that can be quantified by immunoassay (Leers et al., 1999). Caspase-cleaved K18 is much lower after APAP overdose in humans than total K18 (Antoine et al., 2013; Craig et al., 2011). Finally, caspase activity can also be measured in circulation as a biomarker of apoptosis (Lorente et al., 2016; McGill et al., 2012), and it is undetectable in APAP overdose patients (McGill et al., 2012). Together, those data confirm evidence in mice (Gujral, Knight, Farhood, Bajt, & Jaeschke, 2003), in the metabolically competent human hepatocyte cell line HepaRG (McGill et al., 2011) and in primary human hepatocytes (Xie et al., 2014) that oncotic necrosis is the dominant form of cell death in APAP hepatotoxicity and possibly other causes of DILI. Certain cytokines are also increased in circulation in patients with either APAP or non-APAP DILI and also signal inflammation (Bonkovsky et al., 2018; James, 2005, 2001). However, some of these increases of pro-inflammatory cytokines such as IL-1β in APAP overdose patients are minimal (Woolbright & Jaeschke, 2017), which is in agreement with previous animal studies (Williams, Farhood, & Jaeschke, 2010). Other possible biomarkers of inflammation include osteopontin and macrophage colony-stimulating factor receptor (Church et al., 2018), though they require further study for that purpose.

GLDH and mtDNA are considered by many to be biomarkers of mitochondrial damage (McGill & Jaeschke, 2014). Both are localized to the mitochondrial matrix, and are likely only liberated when there is severe mitochondrial damage sufficient to rupture the mitochondrial membranes. It has been demonstrated that both are higher in circulation of mice after APAP overdose than after furosemide overdose (McGill et al., 2012). APAP and furosemide cause a very similar pattern of centrilobular necrosis (McGill et al., 2012), but furosemide does so without affecting mitochondrial function (Wong, Card, & Racz, 2000). Thus, the discovery that GLDH and mtDNA are elevated after APAP overdose in humans indicates that mitochondrial damage occurs in humans during APAP DILI similar to mice (McGill et al., 2012). Consistent with that, there is evidence that long-chain acylcarnitines are biomarkers of mitochondrial dysfunction, and they are also elevated in circulation after APAP overdose in mice and humans (Bhattacharyya et al., 2014; Chen, Krausz, Shah, Idle, & Gonzalez, 2009; McGill, Li, et al., 2014; McGill, Staggs, et al., 2014). Finally, carbamoyl phosphate synthetase-1, another mitochondrial matrix enzyme, is also elevated in APAP hepatotoxicity (Weerasinghe, Jang, Fontana, & Omary, 2014).

Nuclear DNA fragments and nucleosomes may also have mechanistic value. Both nuclear and mitochondrial DNA can act as DAMPs via toll-like receptors and other receptors (Magna & Pisetsky, 2016). Also, in the case of APAP hepatotoxicity, nuclear DNA fragmentation is caused by endonucleases released from damaged mitochondria (Bajt, Cover, Lemasters, &

Jaeschke, 2006), so nuclear DNA fragments and nucleosomes may also indicate mitochondrial damage in some contexts. Nuclear DNA fragments are elevated in circulation of APAP overdose patients with liver injury (Craig et al., 2011; McGill et al., 2012; McGill, Li, et al., 2014; McGill, Staggs, et al., 2014).

7. Conclusion

Numerous circulating and genetic biomarkers show promise for use in DILI. APAP-CYS is likely useful for diagnosis of APAP overdose. HMGB1 and K18 may have modest prognostic value to determine likelihood of later injury in early-presenting APAP overdose patients, while miR-122 could be more useful for that purpose as well as for early identification of non-APAP DILI. Work to identify predictive biomarkers, like HLA B*5701 for abacavir toxicity, will continue and will hopefully yield great rewards despite the challenge of low prevalence. Finally, insights into pathophysiological mechanisms provided by certain biomarkers, like GLDH and K18, could aid development of new treatments for DILI and ALF. In fact, both the US FDA and the European Medicines Agency have expressed support for many of the biomarkers discussed here in the form of letters of support for further research and development.

There are several major areas in which advances are still needed. These include (1) establishment or validation of reference intervals or medical decision limits, respectively, for biomarkers in all categories; (2) identification of liver-specific biomarkers in all categories; (3) identification of DILI-specific, but not drug-specific, biomarkers for general DILI diagnosis; and (4) identification of better biomarkers for prediction of mortality or survival in drug hepatotoxicity and ALF.

Acknowledgments

Work in the authors' laboratories was supported by a Pinnacle Research Award from the American Association for the Study of Liver Diseases (AASLD) Foundation, the National Institutes of Health grant R01 DK102142, and the National Institute of General Medical Sciences (P20 GM103549 and P30 GM118247) from the National Institutes of Health.

Conflict of interest

M.R.M. is a consultant for Acetaminophen Toxicity Diagnostics, Inc., which is developing a diagnostic test for APAP overdose. The authors declare that they have no other conflicts of interest.

References

Alfirevic, A., & Pirmohamed, M. (2012). Predictive genetic testing for drug-induced liver injury: Considerations of clinical utility. *Clinical Pharmacology and Therapeutics*, *92*, 376–380.

Alonso, E. M., James, L. P., Zhang, S., Squires, R. H., & Pediatric Acute Liver Failure Study Group. (2015). Acetaminophen adducts detected in serum of pediatric patients with acute liver failure. *Journal of Pediatric Gastroenterology and Nutrition*, *61*, 102–107.

Andersson, U., Yang, H., & Harris, H. (2018). High-mobility group box 1 protein (HMGB1) operates as an alarmin outside as well as inside cells. *Seminars in Immunology*, *38*, 40–48. https://doi.org/10.1016/j.smim.2018.02.011.

Antoine, D. J., Dear, J. W., Lewis, P. S., Platt, V., Coyle, J., Masson, M., et al. (2013). Mechanistic biomarkers provide early and sensitive detection of acetaminophen-induced acute liver injury at first presentation to hospital. *Hepatology*, *58*, 777–787.

Antoine, D. J., Jenkins, R. E., Dear, J. W., Williams, D. P., McGill, M. R., Sharpe, M. R., et al. (2012). Molecular forms of HMGB1 and keratin-18 as mechanistic biomarkers for mode of cell death and prognosis during clinical acetaminophen hepatotoxicity. *Journal of Hepatology*, *56*, 1070–1079.

Bajt, M. L., Cover, C., Lemasters, J. J., & Jaeschke, H. (2006). Nuclear translocation of endonuclease G and apoptosis-inducing factor during acetaminophen-induced liver cell injury. *Toxicological Sciences*, *94*, 217–225.

Basta, G., Del Turco, S., Navarra, T., Lee, W. M., & Acute Liver Failure Study Group. (2015). Circulating levels of soluble receptor for advanced glycation end products and ligands of the receptor for advanced glycation end products in patients with acute liver failure. *Liver Transplantation*, *21*, 847–854.

Bhattacharyya, S., Yan, K., Pence, L., Simpson, P. M., Gill, P., Letzig, L. G., et al. (2014). Targeted liquid chromatography-mass spectrometry analysis of serum acylcarnitines in acetaminophen toxicity in children. *Biomarkers in Medicine*, *8*, 147–159.

Björnsson, H. K., Olafsson, S., Bermann, O. M., & Björnsson, S. (2016). A prospective study on the causes of notably raised alanine aminotransferase (ALT). *Scandinavian Journal of Gastroenterology*, *51*, 594–600.

Bonaldi, T., Talamo, F., Scaffidi, P., Ferrera, D., Porto, A., Bachi, A., et al. (2003). Monocytic cells hyperacetylate chromatin protein HMGB1 to redirect it towards secretion. *The EMBO Journal*, *22*, 5551–5560.

Bonkovsky, H. L., Barnhart, H. X., Foureau, D. M., Steuerwald, N., Lee, W. M., Gu, J., et al. (2018). Cytokine profiles in acute liver injury—Results from the US Drug-Induced Liver Injury Network (DILIN) and the Acute Liver Failure Study Group. *PLoS One*, *13*, e0206389.

Breu, A. C., Patwardhan, V. R., Nayor, J., Ringwala, J. N., Devore, Z. G., Ganatra, R. B., et al. (2018). A multicenter study into causes of severe acute liver injury. *Clinical Gastroenterology and Hepatology*. https://doi.org/10.1016/j.cgh.2018.08.016. in press.

Chen, M., Borlak, J., & Tong, W. (2014). Predicting idiosyncratic drug-induced liver injury: Some recent advances. *Expert Review of Gastroenterology & Hepatology*, *8*, 721–723.

Chen, C., Krausz, K. W., Shah, Y. M., Idle, J. R., & Gonzalez, F. J. (2009). Serum metabolomics reveals irreversible inhibition of fatty acid beta-oxidation through the suppression of PPARalpha activation as a contributing mechanism of acetaminophen-induced hepatotoxicity. *Chemical Research in Toxicology*, *22*, 699–707.

Church, R. J., Kullak-Ublick, G. A., Aubrecht, J., Bonkovsky, H. K., Chalasani, N., Fontana, R. J., et al. (2018). Candidate biomarkers for the diagnosis and prognosis of drug-induced liver injury: An international collaborative effort. *Hepatology*, *69*, 760–773. https://doi.org/10.1002/hep.29802.

Church, R. J., & Watkins, P. B. (2018). Serum biomarkers of drug-induced liver injury: Current status and future directions. *Journal of Digestive Diseases*, *20*, 2–10. https://doi.org/10.1111/1751-2980.12684.

Cook, S. F., King, A. D., Chang, Y., Murray, G. J., Norris, H. R., Dart, R. C., et al. (2015). Quantification of a biomarker of acetaminophen protein adducts in human serum by high-performance liquid chromatography-electrospray ionization-tandem mass spectrometry: Clinical and animal model applications. *Journal of Chromatography. B, Analytical Technologies in the Biomedical and Life Sciences*, *985*, 131–141.

Craig, D. G., Lee, P., Pryde, E. A., Masterton, G. S., Hayes, P. C., & Simpson, K. J. (2011). Circulating apoptotic and necrotic cell death markers in patients with acute liver injury. *Liver International*, *31*, 1127–1136.

Daly, A. K., Aithal, G. P., Leathart, J. B., Swainsbury, R. A., Dang, T. S., & Day, C. P. (2007). Genetic susceptibility to diclofenac-induced hepatotoxicity: Contribution of UGT2B7, CYP2C8, and ABCC2 genotypes. *Gastroenterology*, *132*, 272–281.

Dear, J. W., Clarke, J. I., Francis, B., Allen, L., Wraught, J., Shen, J., et al. (2018). Risk stratification after paracetamol overdose using mechanistic biomarkers: Results from two prospective cohort studies. *The Lancet Gastroenterology & Hepatology*, *3*, 104–113.

Devarbhavi, H., Patil, M., Reddy, V. V., Singh, R., Joseph, T., & Ganga, D. (2018). Drug-induced acute liver failure in children and adults: Results of a single-centre study of 128 patients. *Liver International*, *38*, 1322–1329.

Duan, L., Ramachandran, A., Akakpo, J. Y., Weemhoff, J. L., Curry, S. C., & Jaeschke, H. (2019). Role of extracellular vesicles in release of protein adducts after acetaminophen-induced liver injury in mice and humans. *Toxicology Letters*, *301*, 125–132.

Galvin, Z., McDonaugh, A., Ryan, J., & Stewart, S. (2015). Blood alanine aminotransferase levels >1,000 IU/l—Causes and outcomes. *Clinical Medicine (London, England)*, *15*, 244–247.

Gonzalez-Quintela, A., García, J., Campos, J., Perez, L. F., Alende, M. R., Otero, E., et al. (2006). Serum cytokeratins in alcoholic liver disease: Contrasting levels of cytokeratin-18 and cytokeratin-19. *Alcohol*, *38*, 45–49.

Gujral, J. S., Knight, T. R., Farhood, A., Bajt, M. L., & Jaeschke, H. (2003). Mode of cell death after acetaminophen overdose in mice: Apoptosis or oncotic necrosis? *Toxicological Sciences*, *67*, 322–328.

Haas, D. W., Bartlett, J. A., Andersen, J. W., Sanne, I., Wilkinson, G. R., Hinkle, J., et al. (2006). Pharmacogenetics of nevirapine-associated hepatotoxicity: An adult AIDS clinical trials group collaboration. *Clinical Infectious Diseases*, *43*, 783–786.

Heard, K. J., Green, J. L., James, L. P., Judge, B. S., Zolot, L., Rhyee, S., et al. (2011). Acetaminophen-cysteine adducts during therapeutic dosing and following overdose. *BMC Gastroenterology*, *11*, 20.

Hetherington, S., McGuirk, S., Powell, G., Cutrell, A., Naderer, O., Spreen, B., et al. (2001). Hypersensitivity reactions during therapy with the nucleoside reverse transcriptase inhibitor abacavir. *Clinical Therapeutics*, *23*, 1603–1614.

Huang, Y. S., Chern, H. D., Su, W. J., Wu, J. C., Chang, S. C., Chiang, C. H., et al. (2003). Cytochrome P450 2E1 genotype and the susceptibility to antituberculosis drug-induced hepatitis. *Hepatology*, *37*, 924–930.

Huang, Y. S., Su, W. J., Huang, Y. H., Chen, C. Y., Chang, F. Y., Lin, H. C., et al. (2007). Genetic polymorphisms of manganese superoxide dismutase, NAD(P)H: Quinone oxidoreductase, glutathione S-transferase M1 and T1, and the susceptibility to drug-induced liver injury. *Journal of Hepatology*, *47*, 128–134.

Issa, A. M., Phillips, K. A., Van Bebber, S., Nidamarthy, H. G., Lasser, K. E., Haas, J. S., et al. (2007). Drug withdrawals in the United States: A systematic review of the evidence and analysis of trends. *Current Drug Safety*, *2*, 177–185.

James, L. P., Farrar, H. C., Darville, T. L., Sullivan, J. E., Given, T. G., Kearns, G. L., et al. (2001). Elevation of serum interleukin 8 levels in acetaminophen overdose in children and adolescents. *Clinical Pharmacology and Therapeutics*, *70*, 280–286.

James, L. P., Farrar, H. C., Sullivan, J. E., Givens, T. G., Kearns, G. L., Wasserman, G. S., et al. (2001). Measurement of acetaminophen-protein adducts in children and adolescents with acetaminophen overdoses. *Journal of Clinical Pharmacology*, *41*, 846–851.

James, L. P., Letzig, L., Simpson, P. M., Capparelli, E., Roberts, D. W., Hinson, J. A., et al. (2009). Pharmacokinetics of acetaminophen-protein adducts in adults with acetaminophen overdose and acute liver failure. *Drug Metabolism and Disposition*, *37*, 1779–1784.

James, L. P., Simpson, P. M., Farrar, H. C., Kearns, G. L., Wasserman, G. S., Blumer, J. L., et al. (2005). Cytokines and toxicity in acetaminophen overdose. *Journal of Clinical Pharmacology*, *45*, 1165–1171.

Kayano, K., Yasunaga, M., Kubota, M., Takenaka, K., Mori, K., Yamashita, A., et al. (1992). Detection of proliferating hepatocytes by immunohistochemical staining for proliferating cell nuclear antigen (PCNA) in patients with acute hepatic failure. *Liver*, *12*, 132–136.

Khandelwal, N., James, L. P., Sanders, C., Larson, A. M., Lee, W. M., & Acute Liver Failure Study Group. (2011). Unrecognized acetaminophen toxicity as a cause of indeterminate acute liver failure. *Hepatology*, *53*, 567–576.

Krauskopf, J., Caiment, F., Claessen, S. M., Johnson, K. J., Warner, R. L., Schomarker, S. J., et al. (2015). Application of high-throughput sequencing to circulating microRNAs reveals novel biomarkers for drug-induced liver injury. *Toxicological Sciences*, *143*, 268–276.

Lee, W. S. (2005). Etiology, outcome and prognostic indicators of childhood fulminant hepatic failure in the United Kingdom. *Journal of Pediatric Gastroenterology and Nutrition*, *40*, 575–581.

Lee, W. M. (2008). Etiologies of acute liver failure. *Seminars in Liver Disease*, *28*, 142–152.

Lee, W. M. (2012). Recent developments in acute liver failure. *Best Practice & Research. Clinical Gastroenterology*, *26*, 3–16.

Leers, M. P., Kölgen, W., Björklund, V., Bergman, T., Tribbick, G., Persson, B., et al. (1999). Immunocytochemical detection and mapping of a cytokeratin 18 neo-epitope exposed during early apoptosis. *The Journal of Pathology*, *187*, 567–572.

Levine, M., O'Connor, A. D., Padilla-Jones, A., & Gerkin, R. D. (2016). Comparison of prothrombin time and aspartate aminotransferase in predicting hepatotoxicity after acetaminophen overdose. *Journal of Medical Toxicology*, *12*, 100–106.

Lorente, L., Martín, M. M., Ferreres, J., Solé-Violán, J., Labarta, L., Díaz, C., et al. (2016). Serum caspase 3 levels are associated with early mortality in severe septic patients. *Journal of Critical Care*, *34*, 103–106.

Lucena, M. I., García-Martín, E., Andrade, R. J., Martínez, C., Stephens, C., Ruiz, J. D., et al. (2010). Mitochondrial superoxide dismutase and glutathione peroxidase in idiosyncratic drug-induced liver injury. *Hepatology*, *52*, 303–312.

Lutkewitte, A. J., Schweitzer, G. G., Kennon-McGill, S., Clemens, M. M., James, L. P., Jaeschke, H., et al. (2018). Lipin deactivation after acetaminophen overdose causes phosphatidic acid accumulation in liver and plasma in mice and humans and enhances liver regeneration. *Food and Chemical Toxicology*, *115*, 273–283.

Magna, M., & Pisetsky, D. S. (2016). The alarmin properties of DNA and DNA-associated nuclear proteins. *Clinical Therapeutics*, *38*, 1029–1041.

Mallal, S., Nolan, D., Witt, C., Masel, G., Martin, A. M., Moore, C., et al. (2002). Association between presence of HLA-B*5701, HLA-DR7, and HLA-DQ3 and hypersensitivity to HIV-1 reverse-transcriptase inhibitor abacavir. *Lancet*, *359*, 727–732.

Markova, S. M., De Marco, T., Bendjilali, N., Kobashigawa, E. A., Mefford, J., Sodhi, J., et al. (2013). Association of CYP2C9*2 with bosentan-induced liver injury. *Clinical Pharmacology and Therapeutics*, *94*, 678–686.

Marques, P. E., Amaral, S. S., Pires, D. A., Nogueira, L. L., Soriani, F. M., Lima, B. H., et al. (2012). Chemokines and mitochondrial products activate neutrophils to amplify organ injury during mouse acute liver failure. *Hepatology, 56*, 1971–1982.

McCrae, J. C., Sharkey, N., Webb, D. J., Vliegenthart, A. D., & Dear, J. W. (2016). Ethanol consumption produces a small increase in circulating miR-122 in healthy individuals. *Clinical Toxicology (Philadelphia, Pa), 54*, 53–55.

McGill, M. R. (2016). The past and present of serum aminotransferases and the future of liver injury biomarkers. *EXCLI Journal, 15*, 817–828.

McGill, M. R., & Jaeschke, H. (2014). Mechanistic biomarkers in acetaminophen-induced hepatotoxicity and acute liver failure: From preclinical models to patients. *Expert Opinion on Drug Metabolism & Toxicology, 10*, 1005–1017.

McGill, M. R., & Jaeschke, H. (2018). Biomarkers of drug-induced liver injury: Progress and utility in research, medicine, and regulation. *Expert Review of Molecular Diagnostics, 18*, 797–807.

McGill, M. R., Lebosky, M., Norris, H. R., Slawson, M. H., Bajt, M. L., Xie, T., et al. (2013). Plasma and liver acetaminophen-protein adduct levels in mice after acetaminophen treatment: Dose-response, mechanisms, and clinical implications. *Toxicology and Applied Pharmacology, 269*, 240–249.

McGill, M. R., Li, F., Sharpe, M. R., Williams, C. D., Curry, S. C., Ma, X., et al. (2014). Circulating acylcarnitines as biomarkers of mitochondrial dysfunction after acetaminophen overdose in mice and humans. *Archives of Toxicology, 88*, 391–401.

McGill, M. R., Sharpe, M. R., Williams, C. D., Taha, M., Curry, S. C., & Jaeschke, H. (2012). The mechanism underlying acetaminophen-induced hepatotoxicity in humans and mice involves mitochondrial damage and nuclear DNA fragmentation. *The Journal of Clinical Investigation, 122*, 1574–1583.

McGill, M. R., Staggs, V. S., Sharpe, M. R., Lee, W. M., Jaeschke, H., & Acute Liver Failure Study Group. (2014). Serum mitochondrial biomarkers and damage-associated molecular patterns are higher in acetaminophen overdose patients with poor outcome. *Hepatology, 60*, 1336–1345.

McGill, M. R., Yan, H. M., Ramachandran, A., Murray, G. J., Rollins, D. E., & Jaeschke, H. (2011). HepaRG cells: A human model to study mechanisms of acetaminophen hepatotoxicity. *Hepatology, 53*, 974–982.

Mosedale, M., & Watkins, P. B. (2017). Drug-induced liver injury: Advances in mechanistic understanding that will inform risk management. *Clinical Pharmacology and Therapeutics, 101*, 469–480.

Muldrew, K. L., James, L. P., Coop, L., McCullough, S. S., Hendrickson, H. P., Hinson, J. A., et al. (2002). Determination of acetaminophen-protein adducts in mouse liver and serum and human serum after hepatotoxic doses of acetaminophen using high-performance liquid chromatography with electrochemical detection. *Drug Metabolism and Disposition, 30*, 446–451.

O'Grady, J. G., Alexander, G. J., Hayllar, K. M., & Williams, R. (1989). Early indicators of prognosis in fulminant hepatic failure. *Gastroenterology, 97*, 439–445.

Olson, H., Betton, G., Robinson, D., Thomas, K., Monro, A., Kolaja, G., et al. (2000). Concordance of the toxicity of pharmaceuticals in humans and in animals. *Regulatory Toxicology and Pharmacology, 32*, 56–67.

Onakpoya, I. J., Heneghan, C. J., & Aronson, J. K. (2016). Post-marketing withdrawal of 462 medicinal products because of adverse drug reactions: A systematic review of the world literature. *BMC Medicine, 14*, 10.

Pumford, N. R., Hinson, J. A., Potter, D. W., Rowland, K. L., Benson, R. W., & Roberts, D. W. (1989). Immunochemical quantitation of 3-(cystein-S-yl)acetaminophen adducts in serum and liver proteins of acetaminophen-treated mice. *The Journal of Pharmacology and Experimental Therapeutics, 248*, 190–196.

Qi, R., Weiland, M., Gao, X. H., Zhou, L., & Mi, Q. S. (2012). Identification of endogenous normalizers for serum microRNAs by microarray profiling: U6 small nuclear RNA is not a reliable normalizer. *Hepatology*, *55*, 1640–1642.

Ramirez, M. L. G., & Salveson, G. S. (2018). A primer on caspase mechanisms. *Seminars in Cell & Developmental Biology*, *82*, 79–85.

Reddy, K. R., Ellerbe, C., Schilsky, M., Stravitz, R. T., Fontana, R. J., Durkalsi, V., et al. (2016). Determinants of outcome among patients with acute liver failure listed for liver transplantation in the United States. *Liver Transplantation*, *22*, 505–515.

Roberts, D. W., Lee, W. M., Hinson, J. A., Bai, S., Swearingen, C. J., Stravitz, R. T., et al. (2017). An immunoassay to rapidly measure acetaminophen protein adducts accurately identifies patients with acute liver injury or failure. *Clinical Gastroenterology and Hepatology*, *15*, 555–562.

Roberts, D. W., Pumford, N. R., Potter, D. W., Benson, R. W., & Hinson, J. A. (1987). A sensitive immunochemical assay for acetaminophen-protein adducts. *The Journal of Pharmacology and Experimental Therapeutics*, *241*, 527–533.

Rudnick, D. A., Dietzen, D. J., Turmelle, Y. P., Shepherd, R., Zhang, S., Belle, S. H., et al. (2009). Serum alpha-NH-butyric acid may predict spontaneous survival in pediatric acute liver failure. *Pediatric Transplantation*, *13*, 223–230.

Rumack, B. H., & Peterson, R. G. (1978). Acetaminophen overdose: Incidence, diagnosis, and management in 416 patients. *Pediatrics*, *62*, 898–903.

Rumack, B. H., Peterson, R. C., Koch, G. G., & Amara, I. A. (1981). Acetaminophen overdose. 662 cases with evaluation of oral acetylcysteine treatment. *Archives of Internal Medicine*, *141*, 380–385.

Russo, M. W., Steuerwald, N., Norton, H. J., Anderson, W. E., Foureau, D., Chalasani, N., et al. (2017). Profiles of miRNAs in serum in severe acute drug induced liver injury and their prognostic significance. *Liver International*, *37*, 757–764.

Sato, Y., Watanabe, H., Kameyama, H., Kobayashi, T., Yamamoto, S., Takeishi, T., et al. (2004). Serum LECT2 level as a prognostic indicator in acute liver failure. *Transplantation Proceedings*, *36*, 2359–2361.

Scaffidi, P., Mistelli, T., & Bianchi, M. E. (2002). Release of chromatin protein HMGB1 by necrotic cells triggers inflammation. *Nature*, *418*, 191–195.

Schmidt, L. E., & Dalhoff, K. (2005). Alpha-fetoprotein is a predictor of outcome in acetaminophen-induced liver injury. *Hepatology*, *41*, 26–31.

Schomaker, S., Warner, R., Bock, J., Johnson, K., Potter, D., Van Winkle, J., et al. (2013). Assessment of emerging biomarkers of liver injury in human subjects. *Toxicological Sciences*, *132*, 276–283.

Senior, J. R. (2014). New biomarkers for drug-induced liver injury: Are they really better? What do they diagnose? *Liver International*, *34*, 325–327.

Smilkstein, M. J., Bronstein, A. C., Linden, C., Augenstein, W. L., Kulig, K. W., & Rumack, B. H. (1991). Acetaminophen overdose: A 48-hour intravenous N-acetylcysteine treatment protocol. *Annals of Emergency Medicine*, *20*, 1058–1063.

Solotke, M. T., Dhruva, S. S., Downing, N. S., Shah, N. D., & Ross, J. S. (2018). New and incremental FDA black box warnings from 2008 to 2015. *Expert Opinion on Drug Safety*, *17*, 117–123.

Starkey Lewis, P. J., Dear, J., Platt, V., Simpson, K. J., Craig, D. G., Antoine, D. J., et al. (2011). Circulating microRNAs as potential markers of human drug-induced liver injury. *Hepatology*, *54*, 1767–1776.

Tang, Y., Zhao, X., Antoine, D. J., Xiao, X., Wang, H., Andersson, U., et al. (2016). Regulation of posttranslational modifications of HMGB1 during immune responses. *Antioxidants & Redox Signaling*, *24*, 620–634.

Thulin, P., Nordahl, G., Gry, M., Yimer, G., Aklilu, E., Makonnen, E., et al. (2014). Keratin-18 and microRNA-122 complement alanine aminotransferase as novel safety biomarkers for drug-induced liver injury in two human cohorts. *Liver International, 34*, 367–378.

United States Food and Drug Administration. (2016). *BEST (Biomarkers, EndpointS, and other Tools) resource glossary*. Silver Spring (MD): Food and Drug Administration (US); Bethesda (MD): National Institutes of Health (US). Retrieved from https://www.ncbi.nlm.nih.gov/books/NBK326791/.

Urban, T. J., Daly, A. K., & Aithal, G. P. (2014). Genetic basis of drug-induced liver injury: Present and future. *Seminars in Liver Disease, 34*, 123–133.

Vliegenthart, A. D. B., Berends, C., Potter, C. M. J., Kersaudy-Kerhoas, M., & Dear, J. W. (2017). MicroRNA-122 can be measured in capillary blood which facilitates point-of-care testing for drug-induced liver injury. *British Journal of Clinical Pharmacology, 83*, 2027–2033.

Ward, J., Kanchagar, C., Veksler-Lublinsky, I., Lee, R. C., McGill, M. R., Jaeschke, H., et al. (2014). Circulating microRNA profiles in human patients with acetaminophen hepatotoxicity or ischemic hepatitis. *Proceedings of the National Academy of Sciences of the United States of America, 111*, 12169–12174.

Watkins, P. B., Kaplowitz, N., Slattery, J. T., Colonese, C. R., Colucci, S. V., Stewart, P. W., et al. (2006). Aminotransferase elevations in healthy adults receiving 4 grams of acetaminophen daily: A randomized controlled trial. *JAMA, 296*, 87–93.

Weemhoff, J. L., Woolbright, B. L., Jenkins, R. E., McGill, M. R., Sharpe, M. R., Olson, J. C., et al. (2017). Plasma biomarkers to study mechanisms of liver injury in patients with hypoxic hepatitis. *Liver International, 37*, 377–384.

Weerasinghe, S. V., Jang, Y. J., Fontana, R. J., & Omary, M. B. (2014). Carbamoyl phosphate synthetase-1 is a rapid turnover biomarker in mouse and human acute liver injury. *American Journal of Physiology. Gastrointestinal and Liver Physiology, 307*, G355–G364.

Williams, C. D., Farhood, A., & Jaeschke, H. (2010). Role of caspase-1 and interleukin-1beta in acetaminophen-induced hepatic inflammation and liver injury. *Toxicology and Applied Pharmacology, 247*, 169–178.

Wong, S. G., Card, J. W., & Racz, W. J. (2000). The role of mitochondrial injury in bromobenzene and furosemide induced hepatotoxicity. *Toxicology Letters, 116*, 171–181.

Woolbright, B. L., Bridges, B. W., Dunn, W., Olson, J. C., Weinman, S. A., & Jaeschke, H. (2017). Cell death and prognosis of mortality in alcoholic hepatitis patients using plasma keratin-18. *Gene Expression, 17*, 301–312.

Woolbright, B. L., & Jaeschke, H. (2017). Role of the inflammasome in acetaminophen-induced liver injury and acute liver failure. *Journal of Hepatology, 66*, 836–848.

Xie, Y., McGill, M. R., Dorko, K., Kumer, S. C., Schmitt, T. M., Forster, J., et al. (2014). Mechanisms of acetaminophen-induced cell death in primary human hepatocytes. *Toxicology and Applied Pharmacology, 279*, 266–274.

Yang, X., Salminen, W. F., Shi, Q., Greenhaw, J., Gill, P. S., Bhattacharyya, S., et al. (2015). Potential of extracellular microRNAs as biomarkers of acetaminophen toxicity in children. *Toxicology and Applied Pharmacology, 284*, 180–187.

Yilmaz, Y., Dolar, E., Ulukaya, E., Akgoz, S., Keskin, M., Kiyici, M., et al. (2007). Soluble forms of extracellular cytokeratin 18 may differentiate simple steatosis from nonalcoholic steatohepatitis. *World Journal of Gastroenterology, 13*, 837–844.

Yimer, G., Amogne, W., Habtewold, A., Makonnen, E., Ueda, N., Suda, A., et al. (2012). High plasma efavirenz level and CYP2B6*6 are associated with efavirenz-based HAART-induced liver injury in the treatment of naïve HIV patients from Ethiopia: A prospective cohort study. *The Pharmacogenomics Journal, 12*, 499–506.

CHAPTER NINE

Mechanisms and biomarkers of liver regeneration after drug-induced liver injury

Melissa M. Clemens*, Mitchell R. McGill[†,‡,1], Udayan Apte[§]

*Interdisciplinary Biomedical Sciences Graduate Program, University of Arkansas for Medical Sciences, Little Rock, AR, United States
[†]Department of Environmental and Occupational Health, Fay W. Boozman College of Public Health, University of Arkansas for Medical Sciences, Little Rock, AR, United States
[‡]Department of Pharmacology and Toxicology, College of Medicine, University of Arkansas for Medical Sciences, Little Rock, AR, United States
[§]Department of Pharmacology, Toxicology, and Therapeutics, University of Kansas Medical Center, Kansas City, KS, United States
[1]Corresponding author: e-mail address: mmcgill@uams.edu

Contents

Abstract

Liver, the major metabolic organ in the body, is known for its remarkable capacity to regenerate. Whereas partial hepatectomy (PHx) is a popular model for the study of liver regeneration, the liver also regenerates after acute injury, but less is known about the mechanisms that drive it.

Recent studies have shown that liver regeneration is critical for survival in acute liver failure (ALF), which is usually due to drug-induced liver injury (DILI). It is sometimes assumed that the signaling pathways involved are similar to those that regulate regeneration after PHx, but there are likely to be critical differences. A better understanding of

Advances in Pharmacology, Volume 85
ISSN 1054-3589
https://doi.org/10.1016/bs.apha.2019.03.001
© 2019 Elsevier Inc.
All rights reserved.

regeneration mechanisms after DILI and hepatotoxicity in general could lead to development of new therapies for ALF patients and new biomarkers to predict patient outcome. Here, we summarize what is known about the mechanisms of liver regeneration and repair after hepatotoxicity. We also review the literature in the emerging field of liver regeneration biomarkers.

Abbreviations

AFP alpha-fetoprotein
ALF acute liver failure
ALI acute liver injury
APAP acetaminophen
CCl_4 carbon tetrachloride
DILI drug-induced liver injury
EGFR endothelial growth factor receptor
GSK glycogen synthase kinase
HGF hepatocyte growth factor
IL-6 interleukin-6
PA phosphatidic acid
PAI-1 plasminogen activator inhibitor 1
PCNA proliferating cell nuclear antigen
PHx partial hepatectomy
TNF tumor necrosis factor
VEGF vascular endothelial growth factor

1. Introduction

The liver is uniquely susceptible to toxic injury. Unlike other organs, it receives most of its blood supply (approximately 80%) from veins. Blood from the spleen, pancreas, stomach, and large intestine drains into the splenic vein which then merges with the superior mesenteric vein from the small intestine to form the hepatic portal vein. This unique arrangement ensures that everything absorbed from the stomach and intestines passes through the liver before reaching systemic circulation. The liver acts a chemical scrubber for the portal blood, catalyzing the conjugation of xenobiotics with highly water-soluble side groups to facilitate their excretion. This anatomy is so important for our health that it is completely conserved across vertebrates, from cyclostomata to placental mammals. Even cephalochordate lancelets possess a portal/liver-like system called the midgut diverticulum (Subbotin, 2017). However, in order to form those soluble conjugates, some chemicals must first pass through an intermediate step in which they form highly reactive metabolites. Those metabolites may bind to proteins or nucleic acids in the hepatocytes causing significant injury. The portal system also means that endotoxins produced by ingested bacteria reach the liver before any other organ, and the liver therefore bears the brunt of those toxins. Finally, the mixing of arterial and venous blood means that the liver is already hypoxic compared to other organs, and any further reduction in oxygen supply (e.g., ischemia) followed by sudden re-oxygenation can be catastrophic.

Fortunately, the liver also has phenomenal capacity for repair and regeneration after injury. This is most strikingly demonstrated in partial hepatectomy (PHx) where as much as 70–80% of the liver is removed and the remaining tissue will enlarge until the original functional mass is restored (Fausto, 2000; Higgins & Anderson, 1931; Michalopoulos, 2017, Sadler, Krahn, Gaur, & Ukomadu, 2007).

It is important to understand the mechanisms of liver repair and regeneration after hepatotoxicity. Most studies of liver regeneration have relied upon the PHx model in rodents introduced by Higgins and Anderson (1931), but the concept of liver regeneration was actually introduced by clinicians who observed that patients with massive acute necrosis and atrophy of the liver can recover normal function over time (Milne, 1909). Importantly, there is strong evidence that regeneration is critical for survival of acute liver failure (ALF), which is usually due to hepatotoxicity. For example, immunostaining for proliferating cell nuclear antigen (PCNA) is greater in liver tissue from ALF survivors than non-survivors (Kayano et al., 1992). While it has been said that the mechanisms of regeneration after acute necrosis are probably similar to PHx (Michalopoulos, 2013, 2014), there are clear differences in the anatomical features of the injury and in subsequent inflammation suggesting that differences in signaling are likely (Fig. 1). A better understanding of the mechanisms involved may lead to new treatments for ALF.

The purpose of this chapter is to review the clinically relevant causes of acute liver injury (ALI) and ALF, and to summarize the mechanisms of regeneration after hepatotoxicity. At the end of this chapter, the reader should be able to (1) list the most common and severe causes of ALI, (2) describe major differences between PHx and hepatotoxicity, (3) discuss the mechanisms of liver repair and regeneration after hepatotoxicity, and (4) discuss biomarkers of liver regeneration and ALF prognosis.

2. Etiology and prognosis of acute liver injury

Ischemic hepatitis is the most common cause of severe ALI in the United States and other developed countries, defined as peak ALT $\geq$ 1000 U/L. It accounts for approximately 50% of all cases (Breu et al., 2018; Galvin,

McDonough, Ryan, & Stewart, 2015). Drug-induced liver injury (DILI) is the second most common cause, at approximately 15% (Breu et al., 2018; Galvin et al., 2015). Other common causes of severe ALI include viral hepatitis (10–15%), hepatobiliary diseases (e.g., gallstones) (5–10%), and autoimmune hepatitis (1–5%) (Breu et al., 2018; Galvin et al., 2015).

Among those etiologies, DILI has the worst prognosis. Although ischemic hepatitis accounts for most cases of ALI, DILI is by far the most common single cause of ALF, responsible for nearly 60% of all cases (Lee, 2008). Furthermore, mortality in DILI-induced ALF is high, ranging from 25% to 75% depending on the causative drug (Larson et al., 2005; Lee, 2008; Ostapowicz et al., 2002; Reddy et al., 2016). While mortality in ischemic hepatitis is also high (approximately 50%) (Tapper, Sengupta, & Bonder, 2015), death is generally thought to be due to the underlying etiology (e.g., cardiovascular disease) and liver injury is often viewed as a secondary issue or merely a complication of the disease.

Acetaminophen (APAP) overdose is far and away the most common cause of DILI and DILI-induced ALF (Breu et al., 2018; Galvin et al., 2015; Lee, 2008). Approximately 50% of DILI cases in the United States are attributed to APAP (Galvin et al., 2015), as well as about 80% of DILI-induced ALF (Lee, 2008). In fact, 80% may be an underestimate. Follow-up studies have revealed that some cases of ALF in which the cause cannot be determined using routine diagnostic tools are actually due to APAP overdose (Ganger et al., 2018). Although prognosis for APAP-induced ALF patients is generally better than for patients with ALF due to other etiologies, the sheer volume of cases means that APAP overdose is also the most common cause of ALF-related death (Ostapowicz et al., 2002). As a result, most studies of liver regeneration after DILI have relied on the mouse model of APAP overdose or samples from APAP overdose patients, though other models have also been used to provide general insight into the regeneration process after hepatotoxicity, or before APAP was recognized as the most common cause of ALF.

3. Major differences between hepatectomy and hepatotoxicity

The most obvious differences between PHx and xenobiotic hepatotoxicity are due to anatomy. While PHx involves the surgical removal of a large portion of the liver, xenobiotic hepatotoxicity causes necrosis that develops in pockets within the tissue. As a result, cell proliferation proceeds differently in the two cases. The process of cell division, which is at the center of liver regeneration, occurs in the remnant lobes after partial hepatectomy. In chemical-induced injury, hepatocytes surrounding the areas of necrosis enter the cell cycle and divide (Apte, Bhushan, & Dadhania, 2017; Leevy, Hollister, Schmid, MacDonald, & Davidson, 1959). Hepatocyte proliferation after PHx is pan-lobular, beginning around the periportal areas and spreading outward in a wave and mainly in total absence of liver injury. The removal of a large piece of the liver in PHx also results in major hemodynamic changes. Loss of normal liver architecture due to necrosis likely also affects blood flow, but probably to a lesser extent. Finally, xenobiotic hepatotoxicity is usually accompanied by extensive sterile inflammation, which is not a consequence of PHx (Michalopoulos, 2013, 2014). Given these major, fundamental differences, it is not at all surprising that regeneration signaling differs at least somewhat between PHx and toxic injury. The major differences in regeneration between PHx and hepatotoxicity are summarized in Fig. 1.

4. Regeneration after drug-induced liver injury

4.1 Carbon tetrachloride hepatotoxicity

Although carbon tetrachloride (CCl_4) is not a drug, it has been used as a model for DILI, and hepatotoxicity in general, for decades (McGill & Jaeschke, 2019). The mechanisms of injury and repair after carbon tetrachloride (CCl_4) hepatotoxicity have been studied since the 1950s (Leevy et al., 1959). The biotransformation of CCl_4 produces toxic products able to cause severe necrosis in the liver. Cytochrome P450s cleave CCl_4 at the carbon–halogen bond, creating the trichloromethyl radical ($CCl3^{\bullet}$) which can react with lipids, proteins, and DNA (Weber, Boll, & Stampfl, 2003). The resulting lipid peroxidation and protein-lipid cross-linking leads to cell dysfunction and cell membrane destruction (Weber et al., 2003).

Several studies indicate that cytokines, presumably secreted in response to liver injury, help to drive regeneration after CCl_4 hepatotoxicity. In the PHx model, serum tumor necrosis factor-alpha (TNFα) increases rapidly (Akerman et al., 1992; Trautwein, Rakermann, Niehof, Rose-John, & Manns, 1996), and inhibition or disruption of TNFα signaling blunts regeneration (Akerman et al., 1992; Yamada, Kirillova, Peschon, & Fausto, 1997).

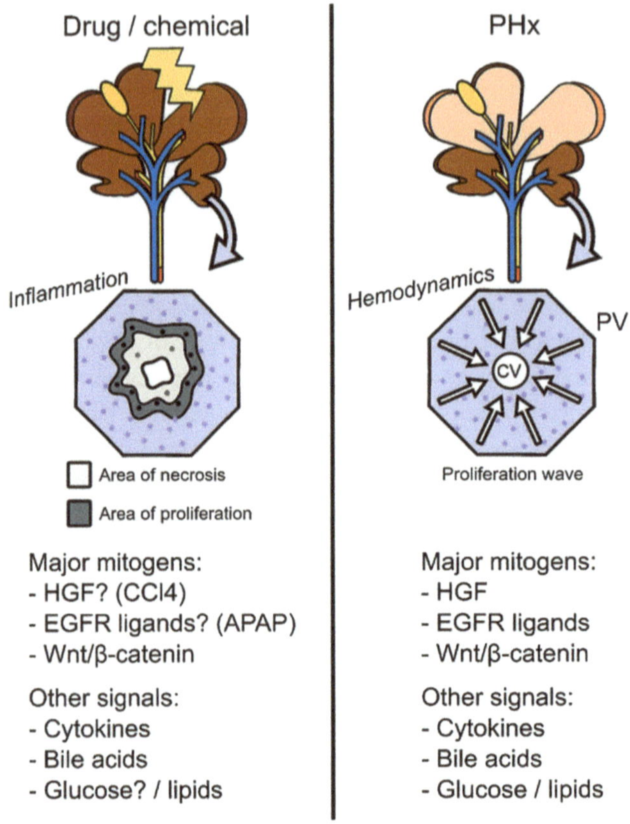

Fig. 1 Major features of regeneration or repair between partial hepatectomy and hepatotoxicity models. In xenobiotic hepatotoxicity, areas of necrosis gradually develop and hepatocytes surrounding those areas begin to proliferate. The necrosis typically results in extensive sterile inflammation. The roles of different mitogens and other signaling mediators appears to be dependent upon the specific hepatotoxicant in question and even on the dose of the hepatotoxicant. In the partial hepatectomy model (PHx), approximately 70% of the total liver mass is surgically removed. Removal of liver tissue is relatively fast, and results in large changes in blood flow and blood pressure in the liver. The most important mitogens in PHx are hepatocyte growth factor (HGF) and other c-Met ligands, epidermal growth factor receptor (EGFR) ligands, and β-catenin. Other signals, especially cytokines like tumor necrosis factor, also have important roles.

Interleukin-6 (IL-6) expression also increases early after PHx, though with a slight delay compared to TNFα (Trautwein et al., 1996). It is thought that the earlier TNFα signaling stimulates IL-6 production through NFκB-regulated transcription, and IL-6 is important for liver regeneration in part through activation of signal transducer and activator of transcription (Stat3). Importantly, Stat3 stimulation and cell proliferation are impaired in IL-6-deficient mice post-PHx (Cressman et al., 1996), while injecting the same mice with IL-6 restores those effects (Cressman et al., 1996). Tumor necrosis factor (TNF) receptor 1 (TNFR1)-deficient mice have reduced Stat3 signaling and significantly delayed regeneration after CCl_4 treatment compared to WT animals (Yamada & Fausto, 1998). Some data also indicate that hepatocyte proliferation is reduced after CCl_4 in liver-specific Stat3 KO mice (Moh et al., 2007). Although it is difficult to directly study the role of IL-6 in regeneration after CCl_4 toxicity due to early protective effects of IL-6 KO in that model, there is some evidence that IL-6 deficiency delays regeneration in a model of chronic CCl_4 toxicity (Río et al., 2008). Altogether, it appears that TNFα and IL-6 signaling are also important for recovery after CCl_4-induced liver injury.

There is also evidence for role of growth factors in regeneration after CCl_4 treatment, as in PHx. For example, direct manipulation of hepatocyte growth factor (HGF) and its receptor c-Met have revealed that HGF is important. Treatment with an antibody against HGF dramatically reduces DNA synthesis after CCl_4-induced injury (Burr, Toole, Chapman, Hines, & Burt, 1998). Interestingly, that effect was not observed in c-Met KO mice, but reduction in necrotic areas during recovery did appear to be delayed in those animals (Huh et al., 2004). Furthermore, mice with Cre adenovirus-driven hepatocyte-specific HGF KO displayed reduced DNA synthesis after CCl_4 treatment, similar to the HGF antibody-treated mice (Phaneuf, Moscioni, LeClair, Raper, & Wilson, 2004). Indirect evidence for the importance of HGF in CCl_4 hepatotoxicity is also available. For example, plasmin is important for maturation and release of HGF from the extracellular matrix (ECM), and plasmin-deficient mice have reduced c-Met signaling after CCl_4 treatment, and DNA synthesis is reduced in plasmin-deficient hepatocytes cultured with HGF (Shanmukhappa, Matte, Degen, & Bezerra, 2009). Overall, it seems clear that HGF is important for regeneration after CCl_4 hepatotoxicity. On the other hand, liver regeneration after CCl_4 treatment is similar between epidermal growth factor receptor (EGFR) KO and WT mice (Scheving, Zhang, Stevenson, Threadgill, & Russell, 2015). That indicates that, unlike the PHx model, EGFR is not very important for regeneration in CCl_4 hepatotoxicity, though it should be noted that combined KO of EGFR and c-Met reduced regeneration at one early time point more than c-Met KO alone (Scheving et al., 2015).

With regard to metabolism, Rao and Mehendale (1989) reported that fructose 1,6-diphosphate treatment can increase regeneration in CCl_4 hepatotoxicity. On the basis of those results and results from similar studies, the authors concluded that fructose aids regeneration by acting as an energy source. Consistent with that, a recent study demonstrated that the energy sensor AMP-activated protein kinase (AMPK) is activated during CCl_4 hepatotoxicity, and treatment with an AMPK inhibitor reduces liver regeneration (Huang et al., 2018). On the other hand, glucose loading and diabetes are both known to reduce recovery in rodents with CCl_4 toxicity (Chanda & Mehendale, 1995).

One of the most interesting results from studies of liver regeneration after hepatotoxicity caused by CCl_4 and other industrial chemicals was the discovery of the phenomenon sometimes referred to as the "threshold effect." Mehendale and coworkers observed that administration of a low dose of CCl_4 protects against lethality of a later large dose by stimulating repair mechanisms and promoting hepatocyte proliferation (Kodavanti, Joshi, Young, Bell, & Mehendale, 1989; Kodavanti, Joshi, Young, Meydrech, & Mehendale, 1989; Thakore & Mehendale, 1991). The initial insult need not be from the same hepatotoxicant. For example, administration of a low dose of thioacetamide protects against APAP hepatotoxicity by increasing hepatocyte proliferation (Chanda, Mangipudy, Warbritton, Bucci, & Mehendale, 1995), likely through Wnt/β-catenin signaling (Dadhania, Bhushan, Apte, & Mehendale, 2017). Numerous other stressors are now known to have the same effect (Apte et al., 2017). They also discovered that pre-treatment with chlordecone abolishes the early phase of hepatocyte proliferation after CCl_4 treatment and increases mortality (Mehendale, 1989). These observations, combined with other discoveries such as the possible role of Ca^{2+}-dependent proteases in the spread of necrosis and inhibition of those proteases by endogenous calpastatin (Limaye et al., 2003, 2006), led to the idea that the outcome of hepatotoxicity is determined by a balance between mechanisms of injury and mechanisms of repair. That idea is supported by the discovery that hepatocyte proliferation increases with increasing severity of hepatotoxicity until a threshold is reached (Anand, Murthy, Mumtaz, & Mehendale, 2004; Mangipudy, Chanda, & Mehendale, 1995; Rao, Mangipudy, & Mehendale, 1997). Beyond the threshold, proliferation is impaired and mortality increases (Anand et al., 2004; Mangipudy et al., 1995; Rao et al., 1997). This observation is also the basis of the incremental dose model of APAP hepatotoxicity mentioned in the next section.

Overall, some mechanisms of regeneration appear to be common between PHx and CCl_4 toxicity, but there may also be major differences. In particular, EGFR signaling may not be as important in the CCl_4 model. Many other mechanisms have yet to be explored in CCl_4 toxicity, and more differences may be revealed over time.

4.2 Acetaminophen hepatotoxicity

The mechanisms of acetaminophen (APAP) hepatotoxicity have been thoroughly investigated, though large gaps in our knowledge remain. The toxicity starts with formation of a reactive metabolite that binds to proteins (Kennon-McGill & McGill, 2018; McGill & Jaeschke, 2013). Binding to mitochondrial proteins in particular causes mitochondrial dysfunction and oxidative stress (McGill, Williams, Xie, Ramachandran, & Jaeschke, 2012; McGill & Jaeschke, 2013; Xie et al., 2015). The initial oxidative stress is thought to activate the c-Jun N-terminal kinases 1/2 (JNK) (Du, Xie, McGill, & Jaeschke, 2015; Gunawan et al., 2006), which then translocate into mitochondria and exacerbate the mitochondrial damage (Hanawa et al., 2008; Ramachandran, Lebofsky, Weinman, & Jaeschke, 2011) leading to loss of mitochondrial membrane potential and decreased respiration (Kon, Kim, Jaeschke, & Lemasters, 2004; Meyers, Beierschmitt, Khairallah, & Cohen, 1988; Ramachandran, Lebofsky, Baines, Lemasters, & Jaeschke, 2011; Reid, Kurten, McCullough, Brock, & Hinson, 2005). The mitochondria then swell and rupture (Placke, Ginsberg, Wyand, & Cohen, 1987), releasing endonucleases that translocate to the nucleus and cleave nuclear DNA (Bajt, Cover, Lemasters, & Jaeschke, 2006). The result is oncotic necrosis of hepatocytes (Gujral, Knight, Farhood, Bajt, & Jaeschke, 2002). Importantly, the mechanisms of injury appear to be the same in mice and humans (McGill, Sharpe, et al., 2012; McGill et al., 2014, 2011; Xie et al., 2014).

The earliest studies of regeneration after APAP overdose in mice revealed that pro-regenerative cytokines play an important role. Although several earlier attempts were made to study the mechanisms of liver regeneration after APAP overdose in rats, we now know that rats are a poor model for APAP hepatotoxicity compared to mice (McGill, Williams, et al., 2012). Those initial mouse studies revealed that IL-6 expression increases early as 4h after APAP overdose (James, Lamps, McCullough, & Hinson, 2003), and Ju et al. (2002) demonstrated that depletion of Kupffer cells with liposomal clodronate reduces expression of TNFα, IL-6, and other cytokines and exacerbates the toxicity at both early and late time points. Shortly thereafter, it was discovered that both IL-6 KO and TNFR KO mice have similar injury compared to wild-type mice at early time points after APAP overdose but delayed recovery later on (James, Kurten, Lamps, McCullough, & Hinson, 2005; James et al., 2003). Furthermore, pretreatment of the IL-6 KO mice with exogenous IL-6 restored hepatocyte proliferation at a late time point (James et al., 2003). Interestingly, it appears that in the absence of IL-6, other cytokines can become upregulated to compensate (James et al., 2003; Masubuchi et al., 2003).

Surprisingly, the role of other signaling pathways in regeneration after APAP hepatotoxicity has only recently been explored. It was demonstrated that β-catenin is activated as early as 1 h after APAP overdose in mice and remains active until at least 6h (Apte et al., 2009). Moreover, the increase in β-catenin activation is preceded by increased phosphorylation (and therefore inactivation) of GSK3β (Apte et al., 2009). Importantly, β-catenin-deficient mice that were induced to express Cyp2e1 had reduced expression of regeneration markers at 24h after APAP despite similar injury (Apte et al., 2009), and staining for nuclear β-catenin was found to correlate with proliferating cell nuclear antigen (PCNA) expression in APAP-induced ALF patients (Apte et al., 2009). Consistent with those data, Bhushan et al. (2014) later used an incremental dosing model to demonstrate that nuclear localization of β-catenin and GSK3β phosphorylation is reduced at a dose of APAP that inhibits liver regeneration, while overexpression of stable β-catenin improves it. Finally, treatment with a highly specific GSK3β inhibitor enhanced liver regeneration after APAP overdose (Bhushan, Poudel, Manley Jr., Roy, & Apte, 2017). Thus, Wnt/β-catenin signaling is clearly important.

Less is known about the importance of growth factors after APAP hepatotoxicity, but some data are available. Similar to PHx, EGFR is activated within 1–6 h after APAP overdose, and treatment with an EGFR inhibitor at a late time point impaired recovery and survival (Bhushan et al., 2017). Also similar to the PHx model, vascular endothelial growth factor (VEGF) increases later after APAP overdose than other growth factors, but inhibition of VEGF signaling also blunts regeneration (Donahower et al., 2010, 2006). Despite those similarities, there do appear to be differences in growth factor signaling between PHx and APAP overdose. Although the role of HGF in regeneration after acetaminophen toxicity has not been directly investigated, there is evidence that it may not be as important as in the PHx model. Deficiency for plasminogen activator inhibitor 1 (PAI-1), which inhibits the plasminogen activators responsible for plasmin activation and therefore

HGF liberation from ECM, unexpectedly increased injury and reduced markers of liver regeneration at multiple time points after APAP treatment (Bajt, Yan, Farhood, & Jaeschke, 2008; Sullivan, Kassel, Jone, Flick, & Luyendyk, 2012). In contrast, inhibition of PAI-1 enhances regeneration after PHx (Watanabe et al., 2007). Although another group reported that PAI-1 KO mice also have reduced regeneration after PHx, no quantitation of regeneration markers was provided to support that claim (Beier et al., 2016). In addition, similar to EGFR, the incremental dose model does not support a role for HGF signaling (Bhushan et al., 2014). Finally, serum HGF values are actually two- to fourfold higher in non-survivors of APAP-induced liver injury than in survivors (Hughes, Zhang, Tsubouchi, Daikuhara, & Williams, 1994), and it is known that over-activation of the HGF receptor c-met can trigger cell death (Zhao et al., 2007). Therefore, it appears that HGF is either not involved in regeneration in APAP hepatotoxicity or at least that it is not a complete mitogen in the APAP model, though further testing is required for verification.

There is some evidence for metabolic signaling in recovery from APAP-induced liver injury. Bile acids are elevated in both mice and humans after APAP overdose (Bhushan et al., 2013; Woolbright et al., 2012), and cholic acid dietary supplementation greatly accelerates regeneration while cholestyramine reduces it (Bhushan et al., 2013). More recently, it has been suggested that phosphatidic acid (PA) and possibly lysophosphatidic acid (LPA) are involved in liver regeneration in the APAP model (Lutkewitte et al., 2018). PA is dramatically elevated in both liver tissue and plasma after APAP overdose in mice and humans due to deactivation of lipin 1 and 2, and inhibition of PA and LPA synthesis reduces expression of regeneration markers at late time points (Lutkewitte et al., 2018), possibly through an effect on Wnt/β-catenin (Clemens et al., 2019). Finally, it has been suggested that β-oxidation is important as an energy source for hepatocyte proliferation after APAP overdose similar to PHx (Bhattacharyya et al., 2013), but that hypothesis has not yet been tested.

Overall, we now know that cytokines, Wnt/β-catenin and EGFR are important for liver regeneration in APAP hepatotoxicity, and emerging data also suggest a role for bile acids and lipid second messengers like PA and LPA. Other factors have also been suggested to play a role, such as β-oxidation and sterile inflammation, but more research is needed in those areas.

However, it appears that HGF may not be as important in APAP hepatotoxicity as in the PHx model.

4.3 Other acute hepatotoxicants

It is clear that regeneration determines outcome after treatment with numerous other hepatotoxicants, including thioacetamide, diallyl sulfide, allyl alcohol, bromobenzene and others (Mehendale, 2005). It is also clear that nutrition, age and other factors have a major influence on liver regeneration in these models (Mehendale, 2005). Unfortunately, it is not yet known if growth factors, cytokines, or metabolic intermediates are important in the mechanisms that lead to hepatic recovery in those models. Furthermore, increases in growth factors like HGF, TGFα and VEGF have been reported in several studies of galactosamine hepatotoxicity (Okajima, Miyazawa, & Kitamura, 1990; Webber, FitzGerald, Brown, Bartlett, & Fausto, 1993), but no mechanistic studies have been done to determine whether or not they play a role in regeneration in that model. Additional research with these models could help us to understand the importance particular regeneration signaling pathways in other forms of acute xenobiotic-induced liver injury. Finally, it could be interesting to study hepatocyte proliferation in a model of idiosyncratic DILI (IDILI), including the recently developed Utrecht-Pohl IDILI model involving breakage of immune tolerance (McGill & Jaeschke, 2019).

4.4 Alcoholic hepatitis

Very little effort has been made to study the role of liver regeneration or hepatocyte proliferation in alcohol toxicity, but some data are available. The proportion of hepatocytes in S-phase increases in rats on the Lieber-DeCarli diet, peaks at approximately 10% after 2 weeks, and then declines back to normal levels while evidence of injury persists (Apte, McCree, & Ramaiah, 2004). Those data indicate that continued ethanol exposure inhibits liver regeneration and recovery from alcohol-associated liver disease, so early progression of the disease may be due in part to failure of regeneration. Consistent with that, it is well known that heavy ethanol consumption can inhibit regeneration after both PHx and acute hepatotoxicity (Chen, Ishac, Dent, Kunos, & Gao, 1998; Diehl, 1999; Duguay, Coutu, Hetu, & Joly, 1982; Juskeviciute et al., 2016; Wands, Carter, Bucher, & Isselbacher, 1979). Furthermore, regeneration and Stat3 signaling appear to be suppressed in patients with alcoholic cirrhosis compared to other cirrhosis etiologies (Horiguchi, Ishac, & Gao, 2007), which suggests a role for IL-6 in regeneration after ethanol-induced hepatotoxicity. Interestingly, experiments with zebrafish suggest that VEGF has a detrimental role in alcohol-associated liver disease through activation of stellate cells (Zhang, Ellis, & Yin, 2016). Finally, recent data demonstrate that augmenter of liver regeneration (ALR) has a role in reducing injury and progression of alcoholic liver disease (Kumar, Wang, Rani, & Gandhi, 2016).

5. Biomarkers of liver regeneration

Biomarkers of liver regeneration may be useful for prediction of survival in ALF, particularly drug-induced ALF. As mentioned, mortality in drug-induced ALF is high. For most ALF patients, a liver transplant is the only life-saving treatment. While *N*-acetylcysteine (NAC) can be used to treat APAP overdose, NAC loses efficacy beyond 24h (Rumack, Peterson, Koch, & Amara, 1981).

Furthermore, the decision to perform a liver transplant must be made quickly, as the median time from onset of ALF to death is only 2–5 days (Reddy et al., 2016). Unfortunately, the current clinical laboratory markers of liver injury do not predict outcome in acute liver injury (Antoine et al., 2012; McGill, 2016; McGill et al., 2014). Better biomarkers could help clinicians making rapid treatment decisions.

Some studies of liver regeneration biomarkers in ALF have already been performed. It has been known for many years that recovery of hepatic function, reflected by markers like prothrombin time (or INR) and bilirubin, is predictive of outcome. In fact, the commonly used Model for End Stage Liver Disease (MELD) score as well as the King's College Criteria for poor prognosis in ALF include both (Malinchoc et al., 2000; O'Grady, Alexander, Hayllar, & Williams, 1989). However, although those markers display good operating characteristics, recovery of liver function typically does not occur until after the peak of injury. Given the rapid progression of ALF, changes are usually too late to be very useful. Thus, novel biomarkers are needed. Schmidt and Dalhoff (2005) reported that circulating α-fetoprotein (AFP), a marker of hepatocyte proliferation, is dramatically elevated in survivors of APAP-induced ALF compared to non-survivors (Schmidt & Dalhoff, 2005). These data were later reproduced in patients with ALF due to other etiologies (Schiødt et al., 2006). Unfortunately, AFP values do not increase until 1–3 days after the peak of liver injury, similar to prothrombin time and bilirubin. Another study found that α-NH-butyric acid is elevated in serum after PHx in mice, and that it is higher in child and adolescent survivors of ALF (Rudnick et al., 2009).

AFP and α-NH-butyric acid have the advantage of already being available in some clinical laboratories. AFP is often measured as a biomarker of hepatocellular carcinoma, while α-NH-butyric acid can be measured in some hospitals that have biochemical genetics laboratories with the capability to screen for and monitor metabolic diseases.

Several biomarkers of regeneration that are not yet widely available may be more useful for prediction of patient outcome than current tests. Data from small studies indicate that serum leukocyte cell-derived chemotaxin 2 (Lect2), which is elevated in mice undergoing regeneration after PHx (Sato et al., 2004b), is far lower in non-survivors of ALF (Sato et al., 2004a). More impressively, Church et al. (2018) recently reported that osteopontin could predict poor outcome in a large cohort of DILI patients. Finally, our lab recently discovered that the lipid phosphatidic acid (PA) is important for liver regeneration after APAP hepatotoxicity, and that it is elevated in serum from APAP overdose patients with liver injury (Lutkewitte et al., 2018). However, it is not yet known if circulating PA values correlate with outcome.

Recently, novel computational methods have been used to aid interpretation of liver injury biomarkers. So far, these methods have primarily been used to understand changes in biomarkers retrospectively, after they have been observed in human subjects (Longo et al., 2017; Woodhead et al., 2017), but it may be possible to predict such changes prospectively. Furthermore, consideration of regeneration has been incorporated into such models to estimate the amount of time needed to restore the hepatocytes lost due to injury (Church & Watkins, 2018; Longo et al., 2017). In the future, it may be possible to use related techniques to predict the extent and kinetics of liver regeneration, and therefore patient outcome, using patient data in real-time from monitoring of serum injury biomarkers.

Overall, the future of liver regeneration biomarkers looks bright, but a better understanding of basic regeneration mechanisms after acute injury such as DILI is needed. Also, larger and more detailed studies of existing regeneration biomarkers are needed to fully evaluate their clinical utility.

6. Conclusion

Liver regeneration after PHx has been thoroughly investigated, but far fewer studies have addressed the mechanisms that drive liver regeneration after DILI. While there is considerable overlap, there are also clear differences such as the relative importance of HGF and EGFR in PHx, APAP, and CCl_4 hepatotoxicity. Mechanistically, additional research is needed on the roles of cell signaling and metabolism in regeneration after toxic injury, as well as on the role of regeneration in alcohol-associated liver disease. Clinically, biomarkers of liver regeneration show promise for prediction of outcome in ALF, but more studies are needed to validate them.

Conflict of interest statement

None of the authors have any conflict of interest to declare.

Acknowledgments

This work was supported in part by a Pinnacle Research Award from the American Association for the Study of Liver Diseases (AASLD) Foundation (M.R.M.), start-up funds from the University of Arkansas for Medical Sciences (M.R.M.), and by National Institutes of Health grants R01 DK098414 (U.A.), P20 GM103549 (U.A.), P30 GM118247 (U.A.), and T32 GM106999 (M.M.C.).

References

Akerman, P., Cote, P., Yang, S. Q., McClain, C., Nelson, S., Bagby, G. J., et al. (1992). Antibodies to tumor necrosis factor-alpha inhibit liver regeneration after partial hepatectomy. *The American Journal of Physiology*, *263*, G579–G585.

Anand, S. S., Murthy, S. N., Mumtaz, M. M., & Mehendale, H. M. (2004). Dose-dependent liver tissue repair in chloroform plus thioacetamide hepatotoxicity. *Environmental Toxicology and Pharmacology*, *18*, 143–148.

Antoine, D. J., Jenkins, R. E., Dear, J. W., Williams, D. P., McGill, M. R., Sharpe, M. R., et al. (2012). Molecular forms of HMGB1 and keratin-18 as mechanistic biomarkers for mode of cell death and prognosis during clinical acetaminophen hepatotoxicity. *Journal of Hepatology*, *56*, 1070–1079.

Apte, U., Bhushan, B., & Dadhania, V. (2017). Hepatic defenses against toxicity: Tissue regeneration and repair. In R. A. Roth (Ed.), *Comprehensive toxicology*. Amsterdam: Elsevier.

Apte, U., McCree, R., & Ramaiah, S. K. (2004). Hepatocyte proliferation is the possible mechanism for the transient decrease in liver injury during steatosis stage of alcoholic liver disease. *Toxicologic Pathology*, *32*, 567–576.

Apte, U., Singh, S., Zeng, G., Cieply, B., Virji, M. A., Wu, T., et al. (2009). Beta-catenin activation promotes liver regeneration after acetaminophen-induced injury. *The American Journal of Pathology*, *175*, 1056–1065.

Bajt, M. L., Cover, C., Lemasters, J. J., & Jaeschke, H. (2006). Nuclear translocation of endonuclease G and apoptosis-induced factor during acetaminophen-induced liver cell injury. *Toxicological Sciences*, *94*, 217–225.

Bajt, M. L., Yan, H. M., Farhood, A., & Jaeschke, H. (2008). Plasminogen activator inhibitor-1 limits liver injury and facilitates regeneration after acetaminophen overdose. *Toxicological Sciences*, *104*, 419–427.

Beier, J. I., Guo, L., Ritzenthaler, J. D., Joshi-Barve, S., Roman, J., & Arteel, G. E. (2016). Fibrin- mediated integrin signaling plays a critical role in hepatic regeneration after partial hepatectomy in mice. *Annals of Hepatology*, *15*, 762–772.

Bhattacharyya, S., Pence, L., Beger, R., Chaudhuri, S., McCullough, S., Yan, K., et al. (2013). Acylcarnitine profiles in acetaminophen toxicity in the mouse: Comparison to toxicity, metabolism and hepatocyte regeneration. *Metabolites*, *3*, 606–622.

Bhushan, B., Borude, P., Edwards, G., Walesky, C., Cleveland, J., Li, F., et al. (2013). Role of bile acids in liver injury and regeneration following acetaminophen overdose. *The American Journal of Pathology*, *183*, 1518–1526.

Bhushan, B., Chavan, H., Borude, P., Xie, Y., Du, K., McGill, M. R., et al. (2017). Dual role of epidermal growth factor receptor in liver injury and regeneration after acetaminophen overdose in mice. *Toxicological Sciences*, *155*, 363–378.

Bhushan, B., Poudel, S., Manley, M. W., Jr., Roy, N., & Apte, U. (2017). Inhibition of glycogen synthase kinase 3 accelerated liver regeneration after acetaminophen-induced hepatotoxicity in mice. *The American Journal of Pathology*, *187*, 543–552.

Bhushan, B., Walesky, C., Manley, M., Gallagher, T., Borude, P., Edwards, G., et al. (2014). Pro-regenerative signaling after acetaminophen-induced acute liver injury in mice identified using a novel incremental dose model. *The American Journal of Pathology*, *184*, 3013–3025.

Breu, A. C., Patwardhan, V. R., Nayor, J., Ringwala, J. N., Devore, Z. G., Ganatra, R. B., et al. (2018). A multicenter study into causes of severe acute liver injury. *Clinical Gastroenterology and Hepatology*. https://doi.org/10.1016/j.cgh.2018.08.016. [Epub ahead of print].

Burr, A. W., Toole, K., Chapman, C., Hines, J. E., & Burt, A. D. (1998). Anti-hepatocyte growth factor antibody inhibits hepatocyte proliferation during liver regeneration. *The Journal of Pathology*, *185*, 298–302.

Chanda, S., Mangipudy, R. S., Warbritton, A., Bucci, T. J., & Mehendale, H. M. (1995). Stimulated hepatic tissue repair underlies heteroprotection by thioacetamide against acetaminophen-induced lethality. *Hepatology*, *21*, 477–486.

Chanda, S., & Mehendale, H. M. (1995). Nutritional impact on the final outcome of liver injury inflicted by model hepatotoxicants: Effect of glucose loading. *The FASEB Journal*, *9*, 240–245.

Chen, J., Ishac, E. J., Dent, P., Kunos, P., & Gao, B. (1998). Effects of ethanol on mitogen-activated protein kinase and stress-activated protein kinase cascades in normal and regenerating liver. *The Biochemical Journal*, *334*, 669–676.

Church, R. J., Kullak-Ublick, G. A., Aubrecht, J., Bonkovsky, H. L., Chalasani, N., Fontana, R. J., et al. (2018). Candidate biomarkers for diagnosis and prognosis of drug-induced liver injury: An international collaborative effort. *Hepatology*, *69*, 760–773. https://doi.org/10.1002/hep.29802. [Epub ahead of print].

Church, R. J., & Watkins, P. B. (2018). In silico modeling to optimize interpretation of liver safety biomarkers in clinical trials. *Experimental Biology and Medicine (Maywood, N.J.)*, *243*, 300–307.

Clemens, M. M., Kennon-McGill, S., Apte, U., James, L. P., Finck, B. N., & McGill, M. R. (2019). The inhibitor of glycerol 3-phosphate acyltransferase FSG67 blunts liver regeneration after acetaminophen overdose by altering GSK3β and Wnt/β-catenin signaling. *Food and Chemical Toxicology*, *125*, 279–288.

Cressman, D. E., Greenbaum, L. E., DeAngelis, R. A., Ciliberto, G., Furth, E. E., Poli, V., et al. (1996). Liver failure and defective hepatocyte regeneration in interleukin-6-deficient mice. *Science*, *274*, 1379–1383.

Dadhania, V. P., Bhushan, B., Apte, U., & Mehendale, H. M. (2017). Wnt/β-catenin signaling drives thioacetamide-mediated heteroprotection against acetaminophen-induced lethal liver injury. *Dose Response*, *15*, 1559325817690287.

Diehl, A. M. (1999). Effect of ethanol on tumor necrosis factor signaling during liver regeneration. *Clinical Biochemistry*, *32*, 571–578.

Donahower, B. C., McCullough, S. S., Hennings, L., Simpson, P. M., Stowe, C. D., Saad, A. G., et al. (2010). Human recombinant vascular endothelial growth factor reduces necrosis and enhances hepatocyte regeneration in a mouse model of acetaminophen toxicity. *The Journal of Pharmacology and Experimental Therapeutics*, *334*, 33–43.

Donahower, B., McCullough, S. S., Kurten, R., Lamps, L. W., Simpson, P., Hinson, J. A., et al. (2006). Vascular endothelial growth factor and hepatocyte regeneration in acetaminophen toxicity. *American Journal of Physiology. Gastrointestinal and Liver Physiology*, *291*, G102–G109.

Du, K., Xie, Y., McGill, M. R., & Jaeschke, H. (2015). Pathophysiological significance of c-jun N-terminal kinase in acetaminophen hepatotoxicity. *Expert Opinion on Drug Metabolism & Toxicology*, *11*, 1769–1779.

Duguay, L., Coutu, D., Hetu, C., & Joly, J. G. (1982). Inhibition of liver regeneration by chronic alcohol administration. *Gut*, *23*, 8–13.

Fausto, N. (2000). Liver regeneration. *Journal of Hepatology*, *32*, 19–31.

Galvin, Z., McDonough, A., Ryan, J., & Stewart, S. (2015). Blood alanine aminotransferase levels >1,000 IU/l—Causes and outcomes. *Clinical Medicine (London, England)*, *15*, 244–247.

Ganger, D. R., Rule, J., Rakela, J., Bass, N., Reuben, A., Stravitz, R. T., et al. (2018). Acute liver failure of indeterminate etiology: A comprehensive systematic approach by an expert committee to establish causality. *The American Journal of Gastroenterology*, *113*, 1319–1328.

Gujral, J. S., Knight, T. R., Farhood, A., Bajt, M. L., & Jaeschke, H. (2002). Mode of cell death after acetaminophen overdose in mice: Apoptosis or oncotic necrosis? *Toxicological Sciences*, *67*, 322–328.

Gunawan, B. K., Liu, Z. X., Han, D., Hanawa, N., Gaarde, W. A., & Kaplowitz, N. (2006). c-Jun N-terminal kinase plays a major role in murine acetaminophen hepatotoxicity. *Gastroenterology*, *131*, 165–178.

Hanawa, N., Shinohara, M., Saberi, B., Gaarde, W. A., Han, D., & Kaplowitz, N. (2008). Role of JNK translocation to mitochondria leading to inhibition of mitochondria bioenergetics in acetaminophen-induced liver injury. *The Journal of Biological Chemistry*, *283*, 13565–13577.

Higgins, G. M., & Anderson, R. M. (1931). Experimental pathology of the liver. *Archives of Pathology*, *12*, 186–202.

Horiguchi, N., Ishac, E. J., & Gao, B. (2007). Liver regeneration is suppressed in alcoholic cirrhosis: Correlation with decreased STAT3 activation. *Alcohol*, *41*, 271–280.

Huang, J., Zhang, D., Lin, L., Jiang, R., Dai, J., Tang, L., et al. (2018). Potential roles of AMP-activated protein kinase in liver regeneration in mice with acute liver injury. *Molecular Medicine Reports*, *17*, 5390–5395.

Hughes, R. D., Zhang, L., Tsubouchi, H., Daikuhara, Y., & Williams, R. (1994). Plasma hepatocyte growth factor and biliprotein levels and outcome in fulminant hepatic failure. *Journal of Hepatology*, *20*, 106–111.

Huh, C. G., Factor, V. M., Sánchez, A., Uchida, K., Conner, E. A., & Thorgeirsson, S. S. (2004). Hepatocyte growth factor/c-met signaling pathway is required for efficient liver regeneration and repair. *Proceedings of the National Academy of Sciences of the United States of America*, *101*, 4477–4482.

James, L. P., Kurten, R. C., Lamps, L. W., McCullough, S., & Hinson, J. A. (2005). Tumour necrosis factor receptor 1 and hepatocyte regeneration in acetaminophen toxicity: A kinetic study of proliferating cell nuclear antigen and cytokine expression. *Basic & Clinical Pharmacology & Toxicology*, *97*, 8–14.

James, L. P., Lamps, L. W., McCullough, S., & Hinson, J. A. (2003). Interleukin 6 and hepatocyte regeneration in acetaminophen toxicity in the mouse. *Biochemical and Biophysical Research Communications*, *309*, 857–863.

Ju, C., Reilly, T. P., Bourdi, M., Radonovich, M. F., Brady, J. N., George, J. W., et al. (2002). Protective role of Kupffer cells in acetaminophen-induced hepatic injury in mice. *Chemical Research in Toxicology*, *15*, 1504–1513.

Juskeviciute, E., Dippold, R. P., Antony, A. N., Swarup, A., Vadigepalli, R., & Hoek, J. B. (2016). Inhibition of miR-21 rescues liver regeneration after partial hepatectomy in ethanol-fed rats. *American Journal of Physiology. Gastrointestinal and Liver Physiology*, *311*, G794–G806.

Kayano, K., Yasunaga, M., Kubota, M., Takenaka, K., Mori, K., Yamashita, A., et al. (1992). Detection of proliferating hepatocytes by immunohistochemical staining for proliferating cell nuclear antigen (PCNA) in patients with acute hepatic failure. *Liver*, *12*, 132–136.

Kennon-McGill, S., & McGill, M. R. (2018). Extrahepatic toxicity of acetaminophen: Critical evaluation of the evidence and proposed mechanisms. *Journal of Clinical and Translational Research*, *3*, 5.

Kodavanti, P. R., Joshi, U. M., Young, R. A., Bell, A. N., & Mehendale, H. M. (1989). Role of hepatocellular regeneration in chlordecone potentiated hepatotoxicity of carbon tetrachloride. *Archives of Toxicology*, *63*, 367–375.

Kodavanti, P. R., Joshi, U. M., Young, R. A., Meydrech, E. F., & Mehendale, H. M. (1989). Protection of hepatotoxic and lethal effects of CCl_4 by partial hepatectomy. *Toxicologic Pathology*, *17*, 494–505.

Kon, K., Kim, J. S., Jaeschke, H., & Lemasters, J. J. (2004). Mitochondrial permeability transition in acetaminophen-induced necrosis and apoptosis of cultured mouse hepatocytes. *Hepatology*, *40*, 1170–1179.

Kumar, S., Wang, J., Rani, R., & Gandhi, C. R. (2016). Hepatic deficiency of augmenter of liver regeneration exacerbates alcohol-induced liver injury and promotes fibrosis in mice. *PLoS One*, *11*, e0147864.

Larson, A. M., Polson, J., Fontana, R. J., Davern, T. J., Lalani, E., Hynan, L. S., et al. (2005). Acetaminophen-induced acute liver failure: results of a United States multicenter, prospective study. *Hepatology*, *42*, 1364–1372.

Lee, W. M. (2008). Etiologies of acute liver failure. *Seminars in Liver Disease*, *28*, 142–152.

Leevy, C. M., Hollister, R. M., Schmid, R., MacDonald, R. A., & Davidson, C. S. (1959). Liver regeneration in experimental carbon tetrachloride intoxication. *Proceedings of the Society for Experimental Biology and Medicine*, *102*, 672–675.

Limaye, P. B., Apte, U. M., Shankar, K., Bucci, T. J., Warbritton, A., & Mehendale, H. M. (2003). Calpain released from dying hepatocytes mediates progression of acute liver injury induced by model hepatotoxicants. *Toxicology and Applied Pharmacology*, *191*, 211–226.

Limaye, P. B., Bhave, V. S., Palkar, P. S., Apte, U. M., Sawant, S. P., Yu, S., et al. (2006). Upregulation of calpastatin in regenerating and developing rat liver: Role in resistance against hepatotoxicity. *Hepatology*, *44*, 379–388.

Longo, D. M., Generaux, G. T., Howell, B. A., Siler, S. Q., Antoine, D. J., Button, D., et al. (2017). Refining liver safety risk assessment: Application of mechanistic modeling and serum biomarkers to cimaglermin alfa (GGF2) clinical trials. *Clinical Pharmacology and Therapeutics*, *102*, 961–969.

Lutkewitte, A. J., Schweitzer, G. G., Kennon-McGill, S., Clemens, M. M., James, L. P., Jaeschke, H., et al. (2018). Lipin deactivation after acetaminophen overdose causes phosphatidic acid accumulation in liver and plasma in mice and humans and enhances liver regeneration. *Food and Chemical Toxicology*, *115*, 273–283.

Malinchoc, M., Kamath, P. S., Gordon, F. D., Peine, C. J., Rank, J., & ter Borg, P. C. (2000). A model to predict poor survival in patients undergoing transjugular intrahepatic portosystemic shunts. *Hepatology*, *31*, 864–871.

Mangipudy, R. S., Chanda, S., & Mehendale, H. M. (1995). Tissue repair response as a function of dose in thioacetamide hepatotoxicity. *Environmental Health Perspectives*, *103*, 260–267.

Masubuchi, Y., Bourdi, M., Reilly, T. P., Graf, M. L., George, J. W., & Pohl, L. R. (2003). Role of interleukin-6 in hepatic heat shock protein expression and protection against acetaminophen-induced liver disease. *Biochemical and Biophysical Research Communications*, *304*, 207–212.

McGill, M. R. (2016). The past and present of serum aminotransferases and the future of liver injury biomarkers. *EXCLI Journal*, *15*, 817–828.

McGill, M. R., & Jaeschke, H. (2013). Metabolism and disposition of acetaminophen: Recent advances in relation to hepatotoxicity and diagnosis. *Pharmaceutical Research*, *30*, 2174–2187.

McGill, M. R., & Jaeschke, H. (2019). Animal models of drug-induced liver injury. *Biochimica et Biophysica Acta—Molecular Basis of Disease*. https://doi.org/10.1016/j.bbadis.2018.08.037. [Epub ahead of print].

McGill, M. R., Sharpe, M. R., Williams, C. D., Taha, M., Curry, S. C., & Jaeschke, H. (2012). The mechanism underlying acetaminophen-induced hepatotoxicity in humans and mice involves mitochondrial damage and nuclear DNA fragmentation. *The Journal of Clinical Investigation*, *122*, 1574–1583.

McGill, M. R., Staggs, V. S., Sharpe, M. R., Lee, W. M., Jaeschke, H., & Acute Liver Failure Study Group. (2014). Serum mitochondrial biomarkers and damage-associated molecular patterns are higher in acetaminophen overdose patients with poor outcome. *Hepatology*, *60*, 1336–1345.

McGill, M. R., Williams, C. D., Xie, Y., Ramachandran, A., & Jaeschke, H. (2012). Acetaminophen-induced liver injury in rats and mice: Comparison of protein adducts, mitochondrial dysfunction, and oxidative stress in the mechanism of toxicity. *Toxicology and Applied Pharmacology*, *264*, 387–394.

McGill, M. R., Yan, H. M., Ramachandran, A., Murray, G. J., Rollins, D. E., & Jaeschke, H. (2011). HepaRG cells: A human model to study mechanisms of acetaminophen hepatotoxicity. *Hepatology*, *53*, 974–982.

Mehendale, H. M. (1989). Mechanism of the lethal interaction of chlordecone and CCl_4 at non-toxic doses. *Toxicology Letters*, *49*, 215–241.

Mehendale, H. M. (2005). Tissue repair: An important determinant of final outcome of toxicant-induced injury. *Toxicologic Pathology*, *33*, 41–51.

Meyers, L. L., Beierschmitt, W. P., Khairallah, E. A., & Cohen, S. D. (1988). Acetaminophen-induced inhibition of hepatic mitochondrial respiration in mice. *Toxicology and Applied Pharmacology*, *93*, 378–387.

Michalopoulos, G. K. (2013). Principles of liver regeneration and growth homeostasis. *Comprehensive Physiology*, *3*, 485–513.

Michalopoulos, G. K. (2014). Advances in liver regeneration. *Expert Review of Gastroenterology & Hepatology*, *8*, 897–907.

Michalopoulos, G. K. (2017). Hepatostat: Liver regeneration and normal liver tissue maintenance. *Hepatology*, *65*, 1384–1392.

Milne, L. S. (1909). The histology of liver tissue regeneration. *The Journal of Pathology and Bacteriology*, *13*, 127–158.

Moh, A., Iwamoto, Y., Chai, G. X., Zhang, S. S., Kano, A., Yang, D. D., et al. (2007). Role of STAT3 in liver regeneration: Survival, DNA synthesis, inflammatory reaction and liver mass recovery. *Laboratory Investigation*, *87*, 1018–1028.

O'Grady, J. G., Alexander, G. J., Hayllar, K. M., & Williams, R. (1989). Early indicators of prognosis in fulminant hepatic failure. *Gastroenterology*, *97*, 439–445.

Okajima, A., Miyazawa, K., & Kitamura, N. (1990). Primary structure of rat hepatocyte growth factor and induction of its mRNA during liver regeneration following hepatic injury. *European Journal of Biochemistry*, *193*, 375–381.

Ostapowicz, G., Fontana, R. J., Schiødt, F. V., Larson, A., Davern, T. J., Han, S. H., et al. (2002). Results of a prospective study of acute liver failure at 17 tertiary care centers in the United States. *Annals of Internal Medicine*, *137*, 947–954.

Phaneuf, D., Moscioni, A. D., LeClair, C., Raper, S. E., & Wilson, J. M. (2004). Generation of a mouse expressing a conditional knockout of the hepatocyte growth factor gene: Demonstration of impaired liver regeneration. *DNA and Cell Biology*, *23*, 592–603.

Placke, M. E., Ginsberg, G. L., Wyand, D. S., & Cohen, S. D. (1987). Ultrastructural changes during acute acetaminophen-induced hepatotoxicity in the mouse: A time and dose study. *Toxicologic Pathology*, *15*, 431–438.

Ramachandran, A., Lebofsky, M., Baines, C. P., Lemasters, J. J., & Jaeschke, H. (2011). Cyclophilin D deficiency protects against acetaminophen-induced oxidant stress and liver injury. *Free Radical Research*, *45*, 156–164.

Ramachandran, A., Lebofsky, M., Weinman, S. A., & Jaeschke, H. (2011). The impact of partial manganese superoxide dismutase (SOD2)-deficiency on mitochondrial oxidant stress, DNA fragmentation and liver injury during acetaminophen hepatotoxicity. *Toxicology and Applied Pharmacology*, *251*, 226–233.

Rao, S. B., Mangipudy, R. S., & Mehendale, H. M. (1997). Tissue injury and repair as parallel and opposing responses to CCl_4 hepatotoxicity: A novel dose-response. *Toxicology*, *118*, 181–193.

Rao, S. B., & Mehendale, H. M. (1989). Protective role of fructose 1,6-bisphosphate during CCl_4 hepatotoxicity in rats. *The Biochemical Journal*, *262*, 721–725.

Reddy, K. R., Ellerbe, C., Schilsky, M., Stravitz, R. T., Fontana, R. J., Durkalsi, V., et al. (2016). Determinants of outcome among patients with acute liver failure listed for liver transplantation in the United States. *Liver Transplantation*, *22*, 505–515.

Reid, A. B., Kurten, R. C., McCullough, S. S., Brock, R. W., & Hinson, J. A. (2005). Mechanisms of acetaminophen-induced hepatotoxicity: Role of oxidative stress and mitochondrial permeability transition in freshly isolated mouse hepatocytes. *The Journal of Pharmacology and Experimental Therapeutics*, *312*, 509–516.

Río, A., Gassull, M. A., Aldeguer, X., Ojanguren, I., Cabré, E., & Fernández, E. (2008). Reduced liver injury in the interleukin-6 knockout mice by chronic carbon tetrachloride administration. *European Journal of Clinical Investigation*, *38*, 306–316.

Rudnick, D. A., Dietzen, D. J., Turmelle, Y. P., Shepherd, R., Zhang, S., Belle, S. H., et al. (2009). Serum alpha-NH-butyric acid may predict spontaneous survival in pediatric acute liver failure. *Pediatric Transplantation*, *13*, 223–230.

Rumack, B. H., Peterson, R. C., Koch, G. G., & Amara, I. A. (1981). Acetaminophen overdose. 662 cases with evaluation of oral acetylcysteine treatment. *Archives of Internal Medicine*, *141*, 380–385.

Sadler, K. C., Krahn, K. N., Gaur, N. A., & Ukomadu, C. (2007). Liver growth in the embryo and during liver regeneration in zebrafish requires the cell cycle regulator, uhrf1. *Proceedings of the National Academy of Sciences of the United States of America*, *104*, 1570–1575.

Sato, Y., Watanabe, H., Kameyama, H., Kobayashi, T., Yamamoto, S., Takeishi, T., et al. (2004a). Serum LECT2 level as a prognostic indicator in acute liver failure. *Transplantation Proceedings*, *36*, 2359–2361.

Sato, Y., Watanabe, H., Kameyama, H., Kobayashi, T., Yamamoto, S., Takeishi, T., et al. (2004b). Changes in serum LECT2 levels during the early period of liver regeneration after adult living related donor liver transplantation. *Transplantation Proceedings*, *36*, 2357–2358.

Scheving, L. A., Zhang, X., Stevenson, M. C., Threadgill, D. W., & Russell, W. E. (2015). Loss of hepatocyte EGFR has no effect alone but exacerbates carbon tetrachloride-induced liver injury and impairs regeneration in hepatocyte Met-deficient mice. *American Journal of Physiology Gastrointestinal and Liver Physiology*, *308*, G364–G377.

Schiødt, F. V., Ostapowicz, G., Murray, N., Satyanarana, R., Zaman, A., Munoz, S., et al. (2006). Alpha-fetoprotein and prognosis in acute liver failure. *Liver Transplantation*, *12*, 1776–1781.

Schmidt, L. E., & Dalhoff, K. (2005). Alpha-fetoprotein is a predictor of outcome in acetaminophen-induced liver injury. *Hepatology, 41*, 26–31.

Shanmukhappa, K., Matte, U., Degen, J. L., & Bezerra, J. A. (2009). Plasmin-mediated proteolysis is required for hepatocyte growth factor activation during liver repair. *The Journal of Biological Chemistry, 284*, 12917–12923.

Subbotin, V. M. (2017). *Arguments on the origin of the vertebrate liver and the Amphioxus hepatic diverticulum: A hypothesis on evolutionary novelties.* Pisma v Vavilovskii Zhurnal. http://www.bionet.nsc.ru/vogis/download/hypothesis/appx1.pdf. Accessed on 09/12/2018.

Sullivan, B. P., Kassel, K. M., Jone, A., Flick, M. J., & Luyendyk, J. P. (2012). Fibrin(ogen)-independent role of plasminogen activators in acetaminophen-induced liver injury. *The American Journal of Pathology, 180*, 2321–2329.

Tapper, E. B., Sengupta, N., & Bonder, A. (2015). The incidence and outcomes of ischemic hepatitis: A systematic review with meta-analysis. *The American Journal of Medicine, 128*, 1314–1321.

Thakore, K. N., & Mehendale, H. M. (1991). Role of hepatocellular regeneration in CCl_4 autoprotection. *Toxicologic Pathology, 19*, 47–58.

Trautwein, C., Rakermann, T., Niehof, M., Rose-John, S., & Manns, M. P. (1996). Acute-phase response factor, increased binding, and target gene transcription during liver regeneration. *Gastroenterology, 110*, 1854–1862.

Wands, J. R., Carter, E. A., Bucher, N. L., & Isselbacher, K. J. (1979). Inhibition of hepatic regeneration in rats by acute and chronic ethanol intoxication. *Gastroenterology, 77*, 528–531.

Watanabe, K., Togo, S., Takahashi, T., Matsuyama, R., Yamamoto, H., Shimizu, T., et al. (2007). PAI-1 plays an important role in liver failure after excessive hepatectomy in the rat. *The Journal of Surgical Research, 143*, 13–99.

Webber, E. M., FitzGerald, M. J., Brown, P. I., Bartlett, M. H., & Fausto, N. (1993). Transforming growth factor-alpha expression during liver regeneration after partial hepatectomy and toxic injury, and potential interactions between transforming growth factor-alpha and hepatocyte growth factor. *Hepatology, 18*, 1422–1431.

Weber, L. W., Boll, M., & Stampfl, A. (2003). Hepatotoxicity and mechanism of action of haloalkanes: Carbon tetrachloride as a toxicological model. *Critical Reviews in Toxicology, 33*, 105–136.

Woodhead, J. L., Brock, W. J., Roth, S. E., Shoaf, S. E., Brouwer, K. L., Church, R., et al. (2017). Application of a mechanistic model to evaluate putative mechanisms of Tolvaptan drug-induced liver injury and identify patient susceptibility factors. *Toxicological Sciences, 155*, 61–74.

Woolbright, B. L., Ramachandran, A., McGill, M. R., Yan, H. M., Bajt, M. L., Sharpe, M. R., et al. (2012). Lysosomal instability and cathepsin B release during acetaminophen hepatotoxicity. *Basic & Clinical Pharmacology & Toxicology, 111*, 417–425.

Xie, Y., McGill, M. R., Dorko, K., Kumer, S. C., Schmitt, T. M., Forster, J., et al. (2014). Mechanisms of acetaminophen-induced cell death in primary human hepatocytes. *Toxicology and Applied Pharmacology, 279*, 266–274.

Xie, Y., McGill, M. R., Du, K., Dorko, K., Kumer, S. C., Schmitt, T. M., et al. (2015). Mitochondrial protein adducts formation and mitochondrial dysfunction during N-acetyl-m-aminophenol (AMAP)-induced hepatotoxicity in primary human hepatocytes. *Toxicology and Applied Pharmacology, 289*, 213–222.

Yamada, Y., & Fausto, N. (1998). Deficient liver regeneration after carbon tetrachloride injury in mice lacking type 1 but not type 2 tumor necrosis factor receptor. *The American Journal of Pathology, 152*, 1577–1589.

Yamada, Y., Kirillova, I., Peschon, J. J., & Fausto, N. (1997). Initiation of liver growth by tumor necrosis factor: Deficient liver regeneration in mice lacking type I tumor necrosis factor receptor. *Proceedings of the National Academy of Sciences of the United States of America, 94*, 1441–1446.

Zhang, C., Ellis, J. L., & Yin, C. (2016). Inhibition of vascular endothelial growth factor signaling facilitates liver repair from acute ethanol-induced injury in zebrafish. *Disease Models & Mechanisms*, *9*, 1383–1396.

Zhao, Y., Difrancesca, D., Wang, X., Zarnegar, R., Michalopoulos, G. K., & Yin, X. M. (2007). Promotion of Fas-mediated apoptosis in Type II cells by high doses of hepatocyte growth factor bypasses the mitochondrial requirement. *Journal of Cellular Physiology*, *213*, 556–563.

Further reading

Anand, S. S., & Mehendale, H. M. (2004). Liver regeneration: A critical toxicodynamic response in predictive toxicology. *Environmental Toxicology and Pharmacology*, *18*, 149–160.

Rao, S. B., & Mehendale, H. M. (1991). Effect of colchicine on hepatobiliary function in CCl_4 treated rats. *Biochemical Pharmacology*, *42*, 2323–2332.

CHAPTER TEN

Evaluation and treatment of acetaminophen toxicity

Erik S. Fisher[*,†,‡], **Steven C. Curry**[*,†,‡,1]
[*]Department of Medical Toxicology, Banner—University Medical Center Phoenix, Phoenix, AZ, United States
[†]Division of Clinical Data Analytics and Decision Support, University of Arizona College of Medicine—Phoenix, Phoenix, AZ, United States
[‡]Division of Medical Toxicology and Precision Medicine, University of Arizona College of Medicine—Phoenix, Phoenix, AZ, United States
[1]Corresponding author: e-mail address: drstcurry@cox.net

Contents

Abstract

A review of the typical clinical course, diagnosis and treatment of acetaminophen toxicity is provided. For an acute overdose, most adults must ingest about 12 g or more acetaminophen (APAP) before risk of serious hepatotoxicity is of concern. A nomogram of serum APAP concentration vs hours post-ingestion can assist in determining risk of liver injury and need for treatment. However, histories concerning the time of ingestion and the amount of drug ingested are usually unreliable. Peak serum transaminase activities usually occur 48–96 h after acute ingestion. It is possible for patients to present in liver failure days after ingestion with undetectable serum APAP concentrations. Patients who have chronically ingested excessive APAP doses and develop hepatotoxicity usually present with such, and renal failure is more common in this population. Current treatment centers on administration of *N*-acetylcysteine (NAC) to prevent hepatotoxicity, though NAC also improves outcomes in patients who present with acute liver failure. When given early after APAP ingestion, NAC's main mechanism of action is to maintain intracellular glutathione stores so to detoxify the electrophilic APAP metabolite, NAPQI. NAC is generally well-tolerated when given intravenously, with the main concern being anaphylactoid reactions. These reactions usually occur during loading doses and are easily treated with discontinuation of the NAC infusion, administration

Advances in Pharmacology, Volume 85
ISSN 1054-3589
https://doi.org/10.1016/bs.apha.2018.12.004
© 2019 Elsevier Inc.
All rights reserved.

of antihistamines, and then restarting the loading dose at a slower infusion rate. There is concern that current NAC dosing is not large enough to adequately treat large APAP ingestions. Patients with acute liver failure may be candidates for orthotopic liver transplantation.

1. Introduction

The nuances of evaluating and treating patients with known or suspected APAP toxicity could compose a book and are beyond the scope of this review. Therefore, a concise overview of typical clinical courses, diagnosis, and treatment of APAP toxicity is provided.

2. Acute acetaminophen ingestions

2.1 Clinical course

Physicians caring for patients who may have acutely ingested toxic quantities of acetaminophen (APAP) are confronted with a mixture of histories and circumstances surrounding those ingestions. Assuming no ongoing APAP use at the time of an acute ingestion, physicians generally become concerned for potential of serious liver injury when adults ingest approximately 12 g APAP or more, or when young children ingest more than about 200 mg APAP per kg body weight. When APAP has been intentionally taken in overdose (e.g., self-harm), or when doses or intentions are unclear, patients are evaluated and serum APAP concentrations are measured (described below). The term hepatotoxicity, in the context of APAP exposure, is currently defined as a serum ALT (alanine aminotransferase) activity greater than 1000 U/L. Lower peaks generally do not represent clinically significant hepatic dysfunction (Rumack, 2002; Rumack & Bateman, 2012).

Traditionally, APAP toxicity has been divided into four clinical stages (Rumack, Peterson, Koch, & Amara, 1981). Stage I is characterized by nausea, vomiting, nonspecific or right upper quadrant abdominal pain, and other nonspecific symptoms that begin within minutes to a few hours of ingestion. However, patients who have ingested potentially fatal amounts of APAP may remain relatively asymptomatic and appear well for the first day or longer. During Stage I, liver function studies such as transaminases, prothrombin time and bilirubin are normal or at baseline. Given the broad availability of APAP-containing products, it is prudent to obtain a serum APAP concentration in patients suspected of any drug overdose. Patients ingesting lethal amounts of APAP may be asymptomatic or have complaints and clinical findings of APAP toxicity masked or confounded by co-ingestants. Most patients who have acutely ingested an excessive dose of APAP and begin receiving treatment with *N*-acetylcysteine (NAC) within about 8 h of ingestion will be protected from developing hepatotoxicity and only rarely will develop acute liver failure.

Stage II marks the beginning of elevated liver function tests. Elevation of serum AST activity usually begins within 24 h of ingestion and rises in ALT activity soon follow or accompany those of AST (aspartate aminotransferase). Rises in transaminases are accompanied by increased prothrombin time (PT) and, at times, by increased serum bilirubin concentrations. In the absence of underlying liver disease, bilirubin concentrations usually remain normal initially, and may never increase in patients who do not progress to fulminant hepatic failure.

Peak hepatic injury characterizes Stage III. Serum transaminases most commonly peak 3–4 days after ingestion. Many patients remain relatively asymptomatic at this stage, but in those patients with more severe liver injury, fulminant hepatic failure (hepatic encephalopathy, hyperbilirubinemia) appears. Potential complications include hepatic encephalopathy, cerebral edema, lactic acidosis, hypoglycemia, vasodilation and shock, profound PT elevation, thrombocytopenia, bleeding, and infection. Death usually results from cerebral edema, septic shock, or, less commonly, hemorrhage.

Stage IV is characterized by recovery in survivors. Transaminase values and PT generally return to normal over a few to 14 days, and there is never resultant cirrhosis or residual hepatic dysfunction in those who survive.

Acetaminophen-induced renal failure from acute tubular necrosis is common in patients who progress to acute hepatic failure (Larson et al., 2005). Recovery of renal function is expected in survivors (Mazer & Perrone, 2008). Pancreatitis and myocardial dysfunction have been described after APAP overdose. Patients who ingest very large amounts of APAP with extremely elevated serum APAP concentrations can present with coma and severe lactic acidosis within hours of ingestion for reasons unrelated to hepatic injury or failure. The acidosis is thought to represent impaired oxidative phosphorylation from APAP's action on the electron transport chain (Fannin et al., 2010). Coma and acidosis usually resolve over 12–36 h. There may not be evidence of liver dysfunction in these patients if NAC therapy is commenced early after ingestion.

2.2 Diagnosis and risk of toxicity

Identification of patients who have taken doses of APAP capable of producing hepatotoxicity depends on the history, measurement of serum APAP concentrations, and consideration of other etiologies of hepatic dysfunction.

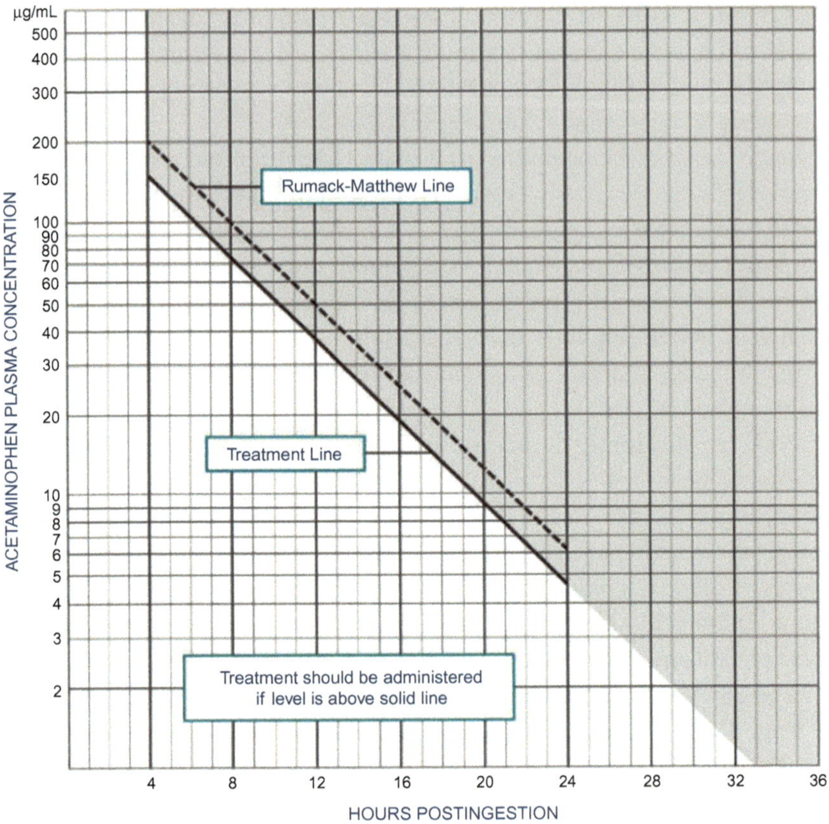

Fig. 1 Rumack-Matthew nomogram. Acetaminophen plasma concentrations vs time postingestion. Patients with levels above the *solid line* should be treated with NAC. Can be used only in patients with single acute ingestions who are not chronically taking acetaminophen. *Source: Wikimedia commons.*

Following a *single, acute* ingestion, patients who present in Stage I are risk-stratified using the Rumack-Matthew nomogram (Fig. 1), on which the serum APAP concentration is plotted against time post-ingestion.

The dotted upper line on the nomogram is meant to separate those patients at risk of developing hepatotoxicity from those who will not, without therapy. In the United States, this nomogram was modified and made more sensitive by creating a treatment line (solid line) 25% below the hepatotoxicity line (Rumack, 2002) to account for inaccurate patient histories and historical issues with measurement of serum APAP concentrations that are no longer relevant. A single serum APAP concentration drawn at least 4h after ingestion is plotted on the nomogram, and if it falls above the treatment line, NAC therapy is commenced. There has previously been theoretical concern for an increased risk of APAP-induced hepatotoxicity in patients with induced CYP2E1 activity such as patient with ketosis, chronic alcohol use, malnutrition, polymorphisms in metabolic pathways, or ingestion of CYP450 inducers. However, the nomogram has a long track record of providing adequate guidance, given its conservative nature.

APAP is available throughout the world in various strengths and in "extended relief," delayed release, suppository, and liquid preparations. However, there is no convincing evidence that use of the nomogram should be modified or that serum APAP levels should be interpreted differently with the use of different APAP products. In 2012 the United Kingdom modified the nomogram to be even more conservative, though many have challenged this decision and consider it unhelpful.

APAP is also available in parenteral form. While acute oral ingestions of APAP are generally considered non-toxic below a dose of 150–200 mg APAP per kg body weight, significant toxicity has been reported in children who received as little as 75 mg/kg parenterally in a therapeutic error. Some authors now recommend antidotal therapy for any patient who acutely receives 60 mg per kg body weight or more of IV APAP (Beringer, Thompson, Parry, & Stoddart, 2011; Berling, Anscombe, & Isbister, 2012). Other evidence suggests that IV APAP may carry a lower risk of toxicity than oral APAP. Regardless, the Rumack-Matthew nomogram is intended for acute oral ingestions and has not been validated as a tool to predict toxicity in the setting of IV APAP exposures.

The nomogram cannot be used in patients who have ingested APAP chronically or in a staggered fashion over, for example, several hours or days. The nomogram also provides no assistance in situations where a reliable time of ingestion cannot be established. Finally, patients who present hours to days after overdose with serum transaminase activity above normal are beyond Stage I and are treated with NAC, regardless of where their APAP level might fall on the nomogram.

In addition to the nomogram, APAP plasma half-life can be used to predict progression to hepatotoxicity. In a prospective study of 112 patients with APAP overdoses treated with NAC, an APAP half-life of >5.5 h had a positive predictive value of 91% for progression to hepatotoxicity (Schiodt, Ott, Christensen, & Bondesen, 2002). A half-life below that cut-off had a negative predictive value of 74%.

In the United States, APAP is among the most common individual causes of acute liver failure (Gill & Sterling, 2001). The main differential diagnoses for patients with serum transaminases elevated into the thousands include drug or toxin-induced hepatic necrosis, ischemic hepatic injury, Wilson Disease, autoimmune hepatitis, and acute viral hepatitis. In a known or highly suspected overdose setting, our experience is that ischemic hepatitis accounts for almost all dramatic elevations of transaminases in the absence of drug- or chemical-induced hepatic injury. Like APAP-induced fulminant hepatic failure, ischemic hepatitis produces the same hepatic histology, similar patterns of liver function test abnormalities, a similar time-course of illness, and is frequently accompanied by renal failure from acute tubular necrosis.

2.3 Treatment

Other than supportive care, the mainstay of treatment consists of administering NAC (Chiew, Gluud, Brok, & Buckley, 2018). Administration of activated charcoal has been shown to reduce APAP absorption, but the clinical benefit of that reduction is uncertain (Chiew et al., 2018). In the United States, the approved dosing for oral NAC is a loading dose of 140 mg NAC per kg body weight followed by 70 mg NAC per kg body weight every 4 h for 17 doses. The approved dosing for IV NAC is a 21-h course comprising a loading dose of 150 mg NAC per kg body weight given over 1 h followed by 50 mg NAC per kg body weight given over 4 h followed by 100 mg NAC per kg body weight given over 16 h. Measurement of transaminases are repeated at the end of the infusion, and if they have risen above the normal range, NAC therapy is continued using an infusion rate of 6.25 mg NAC per kg of body weight per hour. Similarly, many physicians repeat measurement of a serum APAP concentration near the end of the 21-h NAC infusion, and if the serum APAP concentration has not fallen to a low or undetectable range, IV NAC therapy will also be continued. Cases of prolonged APAP absorption or "double bumps" with recurrent rises in serum APAP levels after initial partial declines have been described following large or massive APAP ingestions, sometimes in combination with other drugs that may slow gut motility through anticholinergic actions (Doyon & Klein-Schwartz, 2009; Wang, Monte, Bagdure, & Heard, 2011). Oral NAC and intravenous NAC have demonstrated equivalent efficacy and similar safety profiles (Bebarta et al., 2010; Buckley, Whyte, O'Connell, & Dawson, 1999) but the intravenous route is preferred in many centers, as the course of therapy is significantly shorter (72 h for oral vs 21 h for IV) unless NAC must be continued for aforementioned reasons.

If NAC therapy is commenced within 8 h of ingestion and continued in selected patients as described immediately above, protection against hepatotoxicity is almost assured, and death from APAP-induced liver failure will not occur, even in the small fraction of patients that go on to develop dramatic transaminase elevation (Smilkstein, Knapp, Kulig, & Rumack, 1988). NAC has also been shown to decrease mortality when given to patients who present late after ingestion(s) with established liver failure. For patients who have been placed on prolonged NAC therapy (became ill, persistent serum APAP elevation, etc.), NAC is discontinued when serum APAP concentrations are undetectable, transaminases are clearly falling, the patient is without hepatic encephalopathy, and PT is improving and, typically, less than 25–30 s (Makin, Wendon, & Williams, 1995).

NAC is generally well tolerated and rarely results in serious adverse events. In a multi-center comparison of the safety of PO and IV NAC (Bebarta et al., 2010), the most common adverse events in the PO group were nausea (20%) and vomiting (13%). These effects were less common in the IV group, where the incidence of nausea and vomiting were 7% and 6% respectively. The most concerning adverse events in patients receiving appropriate doses of parenteral NAC are anaphylactoid reactions, which occur in approximately 8% of patients. These reactions generally occur during the initial 150 mg/kg loading dose and, especially, when the dose is given more rapidly than over 60 min. Therefore, it is recommended that patients being treated with IV NAC receive their bolus dose in a monitored setting. Patients who do develop anaphylactoid reactions usually quickly respond to temporarily discontinuing IV NAC, administration of antihistamines, and reinstitution of IV NAC at a lower infusion rate after symptoms have resolved.

Authors have questioned whether currently used NAC dosing strategies allow enough NAC to be delivered during the first day or more following very large APAP ingestions. Apart from continuing infusions of NAC in selected patients, some physicians may choose to administer more NAC initially in a subset of patients, though there are no randomized, controlled trials to guide such therapy at present (Wang et al., 2011).

Patients in fulminant hepatic failure may be considered candidates for liver transplantation. Several severity of illness scales that predict which patients would, on average, benefit from liver transplantation have been described, but none are overall superior to Kings' College Criteria (Table 1), which remains the most widely used.

Table 1 Kings College Criteria for selecting patients for liver transplantation.

King's College Criteria

1. Arterial pH < 7.3 or plasma lactate >3 mM after fluid resuscitation

or

2. All of the following:
   a. Serum creatinine >3.3 mg/dL
   b. Prothrombin time >100 s[a]
   c. Grade III or grade IV hepatic encephalopathy
   The presence of either #1 or #2 parameters predicts a survival rate of less than 20%, and liver transplantation should be considered if the patient is a candidate

[a]Some versions include an international normalized ratio (INR) of greater than 6.5 rather than a prothrombin time. However, the INR normalizes the prothrombin time for a given warfarin concentration, not for the degree of liver failure. Therefore, the use of a prothrombin time is more correct.

3. Chronic APAP oral ingestions

Reasons for chronic excessive APAP dosing are varied and include treatment of acute or chronic pain, abuse of opiate analgesics containing APAP, and unrecognized consumption of multiple products containing APAP. Parents may also unintentionally administer excessive doses to their children. While manufacturers' recommended maximal daily doses range from 3 to 3.9 g for adults in the United States, there is no convincing evidence that hepatotoxicity is likely at less than 6–8 g APAP per day. Claims of hepatotoxicity at doses of 6–8 g per day or less are based on patient recollections of dosage and, in our experience, are unreliable (Curry et al., 2015).

A patient who provides a history of chronic ingestion of excessive APAP dosing over days to weeks is evaluated with measurement of liver function tests and a serum APAP concentration. Those patients with normal AST and ALT activities and serum APAP concentrations within or below the therapeutic range have never been reported to subsequently develop hepatic failure and generally do not require treatment. This principle obviously excludes a patient who has chronically ingested excessive doses of APAP and then has acutely overdosed on APAP shortly before evaluation.

4. Conclusion

Virtually all patients diagnosed with chronic APAP toxicity are recognized as such because they present with various degrees of hepatic dysfunction, whether that was the cause for them to seek medical care or not. Those with dramatic elevations in transaminases after chronic ingestions are more likely to display evidence of renal failure than patients with acute APAP overdose (McClain, Holtzman, Allen, Kromhout, & Shedlofsky, 1988).

Patients with elevated transaminases from chronic APAP ingestions are treated with supportive care and NAC in the same manner as for those with acute ingestions. The time course to recovery after peak illness is the same in the two groups of patients.

Conflict of interest

Dr. Fisher has no conflict of interest to declare.

Dr. Curry has had research supported, in part, by McNeil Consumer Healthcare, a manufacturer of acetaminophen products, within the last 3 years.

References

Bebarta, V. S., Kao, L., Froberg, B., Clark, R. F., Lavonas, E., Qi, M., et al. (2010). A multicenter comparison of the safety of oral versus intravenous acetylcysteine for treatment of acetaminophen overdose. *Clinical Toxicology (Philadelphia, Pa.)*, *48*(5), 424–430.

Beringer, R. M., Thompson, J. P., Parry, S., & Stoddart, P. A. (2011). Intravenous paracetamol overdose: Two case reports and a change to national treatment guidelines. *Archives of Disease in Childhood*, *96*(3), 307–308.

Berling, I., Anscombe, M., & Isbister, G. K. (2012). Intravenous paracetamol toxicity in a malnourished child. *Clinical Toxicology (Philadelphia, Pa.)*, *50*(1), 74–76.

Buckley, N. A., Whyte, I. M., O'Connell, D. L., & Dawson, A. H. (1999). Oral or intravenous N-acetylcysteine: Which is the treatment of choice for acetaminophen (paracetamol) poisoning? *Journal of Toxicology. Clinical Toxicology*, *37*(6), 759–767.

Chiew, A. L., Gluud, C., Brok, J., & Buckley, N. A. (2018). Interventions for paracetamol (acetaminophen) overdose. *Cochrane Database of Systematic Reviews*, *2*, CD003328.

Curry, S. C., Padilla-Jones, A., O'Connor, A. D., Ruha, A. M., Bikin, D. S., Wilkins, D. G., et al. (2015). Prolonged acetaminophen-protein adduct elimination during renal failure, lack of adduct removal by hemodiafiltration, and urinary adduct concentrations after acetaminophen overdose. *Journal of Medical Toxicology*, *11*(2), 169–178.

Doyon, S., & Klein-Schwartz, W. (2009). Hepatotoxicity despite early administration of intravenous N-acetylcysteine for acute acetaminophen overdose. *Academic Emergency Medicine*, *16*(1), 34–39.

Fannin, R. D., Russo, M., O'Connell, T. M., Gerrish, K., Winnike, J. H., Macdonald, J., et al. (2010). Acetaminophen dosing of humans results in blood transcriptome and metabolome changes consistent with impaired oxidative phosphorylation. *Hepatology*, *51*(1), 227–236.

Gill, R. Q., & Sterling, R. K. (2001). Acute liver failure. *Journal of Clinical Gastroenterology*, *33*(3), 191–198.

Larson, A. M., Polson, J., Fontana, R. J., Davern, T. J., Lalani, E., Hynan, L. S., et al. (2005). Acetaminophen-induced acute liver failure: Results of a United States multicenter, prospective study. *Hepatology*, *42*(6), 1364–1372.

Makin, A. J., Wendon, J., & Williams, R. (1995). A 7-year experience of severe acetaminophen-induced hepatotoxicity (1987-1993). *Gastroenterology*, *109*(6), 1907–1916.

Mazer, M., & Perrone, J. (2008). Acetaminophen-induced nephrotoxicity: Pathophysiology, clinical manifestations, and management. *Journal of Medical Toxicology*, *4*(1), 2–6.

McClain, C. J., Holtzman, J., Allen, J., Kromhout, J., & Shedlofsky, S. (1988). Clinical features of acetaminophen toxicity. *Journal of Clinical Gastroenterology*, *10*(1), 76–80.

Rumack, B. H. (2002). Acetaminophen hepatotoxicity: The first 35 years. *Journal of Toxicology Clinical Toxicology*, *40*(1), 3–20.

Rumack, B. H., & Bateman, D. N. (2012). Acetaminophen and acetylcysteine dose and duration: Past, present and future. *Clinical Toxicology (Philadelphia, Pa.)*, *50*(2), 91–98.

Rumack, B. H., Peterson, R. C., Koch, G. G., & Amara, I. A. (1981). Acetaminophen overdose. 662 cases with evaluation of oral acetylcysteine treatment. *Archives of Internal Medicine*, *141*, 380–385[3 Spec No].

Schiodt, F. V., Ott, P., Christensen, E., & Bondesen, S. (2002). The value of plasma acetaminophen half-life in antidote-treated acetaminophen overdosage. *Clinical Pharmacology and Therapeutics*, *71*(4), 221–225.

Smilkstein, M. J., Knapp, G. L., Kulig, K. W., & Rumack, B. H. (1988). Efficacy of oral N-acetylcysteine in the treatment of acetaminophen overdose. Analysis of the national multicenter study (1976 to 1985). *The New England Journal of Medicine*, *319*(24), 1557–1562.

Wang, G. S., Monte, A., Bagdure, D., & Heard, K. (2011). Hepatic failure despite early acetylcysteine following large acetaminophen-diphenhydramine overdose. *Pediatrics*, *127*(4), e1077–e1080.

FSC
www.fsc.org
MIX
Papier | Fördert
gute Waldnutzung
FSC® C083411

Kolibri 360 GmbH
Ferdinand-Jühlke-Straße 7
99095 Erfurt, Deutschland
produktsicherheit@kolibri360.de